Clinics in Developmental Medicine No. 129
CRANIAL HAEMORRHAGE IN THE TERM NEWBORN INFANT

©1993 Mac Keith Press
526/529 High Holborn House, 52–54 High Holborn, London WC1V 6RL

First published in this edition 1994

British Library Cataloguing-in-Publication data:
A catalogue record for this book is available from the British Library

ISSN: 0069 4835

ISBN: 0 901260 98 3

Printed in Great Britain at The Lavenham Press Ltd., Lavenham, Suffolk
Mac Keith Press is supported by **The Spastics Society, London, England**

Clinics in Developmental Medicine No. 129

Cranial Haemorrhage in the Term Newborn Infant

PAUL GOVAERT, Gent University Hospital

With contributions from:

PAUL DEFOORT
Gent University Hospital

JONATHAN S. WIGGLESWORTH
Hammersmith Hospital

1993
Mac Keith Press

Distributed by 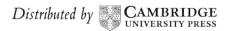 **CAMBRIDGE**
UNIVERSITY PRESS

To
Elliot, Faust and Farah

AUTHORS' AFFILIATIONS

PAUL GOVAERT, MD

Department of Neonatology, Gent University Hospital, Gent, Belgium

PAUL DEFOORT, MD. ScD(Biomed)

Department of Obstetrics, Women's Clinic, Gent University Hospital, Gent, Belgium

JONATHAN S. WIGGLESWORTH, MD, FRCPath

Professor of Perinatal Pathology, Histopathology Department, Royal Postgraduate Medical School, Hammersmith Hospital, London

CONTENTS

PREFACE

This book aims to give an updated account of cranial haemorrhage in the term*
neonate. It was conceived in spite of relatively recent reviews of the topic (*e.g.*
Larroche 1977, Pape and Wigglesworth 1979, Volpe 1987, Friede 1989), because of
the incompleteness of existing descriptions of cranial birth trauma and because
hitherto bleeding unrelated to trauma in term babies has been given less attention
than its counterpart in older children and adults and certainly in comparison with
brain damage in the preterm infant.

An attempt has been made to define separate categories of cranial
haemorrhage from a pathological, pathogenetic, clinical and radiological point of
view. These have been illustrated by case histories of living newborn infants
observed from 1980 onwards at Gent University Hospital in Flanders, Belgium.
Reports of autopsies on stillbirths and neonatal deaths by Professor Jonathan
Wigglesworth at Hammersmith Hospital in London during that span of time were
reviewed for cranial birth trauma. Stress is placed more on findings of practical
importance than on an extensive general discussion of cases. If known from the
available literature or personal observations, the sequence of events leading to a
lesion has been explained to the best of current knowledge.

Malpractice litigation is increasing in this area, and two contributors deal with
separate aspects of medico-legal implications. Professor Wigglesworth gives an
account of his extensive personal experience in sorting out complex perinatal case
histories ending in death or disability; and Dr Paul Defoort provides insight into the
delicate subject of the relation between cranial trauma and instrumental delivery.

In studying the book the reader will note that vacuum extraction is potentially
harmful. However, the frequency with which it is mentioned merely reflects the
popularity of this method of delivery in Flanders, and cannot be used in defence of
forceps extraction. Injury induced by vaginal breech delivery is not described at
length as the spinal cord is deliberately excluded from our field of interest.

Clinicians who daily rely on ultrasound, computerized tomography and
magnetic resonance imaging will agree that interpretation of such images is to a
large extent subjective and dependent on the observer's previous experience. All
these techniques fail in the same way: they create two-dimensional black and white
images of multicoloured three-dimensional lesions within the cranium. Therefore
we have been careful to stress interpretation of disease rather than changes in
density. When available, pathological confirmation of findings in life are referred to
explicitly, despite an obvious lack in the current literature. Magnetic resonance
imaging, still a relatively new and evolving technology, has not been given undue

*See Definitions, *p. xi*.

ix

prominence. It is for others to collect experience with this promising technique in the forthcoming years.

Some entities to be differentiated from haemorrhage and some aetiological aspects have been elaborated on, again focusing on the practical need of the neonatologist in charge. Disorders affecting neonatal basal ganglia, haemorrhagic diathesis and vascular anomalies all constitute complex yet tantalizing areas into which I have tried to pave a way (while admitting the limitations of personal experience). Tumour as a cause of haemorrhage and as a look-alike on sonographic or radiological documents has not been dealt with.

DEFINITIONS OF TERMS

Throughout this book the following definitions have been used.

Term: from 37 to <42 completed weeks of gestation.

Post-term: ≥42 completed weeks of gestation.

Preterm: <37 completed weeks of gestation.

Neonatal period: <28 days from birth.

Perinatal period: from 28 weeks of gestation to <7 days of life. Any perinatal mortality figures (stillbirths plus first-week deaths) quoted refer to this period, although it is realized that certain countries now include stillbirths from 24 weeks of gestation and that international agreement on defining this period has yet to be achieved.

Low birthweight (LBW): <2500g.

Very low birthweight (VLBW): <1500g.

1
THE GENT MATERIAL

The Neonatal Intensive Care Unit at Gent University Hospital (UZ Gent) is a regional tertiary care centre serving two Belgian provinces, East and West Flanders, which together have between 15,000 and 20,000 deliveries annually. Respiratory distress is the main cause of referral to the unit, and up to 120 very low birthweight (VLBW) infants are cared for each year, approximately one third of whom are of extremely low birthweight (ELBW, <1000g). Our interest in cranial birth trauma and asphyxia at term has also meant frequent referral of such problems by some local paediatricians, whereas others select only those infants in need of ventilatory support. *It must be stressed that the present study is not in a position to answer relevant epidemiological questions.* I can claim only that the disease entities seen in our referred cases must to some extent reflect neonatal problems originating in about one third of Flanders.

The study covers a 12–year period (Table 1.1). My special interest in cranial haemorrhage began in 1985; term and post-term newborn infants with severe cranial bleeding were studied prospectively between 1985 and 1991 inclusive. To increase the size of the study cohort, a retrospective search for similar cases was made for the years 1980 to 1984 inclusive. Primary subarachnoid haemorrhage was investigated between 1986 and 1990 until an arbitrary 100 infants had been diagnosed: 62 of these followed instrumental, and four followed breech delivery. The relative importance of intracranial bleeding in term/post-term babies as part of the unit's workload was calculated for a three-year period (1987–89): of 1240 admissions, 18 (1.5 per cent) were term or post-term infants with serious intracranial haemorrhage (six inborn, 12 outborn), and 70 (5.6 per cent) had primary subarachnoid haemorrhage (32 inborn, 38 outborn).

Although by definition they are excluded from these figures, three large pre-term infants (birthweights >2000g, gestational ages 32 to 36 weeks) who had subarachnoid haematomas recognized in life, will be described in a later chapter (see p. 101). This important clinical and pathological entity is not limited to preterm birth, and is rarely recorded in living infants.

As 14 of the 19 neonatal deaths in the group with serious intracranial haemorrhage were due to birth trauma, I have broken down our material into *traumatic* (superficial haemorrhage, Chapter 6) and *non-traumatic* (deep haemorrhage, Chapter 8) causes. Serious intracranial birth trauma has been widely reported, the largest study describing 27 term newborn infants treated by neurosurgery (Romodanov and Brodsky 1987). Available literature and personal findings attest to its continuing importance in perinatal care. An attempt at a

TABLE 1.1
Intracranial haemorrage in term newborn infants: the UZ Gent cohort

	PSAH* 1986–90 (N=100)		Serious haemorrhage 1980–91 (N=59)		Total (N=159)	
	N	%	N	%	N	%
Birthweight						
<1500g	0	0	1	2	2	1
1500 – <2500g	5	5	6	10	11	7
≥2500g	95	95	52	88	147	92
Male	58	58	37	63	95	60
Inborn	59	59	16	27	75	47
Neonatal death	3	3	19	32	22	14

*PSAH = primary subarachnoid haemorrhage.

TABLE 1.2

Traumatic neonatal subdural haemorrhage (UZ Gent 1980–91): type, mode of delivery, associated birth asphyxia and neonatal death*

	Total	Vacuum	Forceps	Breech	Spont.	Caesar.
Convexity SDH	5 (1/1)	3 (0/0)	1 (0/0)	—	1 (1/1)	—
Convexity + basal SDH	3 (1/1)	1 (0/1)	1 (0/0)	1 (1/0)	—	—
Convexity + basal SDH + CTD	8 (2/5)	2 (0/1)	1 (1/1)	2 (0/1)	3 (1/2)	—
Basal SDH	3 (0/0)	3 (0/0)	—	—	—	—
Basal SDH + CTD	9 (5/5)	5 (2/3)	—	3 (2/2)	1 (1/0)	—
CTD	3 (0/0)	1 (0/0)	—	—	1 (0/0)	1 (0/0)

*Data given as: total (birth asphyxia/neonatal death).

Spont. = spontaneous cephalic; Caesar. = emergency caesarean.

SDH = subdural haemorrhage; CTD = centro-tentorial damage.

Birth asphyxia was arbitrarily considered to be present when the Apgar score was <4 at 1 minute and <7 at 5 minutes, and when the umbilical artery pH (if available) was <7.15.

Occipital osteodiastasis was diagnosed in two infants (1 breech, 1 vacuum). *Arterial cerebral stroke* was recognized in five. *Neonatal subgaleal bleeding* was associated in ten. Three infants had simultaneous *intraventricular bleeding*. Two had an intradural haematoma, one presented with sagittal sinus thrombosis and CTD.

definition of birth trauma, viewed from a combined clinical and pathological perspective, is presented—together with similar pathological material accruing over the same 12-year period (1980–91) at Hammersmith Hospital, London—in Chapter 2.

The breakdown of diagnoses is illustrated in Figure 1.1. The anatomical basis for this separation is defined in Chapter 2. Each baby was assigned to only a single diagnostic category; as a multiplicity of different types of haemorrhage is very common in the perinatal period it was often difficult to determine the main

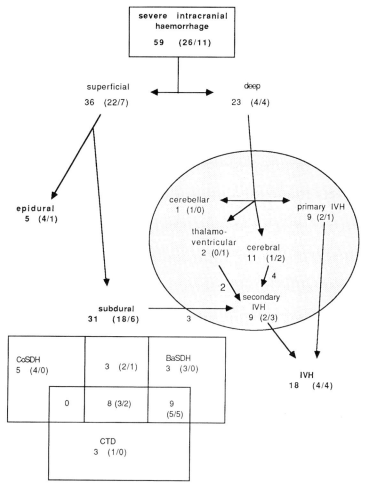

Fig. 1.1. Severe intracranial haemorrhage in 59 term newborn infants seen in the intensive care unit of Gent University Hospital, 1980–91. Numbers in parentheses indicate instrumental/breech deliveries. (IVH = intraventricular haemorrhage; SDH = subdural haemorrhage; CoSDH = convexity SDH; BaSDH = basal SDH; CTD = central tentorial damage.)

diagnosis. Clear guidelines for this algorithmic pattern would be almost impossible to summarize, but all lesions will be defined in the following chapters, emphasis being put on *in vivo* diagnosis and pathogenesis. The mode of delivery in the subdural haemorrhage subgroup is further delineated in Table 1.2, with special emphasis on associated birth asphyxia. The other serious haemorrhages are gathered in Table 1.3, displaying their relation to suspected causes. Next to trauma, birth asphyxia and infection were the main factors associated with intracranial haemorrhage at term (six and four cases respectively) (Fig. 1.2).

3

TABLE 1.3

Serious intracranial haemorrhage other than subdural: type and main association (UZ Gent 1980–91)

Haemorrhage type	Total*	Trauma	Asphyxia	Haemorrhagic diathesis	Infection	Other/?
Epidural	5 (0)	5	—	—	—	—
Primary intra-ventricular	9 (1)	1	2	1	—	0/5
Thalamo-ventricular	2 (0)	1	—	—	1	—
Cerebral	11 (6)	1	4	1	3	1/1
Cerebellar	1 (0)	—	—	—	—	0/1
Total	28 (7)	8	6	2	4	1/7

*Numbers in parentheses show neonatal deaths.

Birth asphyxia was presumed causal in the absence of other aetiological factors. (Criteria for birth asphyxia as in Table 1.2.).

For sake of clarity all infants were entered only once, despite the frequent multiplicity of lesions. One infant had intracerebellar bleeding as well as haemorrhage in the cerebral parenchyma. The newborn infants with thalamo-ventricular (primary thalamic) haemorrhage had an intraventricular clot. One had subgaleal bleeding and one other had an arterial cerebral infarction. One infant had superior sagittal sinus thrombosis associated with deep venous thrombosis and thalamo-ventricular haemorrhage.

Of the two cases of *haemorrhagic diathesis*, a maternal overdose of salicylates near term was responsible in one; the other infant had an unexplained neonatal thrombocytopenia (immune causes being excluded).

The *infections* involved were: cytomegalovirus fetopathy (1), nosocomial gram-negative infection (2), and early-onset group B streptococcal bacteraemia-meningitis (2). All infants with associated infection had some evidence of disseminated intravascular coagulation.

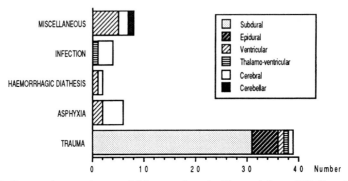

Fig. 1.2. Causes of severe intracranial haemorrhage in 59 term infants, UZ Gent 1980–91.

2
THE HAMMERSMITH MATERIAL

The Hammersmith Hospital Department of Perinatal Pathology is a referral centre for the North West Thames health authority region of London, which is inhabited by about 3.5 million people yielding up to 50,000 deliveries each year.

Between 1980 and 1991 inclusive 57 perinatal necropsies were performed on infants weighing >1000g at birth in whom birth trauma to the central nervous system (CNS) was one of the final diagnoses. (The definition of birth trauma used throughout this study is summarized in Table 2.1.) The gestational age was ⩾37 completed weeks in 31 of these children; 13 were stillborn. All examinations were supervised by Professor J.S. Wigglesworth. There were 23 instances of cranial birth trauma at term in 562 neonatal necropsies (4.1 per cent). The term cohort was subdivided into three categories: (i) *causal*, with mechanical damage as the probable cause of death; (ii) *contributory*, where trauma was obvious but the context suggested other additional mechanisms of perinatal demise; (iii) *irrelevant*, where trauma was considered not to have contributed to the cause of death.

Some general data are shown in Table 2.2. Severe trauma was usually obvious at or near term, whereas in a considerable number of preterm neonates it was an unexpected additional finding. There was no apparent male preponderance. Macrocrania could have played a part in the pathogenesis for only a minority of fetuses, whereas macrosomia (birthweight ⩾4000g) probably contributed to the mechanical problems in 8/31. The peak time of death was within the first day of life (10/31). Fetal distress, suspected because of meconium staining of the liquor or late fetal heart decelerations or bradycardia, was mentioned by the responsible clinician as an indication for speeding up delivery in three, five and four cases respectively for the causal, contributory and irrelevant groups. Delivery modes are detailed in Table 2.3.

Lethal malformation, in many cases stemming from neuromuscular disorders with prenatal onset of abnormal clinical features, is a frequent first diagnosis in fetuses with non-lethal mechanical birth trauma (Quinn *et al*. 1991). To a certain extent traumatic birth lesions are unavoidable in some very easy and rapid spontaneous vertex deliveries and in a number of difficult breech deliveries especially if the aftercoming head is trapped by a contracting cervix. That leaves us with possibly avoidable trauma in a proportion of instrumentally delivered newborn infants. This would imply prior recognition of those situations where delivery will end up in a difficult forceps manoeuvre (in the Hammersmith population, 17/31 perinatal autopsies with birth trauma as a feature), especially extractions with a rotational component (at least half). Most post-mortem reports

TABLE 2.1

Definition of cranial birth trauma

Straightforward trauma
- Skull fracture or fissure, cephalhaematoma, occipital osteodiastasis and its sequelae within the posterior fossa, locking and reverse moulding, growing skull fracture or syndesmosal rupture
- Tentorial and/or falx damage with or without associated subdural haemorrhage above, at, or underneath the cerebellar tent
- Epidural haemorrhage

Conditional trauma
- Subgaleal haemorrhage if primary haemorrhagic diathesis excluded
- Subdural haemorrhage if severe asphyxia, haemorrhagic diathesis, vascular anomaly or tumour excluded
- Parenchymal contusion if primary venous or arterial infarct excluded
- Forward displacement of the tip of the occipital bone if associated with underlying intracranial damage (subarachnoid haemorrhage, superior sagittal sinus thrombosis)
- Primary subarachnoid, intraventricular or thalamo-ventricular haemorrhage or venous cerebral congestion if infection, haemorrhagic diathesis, anticoagulation deficiency, asphyxia and vascular anomalies have been excluded as appropriate
- Typical sequelae such as chronic subarachnoid fluid collections in infancy, chronic infantile subdural haematoma, isolated growth hormone deficiency or syringomyelia in a breech delivered infant, if other causes excluded as appropriate

---

did not contain enough obstetric details to differentiate avoidable and unavoidable birth trauma, but the obstetric profiles of these different groups suffice to give a rough idea of the problem. Certainly, there is indication of an iatrogenic component if an obstetrician, faced with deep transverse arrest in the absence of fetal distress, decides first to try rotational forceps extraction, then vacuum delivery, and when both fail resorts to emergency caesarean section only to deliver a fresh stillborn infant with subgaleal bleeding, skull fracture, bilateral tentorial fraying, falx haemorrhage and both supra- and infratentorial subdural bleeding. There are also obvious risks inherent in the use of any instrumental obstetric traction device, including failure to recognize cephalopelvic disproportion, overestimation of what instruments can achieve, and too much confidence in their innocuity.

Associated trauma outside the CNS contributed to death in at least six infants (Table 2.4). The extent of subgaleal bleeding in three was such that it was probably a sufficient isolated cause of death because of the associated hypovolaemic state, pulmonary hypertension and secondary disseminated intravascular coagulation. The subaponeurotic bleeding would probably not have been lethal given swifter clinical recognition and intervention. In every instance of subgaleal haemorrhage forceps had been applied, although in two the ventouse was used following failed forceps extraction. One baby had forceps applied both vaginally and abdominally at caesarean section. In two cases, transection of the spinal cord (one at the medullo-pontine junction and the other at the level of C1–3) was due to difficult rotational forceps delivery.

TABLE 2.2

General data on 31 term infants with cranial birth trauma autopsied at Hammersmith Hospital 1980–91, by group*

	Causal (N=10)	Contributory (N=10)	Irrelevant (N=11)	Total (N=31)
Nulliparity	6	7	6	19
Male	7	4	6	17
Gestational age 37 – <42 wks	10	8	10	28
≥42 wks	0	2	1	3
Birthweight 1500 – <2500g	1	1	1	3
2500 – <4000g	7	7	6	20
≥4000g	2	2	4	8
OFC[1] at post-mortem >36.5cm	2	2	2	6
Polyhydramnios	1	0	1	2
Lung hypoplasia	0	1	1	2
Lethal malformation	1	1	5	7
Neuromuscular hypotonia and/or arthrogryposis	0	1	0	1
Survival: fresh stillbirth	2	4	2	8
<1 day	4	3	3	10
2–7 days	4	3	3	10
>1 week	0	0	3	3

*See text for definition of groups.
[1]OFC = occipito-frontal head circumference.

TABLE 2.3

Mode of delivery vs. group

	Causal (N=10)	Contributory (N=10)	Irrelevant (N=11)	Total (N=31)
Spontaneous vaginal	2	3	5	10
Vaginal breech	1	2	0	3
(with forceps for head)	(1)	(0)	(0)	(1)
Vaginal forceps	5	4	6	15
(rotational)	(5)	(1)	(3)	(9)
Forceps + vacuum	1	1	0	2
Caesarean	1	0	0	1

TABLE 2.4

Trauma outside the CNS, by group

Trauma type	Causal (N=10)	Contributory (N=10)	Irrelevant (N=11)	Total (N=31)
Subgaleal bleeding	3	0	0	3
Skull fracture	1	0	0	1
Limb fracture	0	2	0	2
Clavicle fracture	0	1	0	1
Liver laceration	1	0	0	1
Cord transection	2	0	0	2

7

TABLE 2.5

Intracranial damage, by group

	Causal (N=10)	Contributory (N=10)	Irrelevant (N=11)	Total (N=31)
Subarachnoid haemorrhage	3	1	2	6
Epidural haemorrhage	0	0	1	1
Convexity SDH	8	7	8	23
Basal SDH	2	3	1	6
Posterior fossa SDH	3	2	2	7
Falx damage	2	1	4	7
Tentorial damage	6	5	6	17
Tentorial tear	4	4	1	9
Occipital osteodiastasis	4	2	1	7
Cerebellar laceration	1	1	0	2
Cerebral haemorrhage	1	0	0	1

SDH = subdural haemorrhage.

From detailed examination of the type of haemorrhage described in these patients (Table 2.5) it became evident that the prototype of mechanical trauma remains tentorial damage. Genuine tears are slightly more common than superficial fraying and isolated intratentorial bleeding together. The epidural variety of haemorrhage is almost non-existent in this population of birth injuries related to breech and forceps delivery. Although descriptions in the post-mortem reports pointed to supratentorial subdural haemorrhage from either ruptured bridging veins (convexity) or tentorial damage (basal convexity), the distinction was not clearly specified in all cases. Posterior fossa subdural bleeding seems to predominate in the causal group, suggesting that in some infants it is important to diagnose this lesion as soon as possible after birth if death is to be prevented by emergency neurosurgical intervention. Striking damage to the falx is less common than injury to the tentorium. Occipital osteodiastasis was closely related to breech delivery, as previously reported (Wigglesworth and Husemeyer 1977). The brunt of force in difficult breech delivery is aimed at the posterior fossa via the base of the occipital squama, whereas in instrumental delivery the moulding of the calvarial bones including the tip of the occipital squama leads primarily to tentorial and falcial stress with subsequent bleeding. Next to tentorial injury, occipital osteodiastasis is a second important hallmark of cranial birth trauma. Primary neonatal subarachnoid haemorrhage does not seem to be a common consequence of forceps or breech delivery, but could be underreported because of its relative unimportance and lack of attraction for perinatal pathologists. Genuine cerebral bleeding or intraventricular haemorrhage are rare manifestations of birth trauma.

3
FATAL CRANIAL BIRTH TRAUMA

It is necessary to express caution when quoting incidence figures for cranial birth trauma, as there has been no standard definition available. However, over the past four decades the reported yearly incidence among liveborn infants of any gestational age has probably dropped from 3/1000 to around 0.5/1000 (Sulamaa and Vara 1952, Nesbitt 1957, Znamenacek *et al.* 1957, Butler and Bonham 1963, Machin 1975, Faix and Donn 1983, Walker 1985, Geirsson 1988). In term firstborn infants it may rise to 1.2/1000 (O'Driscoll *et al.* 1981), while in term infants delivered vaginally by the breech it may be as high as 20.3/1000 (Wigglesworth and Husemeyer 1977). Barson (1983) recorded 1.3 tentorial tears per 1000 live births of all gestational ages. The incidence in term liveborn infants, using a stringent pathological classification, is poorly studied, and gross inadequacies are to be feared if one considers rates deduced from death certificates. Cranial birth trauma is probably more common in LBW infants than in those weighing ≥2500g, while the frequency of mechanical trauma outside the CNS is much higher in the post-term infant (Valdes-Dapena and Arey 1970). In the 1977 Scottish Perinatal Mortality Survey, fatal birth trauma in breech or other deliveries (cord trauma excluded) was recorded in 0.6 per 1000 live and stillbirths weighing ≥1800g (McIlwaine 1980), the incidence doubling in twins. Walker (1985) calculated an incidence for intracranial birth trauma of 0.6 per 1000 deliveries (of all gestational ages) at the Ninewells Hospital, Dundee, in 1980.

Most injuries are associated with instrumental delivery, the tractor itself merely depending on local 'religion' (Fig. 3.1). Improper use of forceps is one of

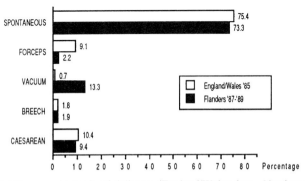

Fig. 3.1. Regional differences in mode of delivery. (England/Wales data—Northern Regional Health Authority 1990; Flanders data—Studiecentrum voor Perinatale Epidemiologie 1987–89.)

TABLE 3.1
Fatal cranial birth trauma at term, 1980–91

	UZ Gent (N=11)	Hammersmith (N=10)	Total (N=21)
Male	7	7	14
Gestational age ⩾42 wks	2	0	2
Birthweight 1500 – <2500g	1	0	1
2500 – <4000g	7	10	17
⩾4000g	2	1	3
Stillbirth	0	2	2
Apgar score <4 at 1 min.	8	7	15
<7 at 5 min.	8	9	17
Subgaleal bleeding	6	3	9
Skull fracture	5	1	6
Supratentorial SDH	7	10	17
Posterior fossa SDH	10	3	13
Tentorial damage	8	6	14
Occipital osteodiastasis	2*	4	6

*At UZ Gent, clinical awareness of the lesion of occipital osteodiastasis did not occur until 1988, so this figure may well be an underestimate.

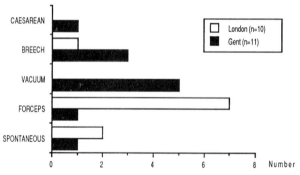

Fig. 3.2. Mode of delivery in fatal cranial birth trauma in term newborn infants.

the three main problems featuring regularly in perinatal obstetric malpractice litigations in the British Isles, together with incorrect use or interpretation of cardiotocography and failure of senior staff to come to the labour ward (Ennis and Vincent 1990).

Within the 12-year period chosen for this study, 11 term and post-term infants who eventually died from mechanical birth trauma were cared for at UZ Gent, their injuries having been suggested during life by the use of ultrasound and CT scan. Data from both the Gent and Hammersmith hospitals are shown in Table 3.1. It should be noted that the respective background populations from which these infants were derived are likely to have been very different. The mode of delivery for the 21 deaths in the two hospitals is shown in Figure 3.2.

4
ANATOMICAL LANDMARKS

The majority both of anatomical reports on intracranial haemorrhage in perinatal autopsies and of studies using CT scan, ultrasound or MRI *in vivo* fail to describe the exact location of the lesions. 'Supratentorial subdural haemorrhage' in some cases refers to the kind of bleeding originating in ruptured bridging veins joining the superior sagittal sinus, but is also used to describe a haematoma under and lateral to the temporal lobe immediately above the tentorium. Blood collecting between the occipital and parietal lobes from a centrally torn tentorium is hardly ever named basal interhemispheric subdural haematoma. Although it can be difficult, and in fact within the posterior fossa often impossible, to recognize anatomical landmarks precisely during life, this excuse cannot be given for post-mortem descriptions.

The importance of correct definition of the sites of blood extravasation is more than merely scientific: some patterns of damage could well relate to specific obstetric events, *e.g.* relative forward displacement of the tip of the occipital

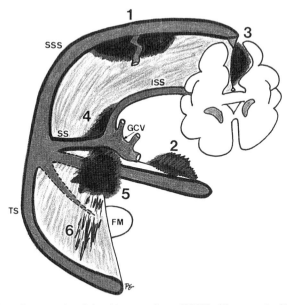

Fig. 4.1. Various sites of traumatic subdural haemorrhage (SDH): (1) convexity SDH; (2) basal SDH; (3) interhemispheric SDH; (4) basal interhemispheric SDH; (5) central tentorial damage with superior posterior fossa SDH; (6) inferior posterior fossa SDH. (SSS = superior sagittal sinus; SS = straight sinus; ISS = inferior sagittal sinus; GCV = great cerebral vein; TS = transverse sinus; FM = foramen magnum.)

TABLE 4.1

Subdural haemorrhage: guidelines for anatomical descriptions

Type	Major site of bleeding	Most likely origin
Supratentorial SDH		
Convexity	Around upper parietal, frontal or occipital lobe(s)	Bridging veins of superior sagittal sinus, large anastomosing veins
Basal	Lateral and inferior to the temporal lobe, extending up along the parietal lobe	Bridging veins of transverse or sigmoid sinus, lateral tentorial injury
Interhemispheric	High between frontal, parietal or occipital lobes along the falx	Falx injury, bridging veins of superior sagittal sinus
Basal interhemispheric	Above the splenium corporis callosi, between basal occipital and parietal lobes	Central tentorial injury or falx damage near the tentorial junction
Posterior fossa SDH		
Superior	Underneath the falco-tentorial junction between great cerebral vein and upper vermis	Cerebellar bridging veins, central tentorial injury (possibly straight sinus or great cerebral vein)
Inferior	Behind and below the cerebellar hemispheres	Occipital osteodiastasis or fracture with cerebellar and/or occipital sinus injury

SDH = subdural haematoma.

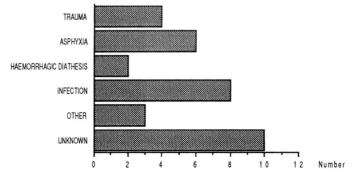

Fig. 4.2. Aetiology of deep intracranial haemorrhage in 33 term neonates, UZ Gent 1980–91.

squama during vacuum extraction and thrombosis of the superior sagittal sinus, primary subarachnoid haemorrhage and difficult high vacuum delivery, or haematoma into the falx and cup placement over the anterior fontanelle.

Based on data available in the literature and on the experience presented here, guidelines for anatomical descriptions of subdural haemorrhage are presented in

12

Figure 4.1 and Table 4.1. The multiplicity of injuries poses difficulties: within one patient several foci of bleeding can occur simultaneously, defying attempts at classification. In spite of this the most practical way to deal with neonatal intracranial haemorrhage is still by segregation into distinct anatomical entities (Volpe 1987). In Chapter 1, arguments have been put foward to justify subdivision of the material for study into two groups, superficial and deep bleeding. Deep intracranial lesions bear some relation to birth trauma, however (Fig. 4.2). Figure 4.3 attempts to summarize the anatomical entities to be discussed in the forthcoming chapters.

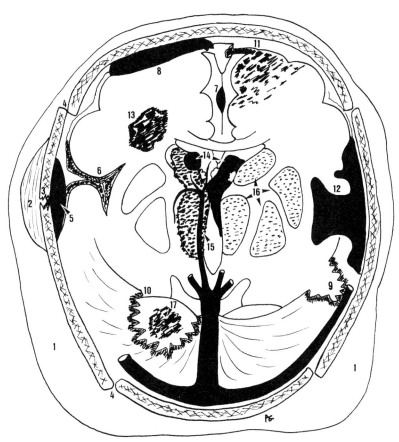

Fig. 4.3. Cranial lesion sites. *Superficial:* (1) neonatal subgaleal bleeding; (2) cephalhaematoma; (3) fractures and fissures; (4) moulding (including occipital osteodiastasis and growing syndesmosal rupture); (5) epidural haemorrhage; (6) primary neonatal subarachnoid haemorrhage; (7) intradural haemorrhage; (8) convexity subdural haematoma; (9) basal subdural haematoma (with subsequent stroke); (10) central tentorial damage (with posterior fossa subdural bleeding); (11) superior sagittal sinus thrombosis. *Deep:* (12) subarachnoid haematoma; (13) (sub)cortical haemorrhage (primary cerebral, haemorrhagic leukomalacia, arterial infarction); (14) intraventricular, subependymal haemorrhage; (15) thalamo-ventricular bleeding (deep venous thrombosis); (16) asphyxial bleeding in basal ganglia, thalamus, brainstem; (17) cerebellar haemorrhage.

5
HISTORICAL ACCOUNT OF THE MAIN MECHANICAL CRANIAL BIRTH INJURIES

Tentorial damage

Tentorial damage was recognized in the 19th century (see Schwartz 1964) but its relevance was pointed out by Beneke (1910) and Holland (1937). Both of these latter authors described anterior and superior displacement of the falco-tentorial junction, following either bitemporal (Beneke) or occipito-frontal (Holland) skull compression. They pointed to the free mesial margin of the tentorium as being highly vulnerable. Kinking, obstruction and thrombosis of the great vein of Galen at its junction with the straight sinus also results. A phenomenon referred to as 'galea-forceps' was depicted by Saunders (1948) in post-mortem experiments with traction on the galea aponeurotica over the anterior fontanelle. This causes direct strain on the falx with convergence of stress-lines toward the fontanelle, which could explain the association between 'frontal' vacuum extraction and falcial haematoma (see p. 50, Table 6.11). Spontaneous vaginal delivery with delayed second stage, midcavity forceps extraction and fundal pressure have all been associated with unilateral tentorial damage (Kehrer 1939). Central tentorial damage is seen in association with occipital osteodiastasis, specifically induced by difficult delivery of the aftercoming head in breech presentation (Wigglesworth and Husemeyer 1977). Tentorial injury has also followed difficult vacuum extraction (Aguero and Alvarez 1962, Plauché 1979, Govaert *et al.* 1990*b*). Lateral minor tentorial lesions are the probable focus of damage and source of bleeding in basal convexity subdural haematoma (Craig 1938, Schreiber 1959). These lesions may predispose to ischaemia within the territory of posterior and middle cerebral arteries (Govaert *et al.* 1992*c*). Welch and Strand (1986) have emphasized that the distribution of haemorrhage found in any one baby may be very complex.

Convexity subdural haemorrhage

Kundrat (1890) suspected that this resulted from interparietal bone displacement (see also Schwartz 1964). Dilatation and thrombosis of the superior sagittal sinus may be associated. Difficult forceps rotation during descent of the head has been suggested as contributory (Craig 1938). Chronic infantile subdural haematoma can be due to birth trauma (see Schwartz 1964).

Occipital osteodiastasis

This is usually the cause of death following difficult breech delivery (Hemsath 1934, Wigglesworth and Husemeyer 1977); it has also been encountered after a cephalic birth in which external pressure was exerted on the mother's abdomen because of slow descent of the fetal head (Roche *et al.* 1990) and following vacuum traction (see p. 32). At the syndesmosal (fibrous) junction of lateral and squamous parts of the occipital bone, a ridge can result from undue force on the occiput, lacerating the occipital sinus and cerebellum, with life-threatening brainstem compression. The boy described by Roche *et al.* survived such injury and was reported to have normal psychomotor development at 3 years.

Forward displacement of the prae-interparietal ossicle
This can disturb the integrity of the superior sagittal sinus with subsequent thrombosis of that vessel (Meier 1938, Govaert *et al.* 1992*e*).

Intracranial arterial hypoperfusion
This can be due to stretch injury of the vertebral artery and its branches (Yates 1959), to uncal herniation with compression of the posterior cerebral artery (Deonna and Prod'hom 1980), to rupture of the internal elastic membrane of the middle cerebral artery (Roessmann and Miller 1980) and to compression and/or vasospasm of the middle cerebral artery in association with basal convexity subdural haematoma (Govaert *et al.* 1992*c*).

Epidural haematoma
This is caused by parieto-temporal bone overlapping, genuine bone fracture or excessive bending of a calvarial bone with rupture of stretched dural vessels (Takagi *et al.* 1978)

Vacuum extraction
Application of vacuum traction over an interosseous fibrous junction can lacerate it with subsequent subgaleal bleeding. This has been recorded for a coronal suture (Hansen *et al.* 1987) and the anterior fontanelle (see p. 20). Proliferation of cerebrofugal arteries into the subgaleal space is an early feature of this complication (Voet *et al.* 1992). By far the most common cause of subgaleal bleeding is difficult vacuum extraction with fibrous injury, bone fracture or rupture of a transosseous emissary vein (Plauché 1980, Govaert *et al.* 1992*d*). Difficult ventouse delivery is a likely cause of minor abnormalities in neurological behaviour within the neonatal period associated with primary subarachnoid haemorrhage (Govaert *et al.* 1990*a*). Cephalhaematoma is more common after vacuum extraction than following forceps or spontaneous vaginal delivery (Plauché 1979). Hansen *et al.* (1987) have described rupture of a coronal suture with formation of a large fronto-parietal subgaleal haematoma.

6
SUPERFICIAL HAEMORRHAGE

Subgaleal bleeding (giant cephalhaematoma, subaponeurotic bleeding)
Anatomical description
A subgaleal haemorrhage forms a fluctuating, boggy collection of blood straddling cranial sutures and fontanelles, extending beyond the margins of artificial or natural caput succedaneum. Pitting oedema and ecchymotic discoloration of the skin develop after a variable interval. Blood spreads into the neck, around the ears—thereby displacing them forward—over the orbital roof into the upper eyelids and on to the root of the nose (Fig. 6.1). Looseness of the mesenchymal tissue in the virtual subaponeurotic space is the reason some haemorrhages become very large, some infants losing over half to three quarters of their total blood volume (Fig. 6.2).

Incidence
Subgaleal haemorrhage is associated with 5 to 10 per 1000 vacuum extractions and rarely complicates spontaneous vaginal delivery or forceps extraction (Plauché 1980, Govaert *et al.* 1992*d*) (Table 6.1). Its occurrence is apparently frequent in Flanders because of the popularity of instrumental delivery with the vacuum extractor: between 10 and 15 per cent of Flemish singletons are born this way.

Pathogenesis
Birth trauma is an obligatory precedent and often the only mechanism: (i) through rupture of the interparietal or fronto-parietal synchondrosis (Lehman *et al.* 1963, see also p. 20); (ii) via a genuine bone fracture (Kozinn *et al.* 1965, Govaert *et al.* 1992*c*); or (iii) by laceration of a transosseous emissary vein (Ahuja *et al.* 1969) (Fig. 6.3). The preceding ventouse delivery is either prolonged, vigorous, jerky, rotational or tangential (Lauridsen *et al.* 1962, Malmström and Jansson 1965, Chalmers 1971, Bird 1982). A series of 27 cases observed at UZ Gent has been previously reported (Govaert *et al.* 1992*d*); in 16 of these the number of ventouse pulls exceeded four, eight of them associated with cup detachments. Associated dystocic features such as persistent occipito-posterior presentation, long first or second stage or fundal pressure are additional risk factors in some but certainly not all vacuum deliveries leading to subgaleal bleeding (Govaert *et al.* 1992*d*). *Purely traumatic* subaponeurotic haematoma will develop in spite of immediate oral or intravenous vitamin K prophylaxis. The variant associated with *haemorrhagic disease of the newborn* due to vitamin K deficiency should be eliminated by routine prophylaxis at birth (Ahuja *et al.* 1969, Kagwa-Nyanzi and Alpidousky 1972). In

16

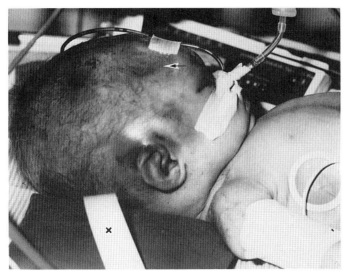

Fig. 6.1. Profile of Case 6.1 on day 1, showing haemorrhagic and oedematous *(arrow)* swelling of the scalp following rotational high vacuum extraction. (The × indicates the tape used for serial head circumference measurements.)

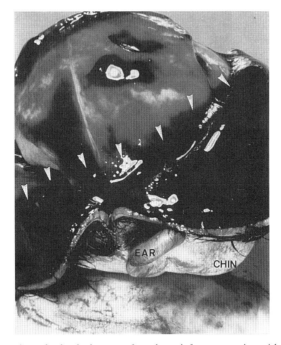

Fig. 6.2. Post-mortem view of subgaleal space of newborn infant presenting with hypovolaemic shock following failed instrumental delivery: *arrowheads* indicate site of scalp reflection. (Courtesy Prof. J.S. Wigglesworth.)

TABLE 6.1

**Subgaleal haemorrhage: rate of occurrence by
method of delivery**

	Literature review* (N=123) %	UZ Gent 1985–92** (N=27) %
Spontaneous vaginal	28	0
Forceps	14	0
Vacuum	49	100
Caesarean	9	0

*Plauché (1980) ** Govaert *et al*. (1992c).

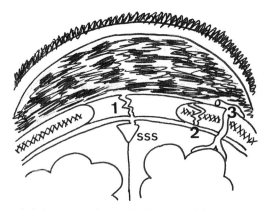

Fig. 6.3. Mechanisms underlying neonatal subgaleal bleeding: (1) rupture of fontanelle and superior sagittal sinus; (2) bone fracture; (3) traction laceration of transosseous emissary vein.

the latter situation the bleeding may accumulate insidiously over the first three days of life. *Haemostatic defect due to hereditary clotting anomaly, e.g.* haemophilia A, is an exceptional cause (Cohen 1978, Rohyans *et al.* 1982). Abnormal clotting studies are frequently secondary to consumption of platelets and coagulation factors within the haemorrhage (Govaert *et al.* 1992*d*). The dynamic changes of coagulation parameters in response to intrahaematoma consumption have been outlined by Easa (1978): in the rebound stage, from two to four days after the onset of bleeding, one may find thrombocytopenia in combination with elevated fibrinogen levels, a high-normal factor VIII and a normal to short partial thromboplastin time.

Clinical setting
The boggy swelling characteristically appears within the first few hours following delivery, the bleeding causing delayed shock with microcardia on chest X-ray and a return to fetal circulation with ensuing death if not recognized and treated urgently

(Levkoff *et al.* 1992). Bilateral large cephalhaematomas may mimic subgaleal bleeding on the first day of life (Pape and Wigglesworth 1979).

Most patients present with a variable combination of the following signs (data derived from the series of cases observed at UZ Gent—Govaert *et al.* 1992*d*): birth asphyxia with an Apgar score <4 at one minute (10/27); pallor and early anaemia (haemoglobin ≤120g/L (14/27); severe metabolic acidosis, as indicated by the need of at least 10mmol sodium bicarbonate on day one (12/27); circulatory collapse with a small heart and enlarged liver (9/27); disseminated intravascular coagulation (8/27); an increase in head circumference of at least 3cm in the first days of life (5/27). Persistent pulmonary hypertension is easily manageable after recognition and treatment of the hypovolaemic state.

Radiological assessment
On uncontrasted CT scan an associated subarachnoid haemorrhage was suspected in all patients, whereas subdural (above or below the tentorium, each in 7/27 infants), intracerebral (5/27), intraventricular (4/27) or epidural bleeding (1/27) was less common (Govaert *et al.* 1992*d*). Also recognized in this population were: two arterial cerebral infarctions, one thrombosis of the superior sagittal sinus, one growing syndesmosal rupture (see below) and one skull base fracture. The severity of intracranial damage roughly correlates with the amount of blood collected in the extracranial spaces on CT scan. Conventional X-ray of the skull and CT scan may show bone fracture in one third of the infants, dehiscence between adjacent bones (Fig. 6.4) in about 60 per cent, and suture diastasis or fragmentation of the superior margin of the parietal bone in a few cases. The bony lesions may sometimes appear grotesque.

Case history
CASE 6.1
This firstborn child (male, outborn) was delivered at 41 weeks of gestation with at least three high rotational vacuum tractions because of persistent occipito-posterior position in the absence of fetal distress. The first stage took 10 hours, the second only 15 minutes. His birthweight was 3210g; Apgar scores were 5 and 7 at one and five minutes respectively; occipito-frontal circumference (OFC) at birth was not recorded. Following an asymptomatic interval of two hours, he developed a 'giant cephalhaematoma' (Fig. 6.1) and became pale with poor peripheral circulation. He deteriorated rapidly and was referred ventilated to our neonatal intensive care unit. On admission, capillary pH was 6.53, P_cco_2 17.8kPa (132mmHg) and base deficit 33mmol/L. In spite of a total volume of transfused blood of 100mL the haemoglobin level was only 120g/L, and chest X-ray showed a small heart. His OFC was 39.5cm. The combined results of ultrasound and CT scan (Fig. 6.5) demonstrated laceration of the right parietal bone with right-sided subdural and cerebral haemorrhage. Complete devastation of the right cerebrum was confirmed at autopsy.

Management and prognosis
Neonatal subgaleal bleeding should be regarded as an emergency necessitating careful monitoring of head circumference, haemoglobin, clotting studies, blood

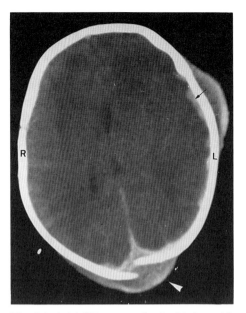

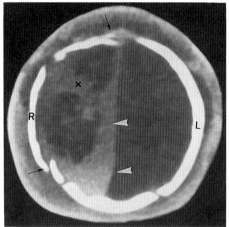

Fig. 6.5. Axial CT scan on day 1 in Case 6.1: several fractures of the right calvarial bone *(arrows)* are visible under an extensive subgaleal haemorrhage; appearances are consistent with right hemisphere contusion (×) and a convexity and interhemispheric subdural haematoma *(arrowheads)*.

Fig. 6.4. Axial CT scan on day 2 of infant with neonatal subgaleal haemorrhage: the parietal bones overlap considerably above the superior sagittal sinus *(arrowhead)*; a small supratentorial possibly subdural haemorrhage is present on the left *(arrow)*.

pressure, blood gases, and heart and liver volume (Pape and Wigglesworth 1979). For urgent transfusion treatment one can estimate the blood loss to approximately 40mL/cm of increased head circumference (Robinson and Rossiter 1968). Extra vitamin K should be administered intravenously, along with appropriate clotting factors. Marked jaundice may develop as haemoglobin is degraded; kernicterus can be prevented by adequate phototherapy. Aspiration of the liquefied contents will only create a risk of infection. A reported mortality rate of 20 to 25 per cent (Plauché 1980) is in agreement with personal experience. The bleeding will resorb within a couple of weeks, and development of residual impairment depends on associated cerebral or skeletal damage.

Growing syndesmosal rupture (cranio-cerebral erosion through suture or fontanelle, pseudomeningocele)

ANATOMICAL DESCRIPTION

Firm connective tissue bridges the gaps between individual bones of the newborn infant's skull and fills the fontanelles. Extreme mechanical birth trauma is capable of interrupting the integrity of this fibrous union and the underlying dural membrane. Simultaneous necrosis by pulsatile arachnoid tissue of the adjacent

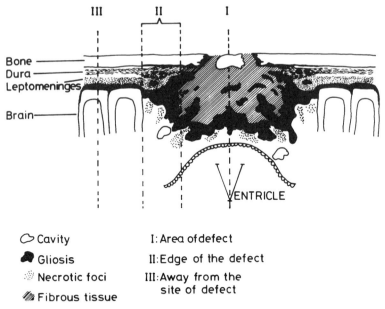

III   II   I

Bone
Dura
Leptomeninges

Brain

VENTRICLE

⌒ Cavity   I: Area of defect

🖤 Gliosis   II: Edge of the defect

⠂⠂ Necrotic foci   III: Away from the
                                  site of defect

▨ Fibrous tissue

Fig. 6.6. Anatomo-pathological description of a cranio-cerebral erosion following calvarial fracture. (Roy *et al.* 1987, by permission.)

cerebral parenchyma, aimed at the ipsilateral ventricle, has been referred to as cranio-cerebral erosion (Roy *et al.* 1987) (Fig. 6.6).

Vacuum extraction may damage the interparietal syndesmosis, and when this occurs the lesion is usually fatal (Lehman *et al.* 1963). Survival with an active syndesmosal cranio-cerebral erosion has been reported only twice (Hansen *et al.* 1987, Voet *et al.* 1992). The former case involved the coronal suture, the latter the anterior fontanelle. Infants have rarely been reported with genuine transosseous growing skull fracture due to birth trauma either during vacuum traction (Von Bucke and Pohl 1964, Vanhaesebrouck *et al.* 1990) or forceps delivery (see Hansen *et al.* 1987).

PATHOGENESIS
The dural breach is always more extensive than the bone gap (Gugliantini *et al.* 1980, Roy *et al.* 1987). Pulsatile CSF together with active fibrogliotic tissue invades the subgaleal space, eroding the brain in the direction of the ipsilateral ventricle. Cystic involvement of neighbouring bone has been well documented. In the girl we recently observed with extensive subgaleal haemorrhage following exceptionally difficult vacuum delivery, (colour) Doppler flow imaging at 2 weeks of age demonstrated early ingrowth of cerebrofugal arteries between the dural gap (Voet *et al.* 1992).

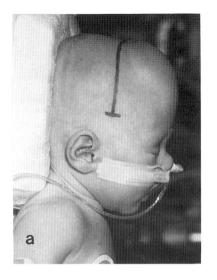

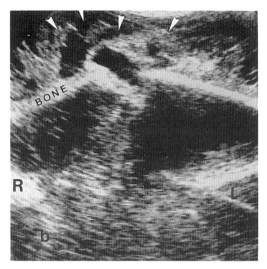

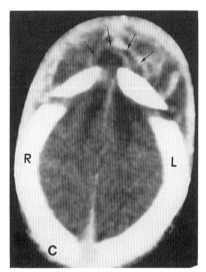

Fig. 6.7. (a) Preoperative view on day 29 of mass bulging above the anterior fontanelle. (b) Coronal ultrasound scan on day 12 of multicystic mass lesion (arrowheads) at the anterior fontanelle growing into the subgaleal space. (c) Axial CT scan on day 12 of cystic mass lesion (arrows) at the anterior fontanelle growing into the subgaleal space: note (sub)cortical hypodensity of frontal parenchyma (most pronounced on the left).

CLINICAL SETTING AND RADIOLOGICAL ASSESSMENT

If associated with birth trauma, subgaleal bleeding seems to be inevitably present (Govaert *et al.* 1992*d*). Within a few weeks one can detect, at first with ultrasound and later with the naked eye, a cystic growth over the injured suture or fontanelle (Fig. 6.7*a,b*). Damage to the subjacent parenchyma can be suspected from its hypodense aspect on CT scan (Fig. 6.7*c*). Inconsolable crying and general hypertonia were late neonatal features in the infant under our care.

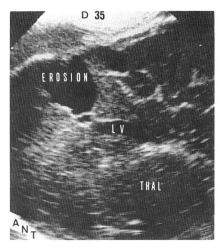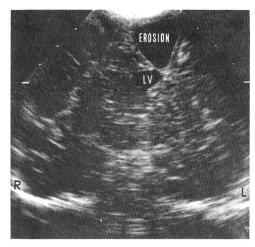

Fig. 6.8. Left parasagittal *(left)* and coronal *(right)* ultrasound scans through the anterior fontanelle on day 35: conical cystic erosion extends from brain surface to left lateral ventricle. (LV = lateral ventricle; THAL = thalamus.)

MANAGEMENT AND PROGNOSIS

Early surgical correction has been advocated in order to prevent active brain erosion (Thompson *et al*. 1973, Roy *et al*. 1987). In our case, despite early diagnosis, surgical removal of the extracranial mass and dural closure at the end of the first month, subsequent brain damage was not prevented (Fig. 6.8). This has tempered our enthusiasm regarding the necessity of early intervention. Removal of the fresh fibrogliotic process within brain tissue, a dangerous enterprise in view of the proximity of the superior sagittal sinus, would probably also have induced a considerable amount of damage.

Cephalhaematoma (external subperiosteal bleeding)
Anatomical description
The bleeding is usually restricted to one skull bone, in about 60 per cent of cases to the right parietal one. Frontal and occipital lesions are less common. Gradual periosteal bone formation at the margins guarantees ready recognition for several weeks or months. Adequate descriptions of the natural history of cephalhaematoma are given by Gresham (1975) and Pape and Wigglesworth (1979).

Incidence
There is little disagreement in the literature on the higher prevalence of cephalhaematoma following instrumental vaginal delivery, with rates of 6 per cent for vacuum extraction and 4 per cent for forceps vs. 2 per cent for spontaneous vaginal delivery (Churchill *et al*. 1966, Zelson *et al*. 1974, Plauché 1979).

23

Pathogenesis
Predisposing factors are male sex, at or near term gestation, nulliparity, private obstetric care, prolonged labour and persistent unusual positions of the fetal head such as occipito-posterior or transverse (Kendall and Woloshin 1952, Churchill *et al*. 1966). In the main, difficult manoeuvres high up in the pelvis, leading to lengthy or repeated extraction attempts, are to be blamed (Fahmy 1971). Occipital cephalhaematoma, though ordinarily seen following breech delivery (Ralis 1975), can be encountered as a sequela of spontaneous vaginal delivery with the occiput posterior (Schwartz 1964) or of vacuum extraction (several personal observations). Tangential forces exerted on the outer periosteum are probably generated by negative traction, causing descent of skin and galea with the calvarium immobilized in the pelvis (Bird 1982). Oblique, rotational and jerky tractions increase the risk. Periosteal dehiscence leads to rupture of emissary veins and subsequent bleeding, arrested only by the rise of pressure within the growing cephalhaematoma. Early liquefaction creates the impression of shifting fluid, whereas hardening of the outer membrane makes an older cephalhaematoma feel like a ping-pong ball.

Clinical setting
This classical birth injury usually becomes obvious on the second day of life. Besides its disfiguring effect on the child's appeareance, even this relatively minor mechanical birth trauma can induce, or hide, some more substantial problems (Table 6.2).

Management and prognosis
Primum non nocere (first do not harm) is the important message. Surgical evacuation is indicated only in the presence of superinfection (Burry and Heller-stein 1966). Aspiration for aesthetic purposes is obsolete. Parents should be warned that the swelling may persist for weeks or months after birth.

Skull trauma during birth
This section briefly reviews bony injury of the cranium inflicted by mechanical birth trauma. Further insight into the obstetric components of skull moulding is provided elsewhere. Details are given only of patterns of damage with limited description in the existing literature.

Moulding
This subject has been well reviewed by Lindgren (1960), Kriewall and McPherson (1981), Amiel-Tison *et al*. (1988) and Svenningsen (1989). Moulding of the fetal skull is generated especially during descent through the pelvis (Sorbe and Dahlgren 1983, Amiel-Tison *et al*. 1988). In cephalic delivery with the occiput anterior, the parietal bones tend to be lifted above frontal and occipital bones (Moloy 1942).

Excessive moulding occurs when labour is prolonged or contractions are too forceful, or when there is malposition of the fetal head or inept instrumental

TABLE 6.2

Complications of cephalhaematoma

Important resorptive jaundice (Fahmy 1971)
Anaemia (Schwartz 1964)
Underlying linear skull fracture in 5% of uni- and 18% of bilateral
    cephalhaematoma (Zelson *et al.* 1974)
Internal cephalhaematoma or epidural haemorrhage (Aoki 1983)
Posterior fossa haematoma with retro-auricular cephalhaematoma (Battle's sign)
    (Young and Zalneraitis 1980)
Osteitis–bacteraemia–meningitis (Ellis *et al.* 1974)
Permanent bony changes (lytic, sclerotic) (Schwartz 1964)
Craniosynostosis (Martinez-Lage *et al.* 1984)

interference. Displacement of the skull bones may cause: (i) bony lesions; (ii) dural membrane injury (falx and/or tentorium); (iii) intracranial hypertension with focal (Von Issel and Bilz 1978) or general brain swelling, possibly with retinal haemorrhage (Neuweiler and Onwudiwe 1967, Critchley 1968, Goetting and Sowa 1990); (iv) congestion of the Galenic venous system (Schwartz 1964); and (v) direct injury of major intracranial vessels (Newton and Gooding 1975). Moulding alone is probably incapable of causing cerebellar herniation, but may lead to uncal herniation (Pryse-Davies and Beard 1973).

Central tentorial damage can occur with any type of moulding, be it vertical, posterior vertical (cephalopelvic disproportion), anterior vertical (brow presentation) or anteroposterior (face or breech presentation). Tearing of the falx is more common in anteroposterior and anterior vertical moulding (Towbin 1977).

The components of skull deformation during vaginal cephalic delivery are depicted in Figure 6.9. The cranium deforms as the result of combined propulsive and resistive forces generated within the birth canal (Fig. 6.10). Propulsive forces are uterine contractions, increased intraperitoneal pressure, fundal pressure and additional instrumental traction. A proportion of these forces, ranging from 25 to 50 per cent, will act as compressive forces (Kelly and Sines 1966, Laufe 1971). Resistive forces are developed at the cervical os, the bony pelvis and the perineum. A complex pattern of skull deformation has been proposed by Kriewall and McPherson (1981), suggesting a physiological sequence of shortening and broadening of the biparietal diameter between cervical dilatation and descent. It was shown that the pressure at the equatorial plane is four times that at the vertex. Near the end of descent the intracranial pressure is about twice the intrauterine one (Eskes *et al.* 1975). The brunt of pressure is sustained by the parietal bone facing the pubic arch (Rempen and Kraus 1991). Brain swelling, as detected with linear ultrasound scanning, is more pronounced on that side (Valkeakari 1973).

Skull X-rays have shown excessive parietal lifting in up to 40 per cent of vacuum deliveries (Hickl *et al.* 1969). The likely mechanism for the vacuum related changes is an increase of galeal traction. The latter was shown to induce falco-

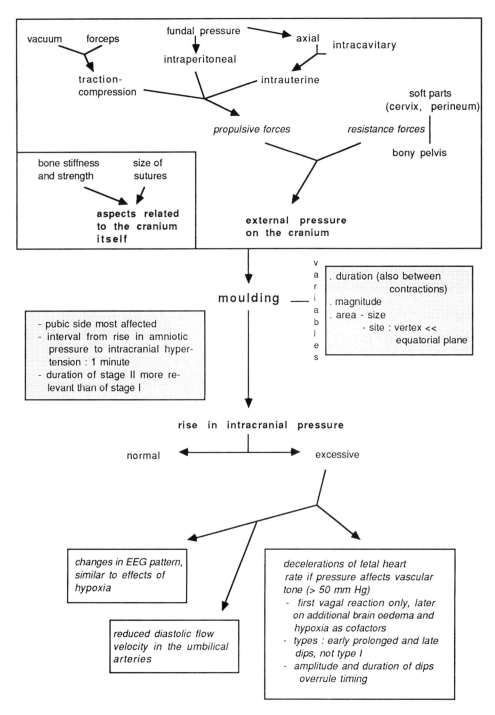

Fig. 6.9. Schematic representation of components and effects of calvarial moulding during delivery.

26

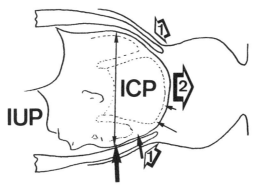

Fig. 6.10. Forces acting on the skull during cephalic vaginal delivery: the net effect of combined propulsive (2) and resistive (1) forces is an increase in intracranial pressure (ICP) above the intrauterine pressure (IUP). Pressure is maximal at the equatorial plane *(graded arrows)*.

tentorial stress (Saunders 1948) and elevation of the parietal bones (Awon 1964).The actual force delivered on the fetal head by the ventouse will depend on the angle of traction, the cup area, the amount of vacuum under the cup, the material used and the individual strength applied by the obstetrician (Thiery 1985). Applying vacuum without traction can lead to fetal bradycardia (Apuzzio *et al.* 1984); it may also also lift a depressed neonatal skull fracture (Tan 1974).

The early neonatal clinical counterpart of moulding has been detailed by Amiel-Tison *et al.* (1988): hyperexcitability and fussiness, or sleepiness and hypotonia with or without neck hyperextension.

Grading the severity of moulding during delivery was correlated with cardiotocographic changes by Stewart and Philpott (1980) (0 separate adjacent bone margins, + touching, ++ reducibly overlapping, +++ fixed overlapping).

An eleborate scoring system worked out by Von Issel and Bilz (1978) was based on clinical examination of the skull. Sorbe and Dahlgren (1983) introduced a photographic method which may prove to be more scientifically reproducible. On standard clinical pictures a moulding index is derived as [(maxillovertical diameter)^2/(biparietal $\times$ suboccipitobregmatic diameter)] (Fig. 6.11). Conventional skull X-rays and CT scans easily demonstrate relative elevation of the parietal bones and forward displacement of the occipital bone. The extent of parietal lift may be such that obvious separation of interlaced lambdoid suture margins is documented (Fig. 6.12).

Bone fissures
This term refers to splintering of bone margins near a suture or fontanelle, usually at the mesial parietal bone limits. They probably result from direct injury underneath the suction cup, as suggested by their close relation to vacuum extraction (Boon 1961, Aguero and Alvarez 1962, Lehman *et al.* 1963).

27

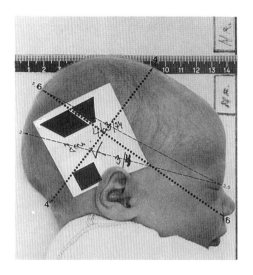
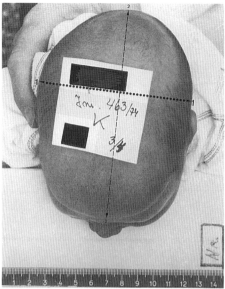

Fig. 6.11. Photographic method of grading severity of moulding shortly after birth. Heavy lines indicate biparietal *(line 1)*, suboccipito-bregmatic *(line 4)* and maxillo-vertical *(line 6)* diameters. (Adapted from Sorbe and Dahlgren 1983, by permission.)

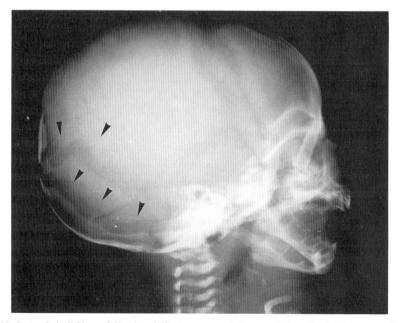

Fig. 6.12. Lateral skull X-ray following difficult vacuum delivery: obvious lambdoid suture diastasis.

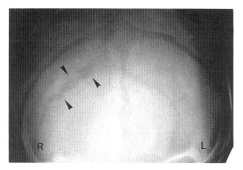

Fig. 6.13. Frontal skull X-ray: linear right occipital bone fracture *(arrowheads)*.

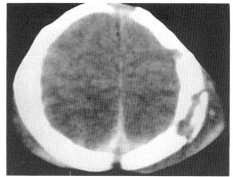

Fig. 6.14. Axial CT scan on day 2 after difficult vacuum delivery: note subarachnoid and subgaleal haemorrhage in addition to left parietal bone fracture.

Calvarial fractures
Within one centre, between 1978 and 1980 skull fractures were recorded in 0.9 per 1000 live births (Cyr *et al.* 1984). Bones of term babies probably fracture more easily because of their increased stiffness (Kriewall and McPherson 1981). *Linear fractures* (Fig. 6.13) are associated with 5 to 25 per cent of all cephalhaematomas (Kendall and Woloshin 1952, Zelson *et al.* 1974). They can occur during forceps or breech delivery, and have been well described following difficult vacuum extraction (Bret and Coiffora 1961, Lehman *et al.* 1963). Some useful data were found in a comparative study of 110 vacuum delivered infants (only seven high- and two mid-pelvic tractions; 55 retinal haemorrhages, three fractures and six fissures) and 103 spontaneous vaginally delivered infants (all with retinal haemorrhage, no fractures and one fissure) (Bachmann *et al.* 1968). In a consecutive series of 27 vacuum deliveries with subgaleal bleeding, six fractures were documented (Govaert *et al.* 1992*c*) (Fig. 6.14).

Depressed fractures are not caused by vacuum delivery and usually originate before descent (Strong *et al.* 1990), although they can follow forceps delivery (Loeser *et al.* 1976), fundal pressure (Kehrer 1939) or breech delivery (Abroms *et al.* 1977). The depressed bones should be elevated, either surgically or with vacuum application (Tan 1974), only if dural or cerebral involvement has been established (Strong *et al.* 1990).

Impression of the prae-interparietal ossicle (the separate ossification centre within the tip of the occipital squama) has previously been reported only by Meier (1938). It involves forward tilting of the upper part of the occipital squama just above the confluence of the sinuses (Fig. 6.15). Direct injury to the superior sagittal sinus is to be expected by this happening (Govaert *et al.* 1992*e*). Six such patterns were observed in the Gent material: three instances of difficult vacuum delivery, two spontaneous vaginal deliveries (one persistent occipito-posterior position, the

29

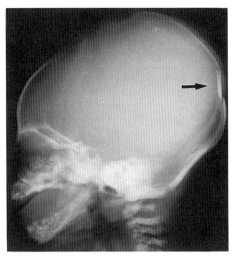

Fig. 6.15. Lateral skull X-ray: forward displacement of prae-interparietal ossicle.

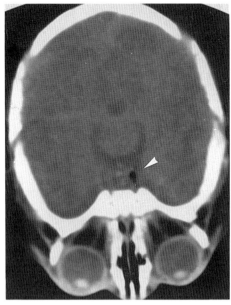

Fig. 6.16. Axial CT scan on day 2: pneumatocele (*arrowhead*) suggestive of basal skull fracture in sphenoid region.

other in an infant with spinal muscular atrophy), and one unexpected breech delivery at home.

Basal skull fractures

These are exceedingly rare and hardly reported on (Natelson and Sayers 1973). One may find associated haemotympanum or facial nerve paralysis. One of the children with subgaleal bleeding in the Gent study had a prepontine pneumatocele on CT scan (Fig. 6.16), suggestive of this lesion.

Locking and reverse moulding

This, hitherto uniformly fatal, phenomenon has been described as the crossing and interfixation of two adjacent calvarial bones, usually both parietals, resulting in a loss of calvarial plasticity and further moulding (Emery 1972). The only alternative to normal bone displacement would then be side to side compression at the basal parietal level, lifting the whole calvarium, and bruising temporo-parietal cerebral parenchyma. Whether or not instrumental delivery can be causal or merely reflects the necessity to expedite delivery because of fetal distress, remains an open question (De la Fuente 1991). As the lesion can be missed on X-ray, careful inspection of the skull is the only certain way to make a diagnosis.

Occipital osteodiastasis

The occipital birth traumas comprise a triad of lesions: (i) occipital osteodiastasis; (ii) genuine occipital bone fracture; (iii) forward displacement of the tip of the occipital squama. Of these, the former is the best described.

Anatomical description
Excessive force exerted on the base of the occipital bone is capable of displacing it inwards at the fibrous junction between squamous and lateral portions in the direction of the posterior fossa. In this process the underlying dura mater, occipital sinus and cerebellar hemispheres are sometimes traumatized as well (Pape and Wigglesworth 1979). Subsequent compression of the brainstem by bony protrusion, haemorrhage or cerebellar coning is often lethal. This squamal movement can actually transect the ponto-medullary junction. Cerebellar emboli to the lungs have been observed along with major lesions (Hauck *et al.* 1990, Wigglesworth 1991). Osteodiastasis is unilateral in about a quarter of cases. Minor degrees are frequently recorded in preterm neonates, not always associated with difficult delivery. In the at- or near-term baby, osteodiastasis automatically infers mechanical birth trauma, as it does at any gestational age if the lesion culminates in vascular or parenchymal damage. The fibrous weak spot turns into bone later in infancy.

Incidence and relation to mode of delivery
Hemsath (1934) documented occipital osteodiastasis (the 'heel of Achilles' of the perinate as he desribed it) in two of 7228 spontaneous vaginal deliveries (0.3 per 1000 total births), in 10 of 858 cephalic forceps deliveries (12/1000) and in 20 of 344 vaginal breech deliveries (58/1000). He was able to trace only four previous reports on this lesion. Wigglesworth and Husemeyer (1977) rediscovered the importance of the event, studying intracranial birth trauma occurring during breech delivery. They registered five instances of occipital osteodiastasis in 17 traumatic deaths out of a total of 32 neonatal autopsies extracted from a population of 477 breech deliveries. When actively and adequately sought for, about one perinatal death in three following breech delivery is associated with occipital osteodiastasis in their experience. A review of cranial birth trauma cases of any gestational age autopsied at Hammersmith Hospital between 1980 and 1991 clearly accentuates the connection between breech delivery and occipital osteodiastasis (5/11) but also with instrumental, mainly forceps, extraction (8/23).

Clinical and pathological details can be summarized for a total of 18 cases: 16 from reports in the literature (eight by Hemsath 1934, five by Wigglesworth and Husemeyer 1977, one by Takagi *et al.* 1982, one by Menezes *et al.* 1983, and one by Roche *et al* 1990), plus two patients observed in Gent. Delivery was spontaneous vaginal in two, by the breech or with version extraction in 11 (six with forceps applied to the aftercoming head), with cephalic forceps extraction in four and by vacuum extraction in one. This lesion has been observed as a complication of difficult tracheal intubation in an infant with a short neck (Wigglesworth 1988).

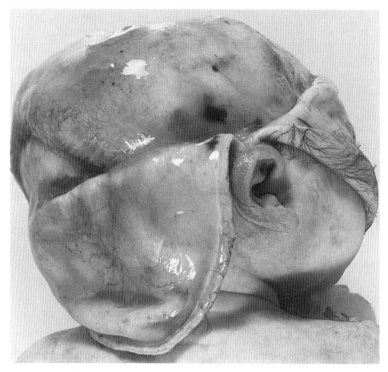

Fig. 6.17. Lateral view of skull of Case 6.2 after opening of subgaleal space at necropsy: the occipital squama is crushed under both parietal bones.

Pathogenesis
Occipital osteodiastasis and extensive occipital bone fractures have similar causes and consequences (Pryse-Davies and Beard 1973, Ralis 1975). In breech delivery they result from impaction of the occiput against the pubic symphysis, which is often inevitable when the aftercoming head is locked above a cervix closing down after passage of the trunk and limbs. According to Hemsath (1934), incorrect application of the forceps blades over the frontal bone and occiput high up in the pelvis is a second important cause. In spontaneous vaginal birth, shoulder dystocia can force the obstetrician to guide delivery with one hand grasping the occiput for support, which may lead to impaction of the occipital bone. Strong fundal pressure is probably sufficient in selected cases (Roche *et al.* 1990). One patient observed in Gent, a firstborn boy, was delivered after lengthy (30 minutes) ventouse traction because of arrest of descent 15 minutes into the second stage of labour.

Clinical setting
As a rule, these children present with severely impaired consciousness without intracranial hypertension. The diagnosis becomes easy, once the neonatologist has

32

TABLE 6.3

Clinical presentation of occipital osteodiastasis, and outcome (N=18)

Clinical feature	N
Birth asphyxia	16
Skull fracture[1]	2
Subgaleal bleeding[2]	2
Tentorial laceration	9
Supratentorial bleeding	
Subdural	11
Ventricular	2
Subcapsular liver bleeding[3]	2
Outcome	
Neonatal death at <1 hr	8
1–12 hrs	3
12–48 hrs	5
Survival[2,4]	2

[1]Wigglesworth and Husemeyer (1977).
[2]Roche *et al.* (1990) and personal case.
[3]Hemsath (1934) and personal case.
[4]Menezes *et al.* (1983).

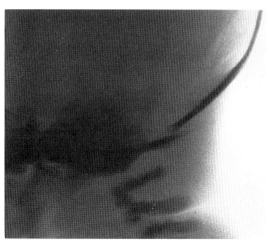

Fig. 6.18. Detail of lateral skull X-ray of Case 6.2 showing inward displacement of occipital squama at junction with lateral occipital bone sections.

acquired enough scepticism to suspect the situation in any neonate with unexplained neurological depression following difficult (breech) delivery. Both newborn infants referred to us in 1990 had palpable forward displacement of the superior part of the occipital squama as well (Fig. 6.17) The actual bony displacement is often hidden by muscle contusion. Associated clinical features and outcome data are presented in Table 6.3.

Radiological assessment
Lateral skull X-ray will document this lesion (Fig. 6.18), unless an increase in tension within the posterior fossa has pushed the bone back where it came from. CT or MRI scan illustrate the peritentorial and pericerebellar haemorrhage; coronal imaging facilitates recognition of the pattern of damage. The displacement of bone into the posterior fossa can also be demonstrated by ultrasound. Post-mortem confirmation requires careful initial dissection of the occipital region (Wigglesworth and Husemeyer 1977, Pape and Wigglesworth 1979).

Case history
CASE 6.2
The breech presentation of this boy (delivered at 37 weeks of gestation, birthweight 2700g) was only recognized after labour had begun. At a cervical dilatation of 8cm it was decided to continue with vaginal delivery despite fetal bradycardia. Following swift passage of trunk and limbs the cervix closed down on the neck, not relaxing until after failed attempts to extract the head with forcep blades and fundal pressure. The Apgar score was only 1 at both

one and five minutes. The child was referred 18 hours later with oliguria and persistent fetal circulation. He was stuporous with minimal reaction to pain, hypotonia, equal pupils and a fontanelle of normal tension. The occipital squama was clearly pushed in underneath the parietal bones (Fig. 6.17). The ultrasound appearance was compatible with severe bleeding in the region of the vein of Galen; a lateral skull X-ray confirmed occipital osteodiastasis (Fig. 6.18), and pericerebellar haemorrhage was documented with CT scan. Stabilization was initially quite easy after correction of associated anaemia and metabolic acidosis. However, a few hours later haemoperitoneum—thought to be both perihepatic and perisplenic in origin—developed and caused intractable hypovolaemic shock. Within minutes following incision of the abdominal wall the boy became exsanguinated from an extensive laceration of the right liver lobe. At necropsy pericerebellar subdural haemorrhage and bilateral complete tentorial tears were additional findings. In the absence of liver trauma, the brain events would probably not have been fatal.

Management and prognosis
Most infants with diastasis severe enough to injure the cerebellum die in the neonatal period. Minor bleeding may either create a therapeutic window for suboccipital craniotomy if necessary (Menezes *et al.* 1983, Govaert *et al.* 1990*b*), or heal spontaneously (Roche *et al.* 1990). Survivors with cerebellar injury could be found either within the group of disabled children with ataxic cerebral palsy (Wigglesworth and Husemeyer 1977) or among patients with growth hormone deficiency and syringomyelia following breech delivery (Fujita *et al.* 1992).

Epidural haematoma (cephalhematoma internum, internal subperiosteal bleeding)
Anatomical description
Epidural collections of blood are located between any calvarial bone and its inner periosteum or between the periosteal membrane and the underlying outer dural fibrous stratum. As with cephalhaematoma, some epidural haemorrhages are confined to one skull bone, either above (Takagi *et al.* 1978) or below (Esparza *et al.* 1982) the cerebellar tent. The frontal variant must be exceptionally rare in the neonatal period. If extravasation follows laceration of the middle meningeal artery or a large venous sinus the bleeding may rapidly attain life-threatening dimensions both as a space-occupying lesion and as a cause of serious hypovolaemia (Choux *et al.* 1975, Gama and Fenichel 1985). Damage to small venous channels alone —emissary veins or dural vessels—will lead to moderate or mild bleeding, detectable only on CT or MRI scan against the appropriate anamnestic background. However, venous haemorrhage with associated haemostatic failure could become a major problem (Cooper and Lynch 1979).

Incidence
The rarity of this event is illustrated by its absence from several classic reports on intracranial bleeding in perinatal autopsies: no such lesion was found in 186 tentorial injuries (Holland 1937, Craig 1938, Gröntoft 1953). Larroche (1977) mentioned one epidural haematoma with associated parietal fracture in a cohort of

700 perinatal autopsies. Valdes-Dapena and Arey (1970) recorded one epidural haemorrhage in six cases of fatal cranial birth trauma coming from a population of 17,022 liveborn infants weighing >2500g. In a series of papers between 1980 and 1988 on a total of 383 intracranial haemorrhagic lesions diagnosed in living term neonates (Flodmark *et al.* 1980*a,b*; Guekos-Thöni *et al.* 1980; Leblanc and O'Gorman 1980; Ludwig *et al.* 1980; Brockerhoff *et al.* 1981; Fenichel *et al.* 1984; Pierre-Kahn *et al.* 1985; Welch and Strand 1986; Romodanov and Brodsky 1987; Sachs et al. 1987, Oelberg *et al.* 1988) only two epidural haemorrhages were reported (Flodmark *et al.* 1980*b*, Leblanc and O'Gorman 1980); of the rest, 4.4 per cent were cerebellar, 8.9 per cent posterior fossa subdural, 9.1 per cent cerebral parenchymal or in the basal ganglia, 15.1 per cent intraventricular, 24.8 per cent supratentorial subdural, and 37.0 per cent subarachnoid. Within a consecutive series of 31 term infants with cranial birth trauma autopsied between 1980 and 1990 at Hammersmith Hospital, epidural haematoma was not recorded.

Aoki (1990), reviewing the available literature from 1922 on, gathered 28 instances of neonatal epidural haemorrhage, the majority of Japanese origin. At least eight additional descriptions can be traced (Naujoks 1934, Saint-Anne Dargassies 1957, Tank *et al.* 1971, Natelson and Sayers 1973). Whatever the exact number of reported cases, their scarcity is in slight contrast with personal observation of five cases in Gent between 1988 and 1991 (Table 6.4). This can probably be explained by our eagerness during the latter part of the 1980s to undertake CT scanning of the cranium in neurologically distressed neonates following difficult vacuum extraction, resulting in recognition of an epidural haemorrhage in four infants over a three year period. Most reported cases have been ascribed to traumatic forceps traction (Saint-Anne Dargassies 1957, Takagi *et al.* 1978, Gama and Fenichel 1985), but breech delivery was responsible in a few (Tank *et al.* 1971, Takagi *et al.* 1978) and vacuum extraction in one other (Aoki 1990). Spontaneous vaginal delivery preceded the event in a newborn infant with an early neonatal haemorrhagic diathesis (Merry and Stuart 1979).

Pathogenesis
The rarity of epidural bleeding before the age of 1 year, even following events as predisposing to trauma as vaginal birth, is in part explained by skull pliability and by firm attachment of the dural membrane to skull sutures (Choux *et al.* 1986). At least three different mechanisms can lead to it. The first was suspected by Lefkowitz (1936) and can be referred to as 'parieto-temporal osteodiastasis': unusual separation between these bones could cause the upper temporal margin to act like a fracture and injure the dural vessels. The second way has been recognized in over half the neonatal cases: irregular sharp bone edges along a genuine fracture lacerate the middle meningeal artery (Gama and Fenichel 1985) or one of its branches, or damage an important underlying sinus. Lack of a real groove for the meningeal vessels to rest in clarifies why skull fractures in the neonate are not often complicated by epidural haemorrhage (Takagi *et al.* 1978). The absence of a

TABLE 6.4
Neonatal epidural haemorrhage, UZ Gent 1988–91 (N=5)

	Case number				
	1	2	3	4	5
Sex	M	F	M	M	M
Inborn	+	+	−	−	−
Gestational age (wks)	39	38	40	39	40
Parity	2	1	?	1	1
Birthweight (g)	2950	3300	3100	2350	3550
OFC (cm)	34	36	33	35	33
Delivery					
Stage I (hrs)	5	25	?	?	21
Stage II (mins)	22	55	40	30	60
Late fetal heart					
decelerations	+	−	+	+	−
Fundal pressure	−	+	+	+	?
Breech	−	−	−	+	−
Vacuum	+	+	+	−	+
Number	3	5	15	−	6
Detachments	−	+	+	−	+
Elective	+	−	−	−	−
Apgar score @ 1/5 mins	2/8	8/10	4/6	1/4	4/6
Umbilical artery pH	7.16	7.27	?	?	?
Pericranial trauma					
Cephalhaematoma	+	−	−	−	+
Subgaleal haemorrhage	−	+	+	−	−
Fracture					
Bone	par.	occip.	par.	par.	par.
Side	R	R	L	R	R
Tense fontanelle	−	−	−	+	−
Seizures	−	−	−	−	+
Intracranial lesions					
Subarachnoid haemorrhage	+	+	+	+	+
Epidural haemorrhage					
Side	R	R	R	R	R
Location	par.	par-occ.	par.	par.	par.
Above insula	+	−	+	−	−
Depth (mm)	8	6	2	13	5
Length (mm)	32	28	8	66	25
Differential density	−	+	−	−	−
Midline shift	−	−	−	+	−
Arterial ischaemia	−	−	−	+*	−
Treatment	−	−	−	+**	−
Development					
Normal	+	+	+	−	?
Cerebral palsy	−	−	−	−	?
Prader–Willi syndrome	−	−	−	+	−

*Region of the right posterior cerebral artery.
**Tapping through the lambdoid suture.

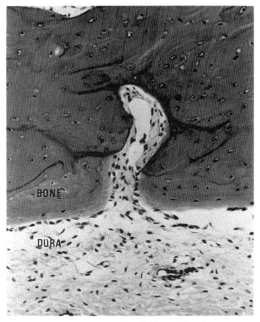

Fig. 6.19. Histological section through neonatal calvarial bone showing entrance of an inner dural vessel into bone substance. (Takagi *et al*. 1978, by permission.)

fracture in an important number of cases is explained by the third method, whereby bending of the moulded bone causes detachment of the dural membrane from its centre. This dehiscence can disrupt fibrovascular connections between dura and bone (Takagi *et al*. 1978) (Fig. 6.19). An interesting observation, of practical importance in relation to treatment, is the early liquefaction of the blood collection, sometimes within 24 hours after birth (personal observation). This phenomenon, noted by Aoki, is comparable to the early liquefaction of a cephalhaematoma, and it is suggested that communication between an external and an internal cephalhaematoma can on occasion lead to it (Aoki 1983, 1990).

Clinical setting
Difficult delivery is obligatory, except in the case of haemorrhagic diathesis, *e.g.* vitamin K deficiency, in exceptional situations (Cooper and Lynch 1979, Lam *et al*. 1991). The mothers are usually primiparous. Fetal and/or birth asphyxia are not constant. As with other types of neonatal intracranial bleeding, male sex clearly dominates in the cases reviewed. Major neurological disturbances (rarely following an apparently normal interval), such as coma or stupor, severe hypotonia, apnoea, fixed bradycardia and a tense fontanelle, are one possible presenting symptom complex. In cases with extensive bleeding, life-threatening intracranial hyperten-

sion warrants neurosurgical intervention, especially if uncal herniation is suggested by unilateral mydriasis. Because the neonatal skull is distensible, significant bleeding may initially present as anaemia and obstructive hydrocephalus (Merry and Stuart 1979). However, the majority of infants with epidural haemorrhage are probably to be found among babies with cephalhaematoma or mild subgaleal bleeding with few or no other signs; others may show respiratory grunting, pallor, grimacing on handling or opisthotonic posturing. Features such as fever (Gama and Fenichel 1985), seizures or hemiparesis are exceptional. One of the Gent patients had Prader–Willi syndrome: the accompanying hypotonia has a well-recognized association with breech presentation and subsequent birth trauma. Some epidural haematomas have been a chance finding during CT scanning for other lesions (Aoki 1983, Gouyon *et al.* 1985). Skull fracture was present in all the Gent patients, though several authors suggest it is absent in up to 50 per cent of cases (Takagi *et al.* 1978, Choux 1986). All the reports I could trace in the literature of epidural haemorrhage following vacuum delivery recorded bone fracture.

Radiological assessment
Conventional skull X-rays usually illustrate a linear fracture of the parietal or occipital bone or, less commonly, a depressed one (Aoki 1983). Temporo-parietal osteodiastasis is indirectly suggested by obvious parietal bone lifting. Even though ultrasound examination will not detect a small haematoma located within the concave curve of a skull bone, obvious haemorrhages are readily demonstrated mainly because of hypodensity due to partial liquefaction (Lam *et al.* 1991). CT, and probably MRI, scans are the only reliable diagnostic tools. Typically the haematoma is biconcave like a lens and has very neat margins (Fig. 6.20). As stipulated in the definition, some of them cross suture lines because they are situated between the periosteum and outer dural layer. Bone window setting on CT scan helps to document associated osseous lesions (Fig. 6.21). The most intriguing phenomenon is a tendency to liquefy rapidly (in about one third of cases) leading to a differential density within the collection (Aoki 1990). Uncal herniation can sometimes be suspected because of hypodensity of the brain parenchyma perfused by the ipsilateral posterior or middle cerebral artery (see section on arterial cerebral occlusion following birth trauma, p. 62). The only haematoma associated with severe neurological problems and arterial cerebral hypoperfusion in our series had a depth >10mm, a width >50mm, was situated below the level of the insula and caused midline shift. Comparable measurements from other reports are not available, but may be surmised according to whether treatment was surgical or conservative.

Case history
CASE 6.3
This boy, whose mother was a primipara, was born at 39 weeks of gestation by the breech, fundal pressure being exerted to deliver the aftercoming head. His birthweight was 2350g,

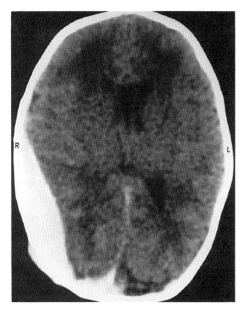 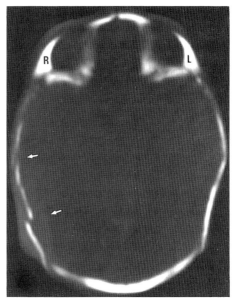

Fig. 6.20. Axial CT scan on day 2 in Case 6.3: a large biconvex epidural haematoma against the right parietal bone is shifting the midline.

Fig. 6.21. Axial CT scan with bone window setting on day 2 in Case 6.3: note multiple right parietal bone fractures *(arrows)*.

and Apgar scores were 1 and 4 at one and five minutes respectively. Pallor, hypotonia and lethargy developed on the first day. He was referred with a tense fontanelle and because an extracerebral haemorrhage had been suspected on CT scan (Fig. 6.20). Neither seizures nor inequality of the pupils had been observed. His heart rate was steady at around 120 bpm. The lentiform extraparenchymal density on CT and ultrasound scans was pathognomonic of epidural haematoma with partial liquefaction. Plain X-rays and CT scan with bone window setting documented an underlying parietal bone fracture on the right (Fig. 6.21). Hypodensity of the ipsilateral occipito-temporal brain parenchyma suggested impending arterial ischaemia and prompted neurosurgical intervention on day 3. The haematoma was aspirated under local anaesthesia through a dural incision via the lateral lambdoid suture. In the immediate postsurgical period the fontanelle lost its increased tension, and the shifted midline, as shown by ultrasound, returned to the original position. A residual epidural hygroma resorbed over the ensuing weeks. Slow neurological recovery, with profound hypotonia and distinct facial dysmorphic features, was shown to be due to underlying Prader–Willi syndrome with characteristic karyotypic abnormalities.

Management and prognosis

Most epidural haemorrhages do not present with intracranial hypertension, and heal spontaneously. Three major indications for surgical intervention are: (i) displacement of a bone fragment into the cerebral parenchyma; (ii) growing skull fracture; (iii) life-threatening acute intracranial hypertension (Choux 1986). Some lesions, especially those with associated fracture, can only be approached safely with craniotomy (Gama and Fenichel 1985). In the same intervention a cephalhaematoma can be surgically drained. Tapping through a suture—either coronal or lambdoid—under local anaesthesia (as in our case 4, see Table 6.4) or through a burr hole is the alternative method (Aoki 1990). Irrespective of the density on CT scan, this percutaneous approach has been advocated as the warranted first treatment method. Within the present small series, no neurological sequelae related to the intracranial injury were found.

Primary subarachnoid haemorrhage

Anatomical description

This diagnosis is reserved for neonates without major intracranial bleeding such as periventricular, subdural or parenchymal, but presenting with a thin film of extravasated blood retained within the arachnoid web and usually distributed over the occipito-parietal cerebrum, in the sylvian clefts, in basal cisterns, and around the cerebellum and/or brainstem (Larroche 1977, Pape and Wigglesworth 1979). Primary subarachnoid haemorrhage (PSAH) appears to be the result of either damaged arachnoid veins or involuting leptomeningeal anastomoses (Schwartz 1964). Capillary and venous hypertension due to asphyxia of any cause is a robust pathogenetic hypothesis (Volpe 1987). The lesion, important because of its high incidence, will be discussed at length in this section. It has to be differentiated from secondary subarachnoid bleeding due to cerebral infarction, intraventricular bleeding and subsequent leakage out of the fourth ventricle, parenchymal haemorrhage or underlying a subdural haematoma.

Incidence and relation to obstetric history

Among a series of reports on a total of 353 living term newborn infants with intracranial haemorrhage studied by CT, in 37 per cent the only diagnosis was primary subarachnoid haemorrhage, indicating that this may well be the most common kind of haemorrhagic lesion of the term newborn brain (Flodmark *et al.* 1980*b*, Guekos-Thöni *et al.* 1980, Leblanc and O'Gorman 1980, Ludwig *et al.* 1980, Brockerhoff *et al.* 1981, Fenichel *et al.* 1984, Pierre-Kahn *et al.* 1985, Welch and Strand 1986, Romodanov and Brodsky 1987, Sachs *et al.* 1987, Oelberg *et al.* 1988). Examination of lumbar CSF, before the advent of modern imaging, led clinicians to suspect an incidence of 10 per cent of meningeal haemorrhage following spontaneous vaginal delivery (Sharpe and Maclaire 1924). As the number of erythrocytes in CSF is slightly higher following ventouse than spontaneous parturition, this suggests minor bleeding to be quite common (Blennow *et al.* 1977). Although the matter is still open to debate, the observation of retinal haemorrhage —probably similar in pathogenesis to the subarachnoid type—in up to 20 per cent of spontaneous and 40 per cent of instrumental (forceps or ventouse) deliveries confirms this suspicion of a very high incidence of subarachnoid bleeding following vaginal birth (Critchley 1968, Svenningsen and Eidal 1988). In my experience, subarachnoid haemorrhage is the most common lesion in term infants with

TABLE 6.5

Associated trauma in 100 term infants with subarachnoid haemorrhage

Lesion	N	Mode of delivery
Skull fracture	2	2 vacuum (1 parietal, 1 basal skull)
Humerus fracture	2	1 vacuum, 1 breech
Clavicle fracture	2	Both spontaneous vaginal
Subgaleal bleeding	11	All vacuum

intracranial haemorrhage. As nearly all such infants live, it is vital to recall that there is very limited pathological correlation of CT findings: observations could be related to venous congestion or intradural haemorrhage as well as subarachnoid bleeding.

In order to study the obstetric precedents of PSAH, a consecutive series of 100 infants with PSAH was collected at UZ Gent (28 referred in 1986, 38 in 1987, 20 in 1988 and seven each in 1989 and 1990). 59 were inborn. Except for one post-term baby, all were delivered at term. The mean birthweight was 3260g (range 1970–4680g), with five <2500g and five >4000g. Male sex predominated (58 vs. 42). Neonatal death was recorded in two: one due to postpartum asphyxia, the other to sudden infant death syndrome. Extracranial trauma was infrequent, except for subaponeurotic bleeding which was diagnosed in 11 babies, all of whom were delivered by vacuum extraction (Table 6.5). For inborn infants ventouse delivery was performed with a 5cm diameter Malmström or Bird cup, with pressure elevated to 1kg/cm^2 in a single step over a few seconds. Extractions were never performed before full cervical dilatation.

Separating cases into those associated with trauma or asphyxia (excluding asphyxia if the Apgar score was ⩾4 at one minute and ⩾7 at five minutes, and if the umbilical artery pH, where available, was >7.15), there were 49 traumatic versus 51 asphyxial instances of PSAH. 19 of 42 inborn infants with a registered umbilical artery pH had a value ⩽7.15. Applying these arbitrary criteria (which were slightly different for this study than those given previously), the distribution in relation to mode of delivery is shown in Table 6.6 and Figure 6.22. The second stage was <15 minutes in 17 of 70 with well documented deliveries, and >60 minutes also in 17/70. A short second stage may have been contributory to the genesis of PSAH in eight of the 12 infants born by spontaneous vaginal delivery without birth asphyxia and in two of the 29 traumatic cases delivered by vacuum extraction. Five emergency caesarean sections were performed following attempted vacuum extraction with three to seven pulls, three of these infants suffering birth asphyxia.

For a cohort of 13 inborn infants with ventouse delivery and an umbilical artery pH >7.2, the mean number of vacuum tractions was 3.3 (range c to seven) and the duration of the second stage was short in one and 'normal   5 to 60 minutes) in nine. The only infant in this group with an Apgar score < at five minutes suffered from acute hypovolaemia following feto-maternal haemo   hage.

41

TABLE 6.6

**Mode of delivery in 100 term infants with primary subarachnoid
haemorrhage: trauma vs. birth asphyxia ± trauma**

Mode of delivery	Trauma alone (N=49)	Asphyxia ± trauma (N=51)
Spontaneous vaginal	12	10
Breech	1	3
Forceps	4	1
Vacuum	29	27
Elective caesarean	0	2
Emergency caesarean	3	8

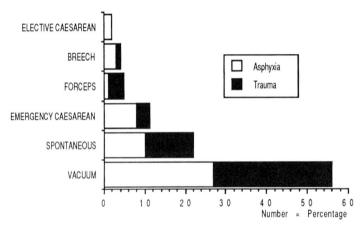

Fig. 6.22. Mode of delivery vs. percentage with birth asphyxia/trauma.

To determine the importance or irrelevance of the ventouse an *imaginary
reference population* was constructed, derived from personal data from the
obstetrics department at UZ Gent, combined with available data on the Flemish
region. The reference data were compiled by adding two thirds of outborn to one
third of inborn values, the distribution of place of birth in infants admitted to our
neonatal ward (Table 6.7). Using the chi-square method it was found that
significantly more infants with PSAH underwent ventouse extraction than were
born by spontaneous vaginal delivery (p<0.001). This difference remains
significant even if the reference population is constructed from 60 per cent inborn
and 40 per cent outborn fractions, the actual relation within the group with PSAH.
Possible causative mechanisms in the vacuum extraction subgroup are summarized
in Table 6.8. Within the population of vacuum deliveries without severe asphyxia at
least eight children had difficult instrumental delivery as the only recognized
mechanical risk factor, assuming that three tractions or less suggest an easy outlet

TABLE 6.7

Incidence of primary subarachnoid haemorrhage (PSAH) vs. mode of delivery:
comparison with an imaginary reference population†

Mode of delivery	UZ Gent 1986* (N=834) %	Flanders 1987–89** (N=117,028) %	Imaginary reference population %	PSAH 1986–90 (N=100) %
Spontaneous vaginal	44.0	73.3	63.6	22.0
Breech	4.2	1.9	2.7	4.0
Forceps	0.3	2.2	1.6	5.0
Vacuum	45.0	13.3	23.9	56.0
Caesarean section	7.0	9.4	8.6	13.0

†See text for composition.
*All birthweights >1000g. **Singletons only.

TABLE 6.8

Possible causative mechanisms in 56 vacuum delivered term infants with
primary subarachnoid haemorrhage

Feature	Trauma alone (N=30)	Asphyxia ± trauma (N=26)
POP or DTA	6	0
POP + long stage II	0	2
Long stage II alone	4	2
Long stage II, >4000g	0	2
>4000g alone	0	2
Short stage II	2	7
Vacuum alone: 0–3 tractions	10	3
4–10 tractions	8	8

POP = persistent occipito-posterior position.
DTA = deep transverse arrest.
Long second stage: >60 minutes.
Short second stage: <15 minutes.

ventouse delivery. Although the exact position of the fetal head at the onset of
traction cannot be traced in all cases, most of those with more than three pulls
started high- or midpelvic. In the subgroup with vacuum delivery and associated
birth asphyxia as defined before, 24 of 27 had additional mechanical problems.

The incidence of PSAH in the inborn term population at UZ Gent is estimated
to be around 20 per 1000 liveborn infants. The majority are associated with
mechanically difficult parturition in the absence of asphyxia, in agreement with
previous findings by Blennow *et al.* (1977). A surprisingly similar incidence was
reported in a prospective study on intracranial haemorrhage by Brand and Saling
(1988): they recorded 10.1 traumatic PSAH cases per 1000 term livebirths and 56.7
per 1000 term instrumental deliveries. In that study too, trauma was more

frequently associated than asphyxia, the latter occurring in 6.4 per 1000 term liveborn infants. Delivery modes specifically implicated in PSAH in the absence of asphyxia have not yet been identified. From the literature review referred to above it appears that the majority of infants with PSAH are born by spontaneous vaginal delivery. The present study suggests that difficult vacuum extraction may contribute to its genesis, either alone or as part of a more complex pattern. In addition it seems that a very short second stage is able to induce minor degrees of haemorrhage.

Comparison with data on cerebral irritation contained in the annual clinical reports (1988–90) of the Coombe Lying-In Hospital in Dublin seems to confirm a lower incidence in institutions using forceps as the tool for instrumental delivery (see below). The importance of birth asphyxia is re-emphasized by the present material, although a mechanical component was obvious.

Pathogenesis
The present findings, preliminary data of which have been published (Vanhaese-brouck 1986), add PSAH to a list of possible adverse events of difficult vacuum extraction. As speculated on and partly substantiated in the sections on cephalhaematoma, subgaleal bleeding and skull trauma during birth, the likely mechanism is increased compression of the fetal skull resulting from added tractional force (Moolgaoker *et al.* 1979), first producing venous congestion and then leading to extravasation of red cells. In some instances actual dural fraying or tearing may be added, although this produces intradural and subdural bleeding more readily than subarachnoid haemorrhage. What relative part is played by direct compression or displacement of major sinuses versus a general or focal increase of intracranial pressure as the origin of venous congestion, remains to be determined.

Clinical setting
Between December 1985 and May 1987, 48 consecutively born infants with subarachnoid haemorrhage were scrutinized for clinical details relating to the haemorrhage or its associations. The clinical diagnosis of PSAH was accepted in term neonates with a combination of (i) complicated delivery, (ii) abnormal neuro-logical behaviour, and (iii) an irregular supratentorial posterior interhemispheric density on uncontrasted CT scan of the brain (see below). The delivery was called uncomplicated in the absence of abnormal presentation, instrumental vaginal birth (low outlet manoeuvres excluded), emergency caesarean section, tight nuchal cord and birth asphyxia. The latter was defined as follows: Apgar score <7 at five minutes, and/or endotracheal resuscitation at birth and/or severe metabolic acidosis in the first hours of life (base deficit >10mmol/L), and/or persistent pulmonary hypertension. Association with more severe intracranial bleeding precluded the eponym primary in nine of them. Three different clinical groups were outlined: (i) 10 neonates presenting without birth asphyxia and with an *uncomplicated*

spontaneous vaginal delivery; (ii) 21 having a complicated delivery but no birth asphyxia—the *traumatic* group; and (iii) 17 who had severe birth *asphyxia*. The birth details and clinical data for the three groups are collected in Table 6.9. Babies in the traumatic group were more frequently firstborn than those in the uncomplicated group. Four spontaneous uncomplicated births had a short second stage. The only infant with convulsions in the uncomplicated group had hypocalcaemia due to maternal hyperparathyroidism.

The clinical features in the asphyxia group are self-explanatory. PSAH of traumatic origin presents in the delivery room with pallor, hypotonia and a partial or sluggish Moro reflex. On the neonatal ward these children appear to be in pain, are irritable, moan for several hours—some of them into the second day of life—and tend to lie with their heads retracted. Some alteration of tone plus irritability or grunting was noted in 16 of 18 inborn infants with presumed traumatic PSAH. The state of consciousness (see Table 6.9) accurately reflected the severity of neurological involvement, with the lowest score in the asphyxia and the highest in the uncomplicated group.

The nurses' hourly recordings of heart rates during the first three days of life, where available, were combined to produce a bradycardia index, as described in Table 6.9. Fixed bradycardia was equipresent, in about one third of cases, in each of the three PSAH groups, inferring that it is not related to asphyxia but possibly to the amount or distribution of extravasated subarachnoid blood. Anecdotal data point to the absence of bradycardia in anaemic infants and also show non-correlation with either serum calcium level or Q–Tc interval on ECG. Although control data from healthy neonates are not available, these findings would seem to implicate the haemorrhage itself and not the preceding cause. Comparable slowing of the heartbeat has been recognized in intracranial hypertension due to posterior fossa subdural haemorrhage (Blank *et al.* 1978) and during delivery as a consequence of intracranial hypertension.

Analysis of the clinical signs demonstrates the validity of the concept that there is a fraction of infants with PSAH attributed to asphyxial cerebrovascular congestion. The signs and symptoms recorded in the traumatic group are probably specific for PSAH and/or cerebro-venous congestion. Similar clinical observations have been reported before, describing minor neurological signs and the 'well baby with seizures on the second day of life' as recognizable correlates (Volpe 1987). Cerebral irritation or depression following instrumental delivery has been registered in an equal 3 per cent of both ventouse and forceps extractions (Chiswick and James 1979, Leijon 1980). It is of interest to note that in this study, seizures in the absence of severe asphyxia always occurred within the first 24 hours of life, except for the one hypocalcaemic infant in the uncomplicated group referred to above. Respiratory grunting, hypotonia, opisthotonus and irritability may relate to extravasation of blood in the subarachnoid space.

The 1988–90 annual clinical reports of the Coombe Lying-In Hospital, Dublin, include data on cerebral irritation as defined by the presence of (i) abnormal tone,

TABLE 6.9
Birth and clinical data on 48 term infants with subarachnoid haemorrhage, related to birth group

	Asphyxia (N=17)	Uncomplicated (N=10)	Traumatic (N=21)
Inborn	9	4	16
Firstborn	8	2	16
Male	10	8	10
Epidural analgesia	6	1	13
Delivery			
Spontaneous vaginal	2	6	0
Forceps	2	0	1
Vacuum	10	4 (easy)	18
Emergency caesarean	4	0	3
Mean Apgar score @ 1 min.	2.1	6.5	5.2
@ 5 mins	4.5	8.5	7.2
Endotracheal resuscitation	10	0	1
Mean Moro reflex score[1]	0.5	1.9	1.2
Pale colour at birth	14	2	11
General hypotonia (atonia)	15 (10)	2 (0)	13 (1)
Grunting	5	4	13
Irritability	3	4	7
Opisthotonus	3	3	3
Cyanotic spells	3	4	3
High-pitched cry	6	7	5
Seizures	11	1	5
Subtle	6	1	3
Clonic	6	1	3
Tonic	8	1	2
Hypotension	8	0	1
Assisted ventilation >24 hrs	10	0	1
Total parenteral nutrition: mean			
duration (days)	9.3	2.6	3.7
Mean hospital stay (days)	13	4.3	7.4
Mean consciousness state, days 1–3[2]	2.1	2.8	2.3
Mean state ≤2 on day 1[2]	7	1	5
Fixed bradycardia[3]	5	3	6
Neonatal death	3	0	0
Severe sequelae	3	0	1

[1]The Moro reflex score attributed zero points to an infant without the reflex at birth, 1 point in the event of a weak or asymmetrical reflex, and 2 points if a normal pattern of flexion and abduction was generated.

[2]The state of consciousness was defined as: state 1 for quiet sleep, state 2 for active REM sleep, state 3 for drowsiness, state 4 for a quietly awake infant, state 5 for an active infant, and state 6 for a crying infant.

[3]The bradycardia index was based on heart rate measurements (recorded only at or below state 4) over the first three days of life, scoring zero or 1pt per day for each of three criteria, for a maximum score of 9, as follows: zero points were accorded if the mean heart rate for the day was ≥130 bpm, if the lowest daily rate was ≥110 bpm, and if less than one third of the valid daily checks showed rates <120 bpm; conversely, 1 point was given if the mean heart rate was <130 bpm, if the lowest rate was <110 bpm, and if more than one third of counts were <120 bpm. Bradycardia was defined as fixed with a total score ≥4, and absent with a score of zero. Some measurements were taken for all infants, and the proportion of total possible measurements actually registered was 65 per cent.

and/or (ii) altered primitive reflexes, and/or (iii) seizures. Though without CT correlation, these clinical observations are similar to those described above. There were 46 instances on record of cerebral irritation in term (35/46) or post-term (11/46) neonates, a rate of 2.1 and 4.3 per 1000 term and post-term liveborn infants respectively. Seizures were recorded in 23/46, suggesting that only severe cases of cerebral irritation were taken into account. The incidence of cerebral irritation in firstborn infants of all gestational ages was 2.6/1000, compared with 1.8/1000 for the offspring of paras II–IV and 3.9/1000 for paras V and above. In 15/46 the Apgar score at five minutes was <7; of the remaining cases, seven followed spontaneous vaginal delivery (four with normal duration of labour, three with labour exceeding 12 hours), six followed forceps and six vacuum extraction, one was a breech birth and 11 were delivered by emergency caesarean section. There were 2668 forceps deliveries (13.6 per cent of all deliveries) versus 554 vacuum deliveries (2.8 per cent) during the period under study, but vacuum was used more on indication of fetal distress (58 per cent) than were forceps (51 per cent). 23 infants (1.2 per 1000 live births at or beyond 37 weeks of gestation) had neonatal seizures possibly related to the mode of delivery. Of those, 16/23 had an Apgar score ⩾7 at five minutes.

Radiological assessment
The present cornerstone of diagnosis, interpretation of the uncontrasted CT scan, has been explored and reported in a previous study (Govaert *et al.* 1990*a*). Briefly summarized, PSAH was considered present when irregular densities were found along the posterior interhemispheric cerebral fissure on at least two sections 4mm apart. Additional similar densities were often noticed in the vicinity of the cistern of the great cerebral vein of Galen, along the anterior interhemispheric fissure and covering parasagittal parts of the tentorium cerebelli (Figs. 6.23, 6.24). Although some of these alleged extravasations may actually have been located within the falx or tentorium or—more likely—were simply due to excessive venous congestion (Fig. 6.25) in babies with a normal high haemoglobin level, the strong correlation with difficult delivery and associated abnormal neurological signs lends them their pathological significance. Horie *et al.* (1988) described this 'falx image' in 45 per cent of a cohort of term infants admitted to neonatal care because of abnormal neurological signs and shown to have no abnormal neurological findings on follow-up at age 3 to 5 years; it was found in 13/19 cases on the first day of life, on day 14 in 14/37 cases and on day 28 in 1/17 cases. This gradual disappearance over days to weeks indicates pathological changes in addition to congestion. This lesion cannot be recognized with ultrasound.

Management and prognosis
Management will be purely symptomatic and is inherent to good routine neonatal care. As for long-term sequelae, the lack of systematic follow-up data does not allow comment. A proportion of cases in the present study have been shown to

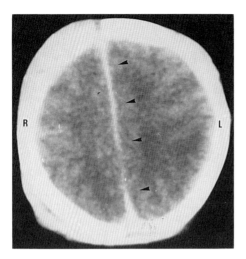

Fig. 6.23. Uncontrasted axial CT scan on day 1 following vacuum delivery (five pulls); note irregular density along falx in anterior and posterior interhemispheric fissure *(arrowheads)*.

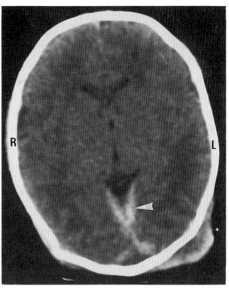

Fig. 6.24. Uncontrasted axial CT scan on day 2 following vacuum delivery in infant with sinus bradycardia and apparent discomfort: note symmetrical density along anterior tentorial margins near vein of Galen *(arrowhead)*.

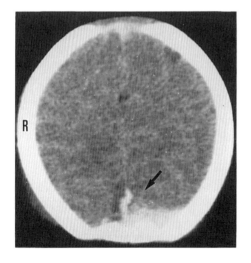

Fig. 6.25. Uncontrasted axial CT scan on day 2 following birth asphyxia with Sarnat grade III encephalopathy (coma and seizures): note pronounced congestion of superior sagittal sinus bridging vein *(arrow)*.

develop enlargement of the subarachnoid spaces and gross motor retardation in infancy (Alvarez *et al.* 1986, Govaert *et al.* 1991). In the acute stage, vasospasm might theoretically induce permanent lesions, a problem discussed in the section on arterial cerebral infarction due to intracranial haemorrhage (p. 62). Damage to the pia mater around birth hypothetically causes marginal glioneuronal heterotopic areas, necrosis in the outer marginal cortex layer and damage to radial glial end-feet (Sarnat 1987). Repeated subarachnoid bleeding in adults may lead to superficial siderosis affecting mainly the cerebellum and the nuclei of the VIIIth cranial nerve (Koeppen and Dentinger 1988). Volpe (1987) refers to epilepsy as a likely corollary, although confirmatory reports are lacking. One term infant with PSAH following vacuum extraction reported by Nanba *et al.* (1984), developed focal seizures and had delayed motor and speech development at 33 months of age. School problems were experienced by 10 per cent of infants with grade 1 neurological dysfunction in a classification system used by Amiel-Tison *et al.* (1988): the main cause for this minor cerebral dysfunction was postulated as mechanically difficult delivery. However, it is important to realize that the vast majority of term infants with posterior interhemispheric hyperdensity on CT scan and neurological abnormalities in the neonatal period will be apparently normal at 3 to 5 years of age (Horie *et al.* 1988).

Conclusions
This large collection of patients with suspected PSAH throws new light on the aetiology and clinical presentation of a relatively common neonatal intracranial event. Its retrospective character precludes detailed conclusions regarding clinical signs and symptoms. The lack of systematic follow-up beyond the newborn period, a second flaw in this study, limits its usefulness in developmental terms. Restrictions in the interpretation of CT scans have been outlined.

Given these limitations this study does suggest that (at least at UZ Gent):
• PSAH or marked intracranial venous congestion is a frequent reason for admitting a neonate to intensive care monitoring;
• PSAH is mainly associated with difficult vacuum extraction; although asphyxia can be a solitary association, most deliveries leading to PSAH are complicated by dystocia;
• the purely traumatic variety can be recognised clinically as a combination of some of the following signs: grunting, pallor at birth, partial depression of consciousness and primitive reflexes at birth, irritability, hypotonia, opisthotonus, high pitched cry and fixed slowing of the heartbeat.

Bleeding into the falx (intradural haematoma of the falx)
Anatomical description
As limited tentorial damage is difficult to recognize on CT or MRI scan, it has become practical to identify 'dural' with 'falcial' lesions. If actual dural tearing is associated, which occurs in less than half of the cases with falx damage, haemorrhage tends to be larger and becomes subdural. Major haemorrhages are occasionally retained within the dural leaflets (Kehrer 1939, Larroche 1977). Rupture of large anastomosing vessels between superior and inferior sagittal sinuses is their usual cause (Kehrer 1939). The location of most minor extravasations is close to the superior sagittal sinus or tentorial junction (Craig 1938).

TABLE 6.10

Dural injury at perinatal post-mortem examination in five studies*

Reference	Post-mortem population N	Tentorial damage N	Falx damage N
Saunders (1948)	50	48	4
Sulamaa and Vara (1952)	602	11	26
Nesbitt (1957)	94	11	4
Giordano (1959)**	310	16	1
Wigglesworth (1988)	515	20	7

*For various reasons these studies are not comparable (selection bias, differing definitions of dural damage, etc.).
**In Schwartz (1964).

TABLE 6.11

Intradural haemorrhage diagnosed during life in five term infants (UZ Gent, 1987–91)

Sex	Birthweight (g)	Mode of delivery	Neonatal history
M	3500	Spontaneous vaginal vertex (home)	Seizures, subarachnoid haemorrhage
M	2700	Breech, forceps, fundal pressure	Occipital osteodiastasis, fatal liver laceration
F	3110	Vacuum (8 pulls)	Seizures, persistent fetal circulation
M	3060	Vacuum (4 pulls)	Not available
F	3450	Vacuum (4 pulls)	Basal convexity subdural haemorrhage

Incidence

Limited falcial bleeding without tearing or fraying is infrequently reported because of its apparent innocuity or the overwhelming nature of associated injuries. Several authors have recorded prevalence of tears in the falx at post-mortem examination. In some reports the amount of tentorial damage can even be compared with that of the falx (Table 6.10). Combining the data from the two largest studies (Sulamaa and Vara 1952, Wigglesworth 1988) reveals a prevalence of 3 per 100 perinatal autopsies. According to Ludwig *et al.* (1980), using CT scan for diagnostic purposes, bleeding into the falx is about as frequent as PSAH. From early on and reconfirmed recently, it has been suggested that some of these falcial haemorrhages are observed following normal vaginal deliveries (Schwartz 1964). Other data clearly show an association with forceps delivery (0.49 per cent dural tears versus 0.018 per cent for spontaneous vertex deliveries) (Sulamaa and Vara 1952).

50

Personal observations suggest a link with vacuum delivery (five of seven cases diagnosed between 1988 and 1991). Table 6.11 lists five term newborn infants with intradural haemorrhage. In two others, both preterm second twins with a birthweight between 1500 and 2500g, the cup had been placed over the anterior fontanelle. These observations agree with those of Yllpö (1919) who reported a high incidence of dural lesions in the falx and around the superior sagittal sinus in infants of low birthweight.

Pathogenesis
A dural tear or superficial fraying of its layers is by definition traumatic. As elaborated in the preceding sections on tentorial damage and skull trauma during birth, excessive skull compression—either antero-posterior or latero-lateral—is the main cause. In a recent MRI-based study of three neonates with tentorial tears related to vacuum extraction, it has been suggested that the suction cup and its vacuum exert a direct effect on the falx, pulling it up toward the site of application (Hanigan *et al.* 1990*b*). Although nothing in that report substantiates it, the idea is not original. Saunders (1948), in a detailed description of 50 tentorial injuries at necropsy, tested his observations experimentally by exerting galeal traction on the skull of dead infants. This allowed him to demonstrate obvious falx strain via the scalp only when traction was applied over the anterior fontanelle. Similar forces on chin or occiput did not produce this amount of stress on the falx. Possibly vacuum extraction with the cup over the anterior fontanelle is also capable of lifting the falx directly.

Clinical setting
Signs, similar to those referred to in the section on PSAH, are the presenting features of isolated falx bleeding. If associated with major trauma, the intradural component is obscured by it and by asphyxial features.

Scanning assessment
I have been unable to find or produce ultrasonographically documented diagnoses, although some lesions high up in the falx must be accessible for recognition by ultrasound. Even CT documented falcial haemorrhage in the newborn infant is hard to find; one report correlates CT pictures with limited pathological findings (Ludwig *et al.* 1980). Intradural haemorrhages can be very similar to subarachnoid ones: they can be easy to differentiate in some babies but impossible to exclude in others. The typical image is that of a small focal linear or nodular density along the falx but not extending from bone to bone (or from bone to tentorium on coronal scans) (Fig. 6.26). A CT picture of a large falcial haematoma is shown by Volpe (1987) in a macrosomic infant following difficult breech delivery.

Management and prognosis
Treatment is impossible and unnecessary. The prognosis is unknown.

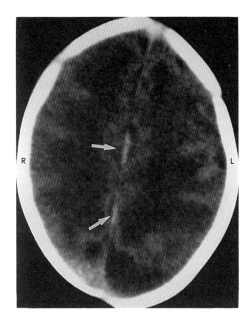

Fig. 6.26. Uncontrasted axial CT scan on day 2 showing two focal linear densities *(arrows)* suggestive of bleeding into the falx.

Acute convexity subdural haemorrhage

Anatomical diagnosis

Extracerebral effusions come in many different forms in early childhood, the differentiation of which is by no means obvious or simple. Based on personal experience and reports in the literature, the following categories are proposed: (i) prenatal subdural haemorrhage (SDH) or antenatal enlargement of the subarachnoid spaces either due to brain shrinkage or associated with disturbed cerebrospinal fluid (CSF) circulation; (ii) acute neonatal subdural haematoma; (iii) chronic subdural effusion of infancy with or without superimposed acute or recent haemorrhage; (iv) chronic subarachnoid fluid collections in macrocephalic infants; (v) acute infantile subdural haematoma of postnatal origin. Full discussion of some aspects is warranted here because of an established association with birth trauma (Schipke *et al.* 1954).

Blood can collect in the neonatal subdural space due to birth trauma, bleeding diathesis or rupture of a dural vascular malformation. In the case of mechanical injury, the vessels involved are either bridging veins crossing the subdural space from cortex to superior sagittal sinus (Kundrat 1890, Ballantyne 1890—in Schwartz 1964) or superficial cerebral veins crossing the dorsolateral cerebral surface including the large anastomosing veins emptying into the superior sagittal or transverse sinuses (Cushing 1905, Larroche 1977). Although the concept is long established, it is still unclear what, during birth moulding, makes the subdural course of those veins vulnerable. Congestion due to increased intracranial pressure

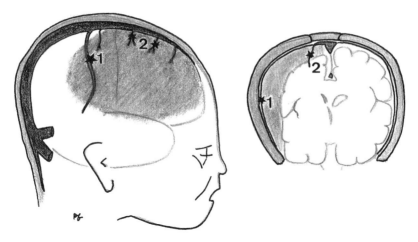

Fig. 6.27. Convexity subdural haematoma results from a ruptured large anastomosing (1) or superior sagittal sinus bridging vein (2); blood mainly collects above the insula, near the sinus.

and/or asphyxial cardiovascular compromise will probably increase that vulner-ability (see section on PSAH). The ensuing collection of blood spreads above the subarachnoid membrane to cover the frontoparietal and even occipital regions on the lateral brain surface with the bulk of coagulum above the sylvian fissure (Fig. 6.27), At autopsy, clot might be attached to the reflected parietal bone flap or lie free on the subarachnoid membrane. Subdural blood will subsequently separate easily from the brain (Larroche 1984). The underlying cerebrum often shows haemorrhagic softening, referred to as contusional (Larroche 1977). As the veins involved in the generation of a convexity SDH are hidden by the clot, absence of bridging veins compared with the intact ones on the unaffected side may be an indirect means of diagnostic confirmation (Pape and Wigglesworth 1977). Bilateral bleeding, affecting only about one neonatal case in five, is uncommon in comparison with infantile subdural hygroma or haematoma. Throughout the existing literature little distinction is made between convexity SDH and basal SDH (detailed in the following section).

Incidence and causation
This type of haemorrhage was regarded as the main consequence of mechanical birth trauma before the discovery, at the beginning of the century, of tentorial stress and related lesions (Beneke 1910 in Schwartz 1964). Craig (1938), not separating convexity from basal haematoma in an overview of 126 neonatal autopsies with intracranial haemorrhage, recorded 20 isolated SDHs (10 in term infants), of which six followed breech delivery and eight forceps extraction. Gröntoft (1953) on the contrary did not observe any convexity SDH in a series of 120 stillbirths and first week deaths with intracranial bleeding; he assumed this

TABLE 6.12

Obstetric profile of 23 term infants with isolated convexity subdural haemorrhage†

	UZ Gent 1980–91 (N=5)	Hammersmith 1980–91 (N=18)
Birth asphyxia*	1	7
Stillbirth	0	5
Mode of delivery		
Spontaneous vaginal	1	5
Breech	0	1
Forceps	1	11**
Vacuum	3	1
Neonatal death	1	18

†The background populations from which these two cohorts are derived are very different (see text).
*Apgar scores <4 at one and <7 at five minutes; umbilical artery pH, if available, <7.15.
**Includes one infant with forceps delivery after failed vacuum extraction.

absence to be partly due to routine vitamin K supplementation. Natelson and Sayers (1973), in a study of 42 neonates with traumatic intracranial haemorrhage diagnosed in life, recorded 10 acute SDHs, at least four of which were of the convexity type as suggested by positive subdural taps.

It has become quite exceptional to publish genuine convexity SDH: Fenichel *et al*. (1984) recorded none in 24 subsequent intracranial bleeds recognized in living term infants. The prevalence in reports on intracranial haemorrhage diagnosed in living term neonates is 23 out of a total of 238 cases reviewed to date (9.7 per cent) (Natelson and Sayers 1973, Flodmark *et al*. 1980*b*, Leblanc and O'Gorman 1980, Pierre-Kahn *et al*. 1985, this report). One explanation for the scarcity of reports on convexity SDH is that in most instances this type of lesion seems to be overshadowed by associated (central or lateral) tentorial damage, occipital osteodiastasis or parenchymal injury. In 31 stillbirths and neonatal deaths of term infants autopsied at Hammersmith Hospital, London, between 1980 and 1991, 18 isolated convexity SDHs were recorded, most of them either irrelevant (7/18) or only contributory (6/18) to the cause of death, with a mere five fatal haemorrhages. In the latter series, occipital osteodiastasis (5/18), falx damage (5/18) and tentorial injury (6/18), all of minor degree, were associated. Only two infants had fatal convexity SDH without tentorial damage. Obstetric histories of these 18 cases, plus five from UZ Gent, are summarized in Table 6.12. As pointed out by Tank *et al*. (1971), breech birth has now become an uncommon cause of convexity SDH, replaced by instrumental delivery as the most important aetiological factor. Compared with other types of SDH, vaginal breech delivery was rarely associated with convexity SDH either in the cases gathered on the neonatal ward at UZ Gent or in the post-mortem series from London. The single Hammersmith case related to assisted birth from the breech with resulting birth asphyxia and occipital osteodiastasis. This lack of an association with breech birth is in disagreement with a report by Abroms *et al.* (1977) in which prevention of convexity SDH was suggested as an indication for caesarean delivery in fetuses presenting by the breech.

Spontaneous vaginal delivery preceded genuine convexity SDH in five Hammersmith cases, three of which were fresh stillbirths: in one the second stage was less than 10 minutes, in two it exceeded one hour; two other infants presented with a persistent occipito-posterior position and normal second stage length. Whereas the instrument used in London to facilitate deliveries associated with convexity SDH was mainly forceps, in Gent it was the vacuum extractor. In two of the five latter instances, both associated with skull fracture, the number of pulls exceeded four.

Clinical setting
Most convexity SDHs seem to attract attention after a minimum interval of 24 hours, in accord with their non-arterial origin (Pierre-Kahn *et al.* 1985, Romodanov and Brodsky 1987, Volpe 1987). Where there is associated severe birth asphyxia, certain signs may be masked by those of hypoxic–ischaemic encephalopathy, or they may be so minor as to escape detection or not cause enough concern to undertake CT scanning.

In its classical presentation it behaves like infantile subdural haematoma with (i) seizures, initially focal, (ii) contralateral paralysis with the eyes deviated toward the paralytic side, (iii) a tense fontanelle, and (iv) retained doll's eye movements reflecting an intact brainstem circuitry (Volpe 1987). Irritability has always been considered somewhat typical of convexity SDH, and unusual alertness, jitteriness and generalized hypertonia may be present (Seitz 1907, Craig 1938). However, most authors agree that the symptomatology of convexity SDH lacks specificity and cannot be distinguished from that of, for instance, posterior fossa SDH (Rydberg 1932, Thorn 1969).

Radiological assessment
The difficulty of clinical recognition is overcome by the use of ultrasound and CT scanning. Major haemorrhages will lead to hypovolaemic shock, anaemia and uncal herniation with ipsilateral mydriasis. On the other hand, residual chronic subdural hygroma and external hydrocephalus in infancy could well be the first, delayed sign of traumatic neonatal convexity SDH.

Angiographic documentation of arterial shifts to confirm the presence of SDH would only be useful now in selected cases with suspicion of an underlying vascular anomaly (Emmanouilides and Hoy 1967, Deonna and Oberson 1974). The same goes for isotope brain scanning (Deonna and Oberson 1974). Surprisingly, it was

55

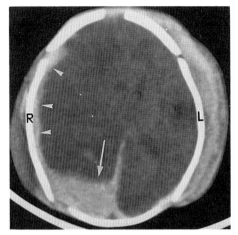

Fig. 6.28. Axial CT scan on day 2 following vacuum extraction of boy with subgaleal bleeding and cardiac arrest at 2 hours: note major convexity subdural haemorrhage *(arrow)* covering right occipital area and shifting the midline, and minor subdural bleeding in right parietal area *(arrowheads)*. At post-mortem examination the superior sagittal sinus was found to be lacerated.

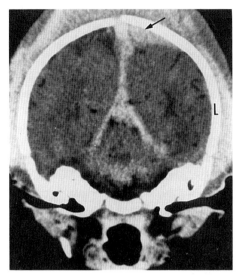

Fig. 6.29. Coronal post-mortem CT scan on day 1 in boy whose death was due to subgaleal haemorrhage and occipital osteodiastasis following vacuum delivery. Note minor convexity subdural haemorrhage to left of superior sagittal sinus *(arrow)*. Gas arteriogram is the result of systemic embolization during resuscitation attempts.

difficult to trace reported ultrasound and CT pictures of neonatal subdural haemorrhage in the vicinity of the superior sagittal sinus. Even in textbooks the pictures used as representative of convexity SDH could well be of the basal convexity variety (Volpe 1987). Two typical CT pictures of minor convexity SDH are shown in Figures 6.28 and 6.29: the major bleeding site is at or above the insula, on coronal sections shown to be related to the superior sagittal sinus or a tributary. All supratentorial haematomas in a recent prospective MRI-based study, were of the basal subdural type (Keeney *et al.* 1991).

Management and prognosis
Diagnostic subdural tapping need no longer be performed if brain imaging is available, but 'needling' of the subdural space is still advocated as the first choice of treatment by some (Romodanov and Brodsky 1987). For details on the method the reader is referred elsewhere (Abroms *et al.* 1977). Only if the clot is too solid, or so posterior that it cannot be reached through the anterior fontanelle, is craniotomy and subsequent temporary drainage the alternative choice (Schipke *et al.* 1954, Romodanov and Brodsky 1987). Suggested 'needle' trajectories for evacuation of subdural haematomas are presented in the ensuing section on basal SDH. The

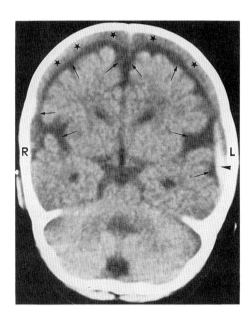

Fig. 6.30. Coronal CT scan of 2-month-old boy with irritability, anaemia, tense fontanelle and seizures. Note chronic hypodense subarachnoid fluid collection *(arrows)* covered by bilateral subacute isodense *(asterisks)* and acute left hyperdense *(arrowhead)* convexity subdural haematoma.

inherent dangers of subdural tapping are (i) creation of fresh sub- or epidural bleeding, (ii) creation of a fistulous track if used repeatedly, (iii) creation of a cerebral convexity implantation epidermoid tumour, (iv) meningitis, and (v) seizures if the brain substance is penetrated (Dunn 1982). Neurosurgeons proclaiming the superiority of emergency craniotomy would only withhold from surgery if the haemorrhage was multifocal or the midline was not shifted (Pierre-Kahn *et al*. 1985). Thus the absolute indication for treatment, either by tapping or craniotomy, is life-threatening intracranial hypertension. Although suggested to be the cause of chronic subdural hygroma (Pape and Wigglesworth 1979), there is no proof of the need to evacuate minor haematomas.

Some 15 per cent of chronic infantile SDHs are engendered by birth trauma, both in my experience (Fig. 6.30) and in that of others (Ingraham and Matson 1954, Mealey 1968, Rabe *et al*. 1968, Till 1968, Hooper 1969, McLaurin *et al*. 1971, Aoki *et al*. 1985). In a subgroup of 35 infants with SDH treated neurosurgically at UZ Gent between 1970 and 1979, 11 had been admitted for neonatal care; 10 deliveries were by instrumental traction (eight vacuum) and four by emergency caesarean section. The presenting signs were intracranial hypertension in 28 of the 35, macrocephaly in 16 and seizures in five. Four children were left with residual brain damage and epilepsy. Convincing documentation of the outcome of isolated convexity SDH in the absence of associated asphyxial brain damage is lacking. Infarction of the adjacent cerebral (sub)cortex by contusion, compression, or venous or arterial ischaemia is a hypothetical mechanism of permanent neurological impairment.

Basal subdural haemorrhage (lateral tentorial injury)

Anatomical description

Basal SDH can be depicted as the neonatal intracranial haemorrhage variant where extravasated blood is collected in the subdural space underneath the temporal and/or occipital lobes. In most cases the bleeding reaches the basal parts of the cerebral convexity, not surmounting the sylvian fissure. Some haemorrhage may also collect between both occipital lobes. It has to be distinguished from convexity SDH related to rupture of superior sagittal sinus bridging veins, the classical presentation of infantile SDH. Severe central tentorial damage can also lead to a collection of clots underneath the cerebrum, but in such cases it is clear that the epicentre of trauma is not in the vicinity of the transverse sinus (Gröntoft 1953). The vessels involved in basal SDH are small veins running in the tentorial leaflets (Craig 1938), cerebral bridging veins draining into the transverse sinus (Schreiber 1959) or the inferior anastomotic vein linking the middle and posterior convexity cerebral drainage to the transverse sinus or great vein of Galen (Larroche 1977). In my experience this event can lead to uncal herniation and ipsilateral arterial ischaemia in the regions of middle or posterior cerebral arteries (Govaert *et al.* 1992*c*).

Incidence

Basal SDH is not explicitly described in recent relevant textbooks (Pape and Wigglesworth 1979, Volpe 1987, Friede 1989). There is evidence, however, that it is not uncommon in relation to mechanical birth injury. Beneke (1910) had stressed the overall dominance of tentorial damage compared with classical convexity SDH. Craig (1938) may have been one of the first to suggest lateral tentorial damage as the main problem in some of his cases, whereas Gröntoft (1953) recorded 25 instances of minor (vs. 38 severe) tentorial injuries associated with predominant bleeding into the middle cranial fossa which was not really considered to be the cause of death. Schreiber (1959) reported 17 neonates with supratentorial SDH, 13 of whom presented with a tense fontanelle and unilateral oculomotor nerve palsy. Subdural punctures were negative in two, but subsequent craniotomy showed the blood to be located under the sylvian fissure. 16 of the 17 haemorrhages were unilateral.

I have been able to compile a total of 21 cases of basal SDH confirmed by CT scan in term infants, including ten from the literature (Ponté *et al.* 1971, Cartwright *et al.* 1979, Guekos-Thöni *et al.* 1980, Meidell *et al.* 1983, Pierre-Khan *et al.* 1985, Romodanov and Brodsky 1987), plus five from UZ Gent and six from Hammersmith Hospital. Details are given in Table 6.13. A typical case was described by Ponté *et al.* (1979): they recorded shifting of the middle cerebral artery by a left basal convexity subdural and intracerebral haematoma, evacuated during craniotomy on the 14th day of life.

Although diagnostic methods *in vivo* are not really comparable with autopsy findings, the combined results from Gent and Hammersmith do indicate that

TABLE 6.13

**Obstetric and clinical data on 21
term infants with basal subdural
haemorrhage***

Sex (M/F/?)	8/9/4
Mode of delivery[1]	
Spontaneous vaginal	7
Breech	3
Forceps	5
Vacuum	4
Caesarean	1
Birthweight >4000g	2
Apgar score <4 @ 1 min.	2
<7 @ 5 mins	6
Side of bleeding (R/L/B)[2]	9/9/3
Craniotomy	3
Arterial stroke	8
Neonatal death	8

*See text.
[1]One infant, who had haemophilia as
underlying haemostatic disorder, was
delivered by emergency caesarean
section after failed vacuum traction.
[2]R = right, L = left, B = bilateral.

bleeding in the lateral tentorial region is not as uncommon as suggested by the scarcity of reported cases. It should be carefully looked for in children surviving mechanically difficult delivery. In a series of 41 newborn infants operated on for intracranial birth trauma over the course of 15 years (Romodanov and Brodsky 1987), 13 had basal SDH versus 13 with classical convexity and 15 with posterior fossa SDH.

Of 31 cases of SDH in term neonates observed at UZ Gent and Hammersmith Hospital between 1980 and 1991, six had basal SDH versus five with convexity SDH and 20 with central tentorial damage.

Reviewing details of the cases presented in Table 6.13, it is clear that— as with convexity SDH—breech presentation does not feature as an important risk factor in contrast with instrumental delivery.

Pathogenesis

The lesion is almost invariably of traumatic nature, although any bleeding tendency can modulate the extent of haemorrhage. Tentorial stress has been outlined in the section on skull trauma during birth. The necropsy findings in the Hammersmith autopsy subgroup indicated tentorial fraying in three (one unilateral, two bilateral) and a genuine unilateral tear in two. This coincides with the proposed aetiology of minor lateral tentorial damage. What differs in the causation between central and lateral tentorial damage is not known. The site of bleeding is not necessarily from the partial tear, but can be a ruptured bridging vein in the surroundings. When following breech delivery the presentation will usually be more dramatic because of the associated posterior fossa haemorrhage, in part explaining classification of those cases outside this selected variety of basal SDH.

Clinical setting
Of the 15 living newborn infants, referred to in the preceding overview, for whom some clinical data were available (nine literature cases and six from Gent), six presented with intracranial hypertension as indicated by a tense anterior fontanelle. Although uncal herniation, indicated by unilateral mydriasis, was only mentioned in two (Schreiber 1959, Ponté *et al.* 1971), documentation of ipsilateral hypoperfusion of the middle cerebral artery in three Belgian infants suggests the importance of the space-occupying effect this kind of bleeding can produce (see sections on arterial cerebral hypoperfusion and intracranial birth trauma). Seizures were recorded in at least seven of 12 neonates, some with associated focal changes on EEG. Unusual episodes of bradycardia with shallow breathing for about one minute were the presenting features on the first day of life in one infant (Meidell *et al.* 1983).

Radiological assessment
I could find no report of associated skull fractures on standard X-rays. Ultrasonography is unsatisfactory for display of this kind of bleeding in proximity to the tentorial leaflet and bone. As mentioned before, angiographic evidence of extracerebral haemorrhage and associated displacement of ipsilateral arteries has been shown in the past (Emmanouilides and Hoy 1967, Ponté *et al.* 1971). On CT scans made using earlier equipment (Fig. 6.31), this type of bleeding was possibly misinterpreted as being of intracerebral nature (Welch and Strand 1986), a problem that should now be overcome by current CT or MRI apparatus. Coronal sections, as with central tentorial damage, will provide images that readily fit our anatomical way of comprehending intracranial lesions (for examples, see section on superficial cerebral venous thrombosis).

Case history
CASE 6.4
This girl was inborn as the fourth child to a 34-year-old woman, with induction of labour at 38 weeks for maternal and obstetric practical reasons. The first stage took 11 hours, whereas the second ended after six minutes with vacuum extraction (four pulls) because of early fetal heart deceleration. The baby's cord was tightly wrapped around the neck twice, and shoulder dystocia was recorded. Birthweight was 3450g and the head circumference was 35cm. Apgar scores were 1 and 6 at one and five minutes. Umbilical artery pH was 7.21. Resuscitation with bag and mask was given for four minutes. We admitted a very pale and hypotonic female with extensive caput formation and laceration of the skin at the cup margins. She showed respiratory grunting for several hours. Her second day haemoglobin was 101g/L (possibly associated with suspected feto-placental haemorrhage, as the placental

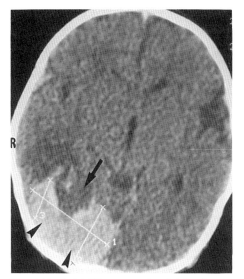 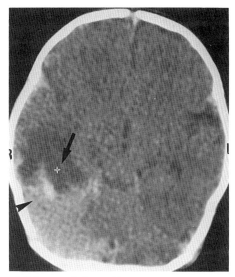

Fig. 6.31. Axial CT scan on day 6 following 'uneventful' forceps delivery (Case 6.6). Note irregular density above right tentorial leaflet, abutting temporal bone *(arrowheads)*; hypodensity within adjacent parenchyma suggests hypoperfusion of posterior branches of ipsilateral middle cerebral artery *(arrow)*.

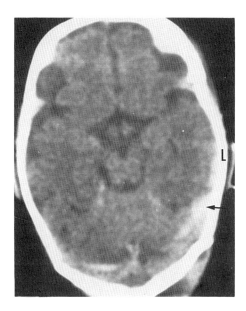

Fig. 6.32. Axial CT scan on day 2 in Case 6.4. Note density within region of left transverse sinus suggestive of basal subdural haematoma *(arrow)*. Other sections showed suspected subarachnoid haemorrhage and bleeding into the falx.

weight was 880g with a negative maternal Kleihauer–Betke test). A CT scan on day 2 documented left basal convexity subdural bleeding and subarachnoid haemorrhage (Fig. 6.32). A coagulation profile was completely normal. We lost this girl from follow-up when her parents moved abroad.

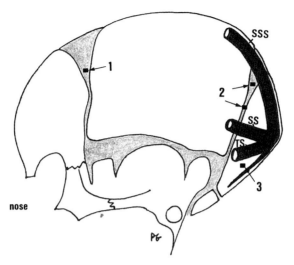

Fig. 6.33. Suggested approach for aspiration of subdural collections: (1) lateral anterior fontanelle for convexity subdural haemorrhage; (2) lambdoid suture or lateral posterior fontanelle for basal subdural haemorrhage; (3) burrhole through lateral occipital squama for posterior fossa subdural haemorrhage. (SSS = superior sagittal sinus; SS = straight sinus; TS = transverse sinus.)

Management and prognosis

In the presence of life-threatening intracranial hypertension a neurosurgical evacuation of some clot is warranted. Apart from classical craniotomy or aspiration through a burr hole, tapping through the lambdoid suture has been proposed as an alternative (Brill *et al.* 1985, Romodanov and Brodsky 1987) (Fig. 6.33). During this procedure care must be taken not to puncture the transverse sinus, which can be done by entering the dura slightly higher than the external occipital protuberance. If not complicated by severe birth asphyxia and arterial ischaemia the outlook may be good (Schreiber 1959).

Arterial cerebral stroke and birth trauma

Anatomical description

In some newborn infants recovering from mechanically difficult delivery, an extracerebral intracranial haemorrhage is associated with hypoperfusion of the ipsilateral territory of posterior and/or middle cerebral artery on CT or MRI scan. A residual triangular cortico-subcortical cavitation on follow-up will prove the advanced degree of ischaemia in those areas. Underlying mechanisms described so far, and an additional one documented within the Gent material, are depicted in Figures 6.34 and 6.35.

Incidence and pathogenesis

Of seven personal observations, five were associated with SDH, one with PSAH

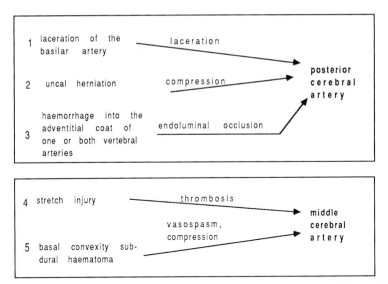

Fig. 6.34. Underlying mechanisms of cranial birth trauma and stroke, as reported by: (1) Krauland (1952); (2) Remillard *et al.* (1974), Deonna and Prod'hom (1980); (3) Yates (1959); (4) Miller *et al.* (1981); (5) Govaert *et al.* (1992c).

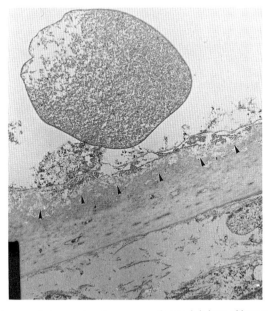

Fig. 6.35. Electron microscopic image showing presumed stretch injury of internal elastic membrane of middle cerebral artery *(arrowheads)* following forceps delivery; in the absence of major intracranial haemorrhage this lesion caused thrombosis of the vessel involved. (Roessman and Miller 1980, by permission.)

and another with epidural haematoma (Govaert *et al*. 1992*c*). Of a combined series of 23 infants with basal SDH as part of their injury (21 term, as described in the preceding section, plus two preterm infants), four had associated stroke as against one of 20 patients with central tentorial damage. The one infant with isolated convexity SDH and necrosis of the area perfused by the posterior middle cerebral artery branches following difficult vacuum delivery had bilateral parietal fractures and cerebral contusion on the involved side.

In addition to these seven personal cases, I have reviewed 10 cases diagnosed *in vivo* reported in the literature (Remillard *et al*. 1974, Deonna and Prod'hom 1980, Roessmann and Miller 1980, Billard *et al*. 1982, Hill *et al*. 1983, Mannino and Trauner 1983, Fenichel *et al*. 1984, Halsey and Stoddard 1984, Hanigan *et al*. 1990*b*). Nine of 15 for whom the sex is noted were male. All were born at term; two had a low birthweight (one LBW, one VLBW). Birth asphyxia was thought to have complicated the picture in only 6/17. On record were four skull fractures (one left, two right, one bilateral), five cephalhaematomas and two subgaleal haemorrhages in eight infants with associated epicranial trauma. One child suffered from a fractured long bone, whereas four had facial nerve palsy (one central, three peripheral due to applied forceps blades). The ischaemic artery, invariably ipsilateral to the haemorrhage if described, was the posterior cerebral in five instances and the middle cerebral in 12. In four (one vacuum and three forceps deliveries) there was no underlying haemorrhage; in another four (one emergency caesarean and three vacuum deliveries) there was a PSAH; in one breech-delivered infant an epidural haemorrhage was recorded; two convexity SDHs were recorded following vacuum delivery; there were three basal SDHs, one each following breech, vacuum and forceps delivery; two cases of central tentorial bleeding were related to a breech and a vacuum delivery; and finally one parenchymal cerebral haemorrhage was associated with precipitate delivery. Of 15 children surviving the neonatal period, seven had cerebral palsy and at least four developed epilepsy.

Three personal cases suggest the existence of a mechanism not yet adequately documented: basal convexity SDH leading to occlusion of the ipsilateral middle cerebral artery or its branches. This vessel obstruction might follow stretch injury and subsequent thrombosis (Roessman and Miller 1980), direct compression by the space-occupying haematoma or arterial embolism. Vasospasm due to the presence of surrounding subarachnoid haemorrhage, as in adults, may well be another mode of genesis. Supporting the latter hypothesis is the observation in a personal case of the absense of ischaemia on day 2 and its subsequent appearance on day 8. The necessity for performing a scan in the second week of life to detect arterial cerebral stroke in infants with seizures, was already recognized by others (Mannino and Trauner 1983). Attenuation of affected zones on uncontrasted CT scan normally presents within 12 to 24 hours following occlusion, rendering unlikely the hypothesis of direct arterial damage in this personal case. Some experimental work on cats supports the idea of erythrocyte-induced perihaemorrhagic vasoconstriction of isolated middle cerebral arteries (Edvinsson *et al*. 1986). MacDonald *et al*. (1991)

studying cerebral arteries *in situ* in monkeys found that oxyhaemoglobin rather than methaemoglobin or bilirubin caused vasospasm following SAH. In addition, spasm of the middle cerebral artery has been reported in older children with head and neck injury (Frantzen *et al.* 1962). Raised potassium levels in CSF have been found in preterm infants with intraventricular haemorrhage and cerebral infarction, raising the possibility that they may contribute to the development of infarction through vasospasm (Stutchfield and Cooke 1989).

The absence of a left-sided predilection, currently observed in neonatal stroke in general, in this series of trauma-related cerebral infarctions (five right and six left middle cerebral arteries involved) is compatible with a local and not an embolic phenomenon (Mannino and Trauner 1984). Whatever the underlying mechanism, both posterior and middle cerebral arteries are vulnerable to occlusion following peritentorial subdural bleeding. In one infant, arterial occlusion of a posterior branch of the middle cerebral artery might have been brought about by contusion of the parenchyma in addition to the above-mentioned proposed mechanisms. Of some importance may be the rarity of this event following breech delivery (only 3/17 reviewed cases) and the possibility of its occurrence after vacuum as well as forceps extraction, confirming the proposed hypothesis of supratentorial injury as an initiator.

Case histories

CASE 6.5
This girl, second of female twins, was outborn at 38 weeks of gestation with three emergency vacuum tractions because of fetal bradycardia. Her Apgar scores were 4 and 6 at one and five minutes. She weighed 2270g at birth and was referred promptly with a diagnosis of subgaleal haemorrhage with hypovolaemic shock. Neither seizures nor signs of intracranial hypertension were apparent. CT scan showed appearances compatible with epicranial bleeding and revealed small ventricles, dehiscence between the left parietal and occipital bone, and a distinct extracerebral haemorrhage overlying the left tentorial leaflet adjacent to the posterior falx and left occipital cerebral lobe (Fig. 6.36*a*). A repeat CT scan on day 8, taken because of focal EEG disturbances, demonstrated residual subdural blood and additional marked hypodensity of the left parieto-temporal area (Fig. 6.36*b*). Doppler ultrasound on the other hand showed symmetrical flow velocities in both middle cerebral arteries. At the age of 6 months the ultrasound image of the brain was symmetrically normal, but detailed neurological examination suggested a mild right spastic hemiplegia.

CASE 6.6
After an uneventful pregnancy this firstborn boy was delivered at term; the vaginal delivery was difficult, complicated by a persistent occipito-posterior position, long second stage (135 minutes) and failed forceps traction. Nevertheless, his Apgar score was 9 at one and five minutes. He weighed 3450g. There were no obvious neonatal problems. Pathological density of the right temporal region on ultrasound prompted CT scanning on the sixth day of life: appearances suggested that the right tentorial leaflet was covered with blood extending into the cerebral parenchyma of temporal and occipital lobes. In front of the bleeding an area of hypodensity could be seen up to the level of the insula (Fig. 6.31). At 6 months he had a normal ultrasound and neuromotor development remained within normal limits.

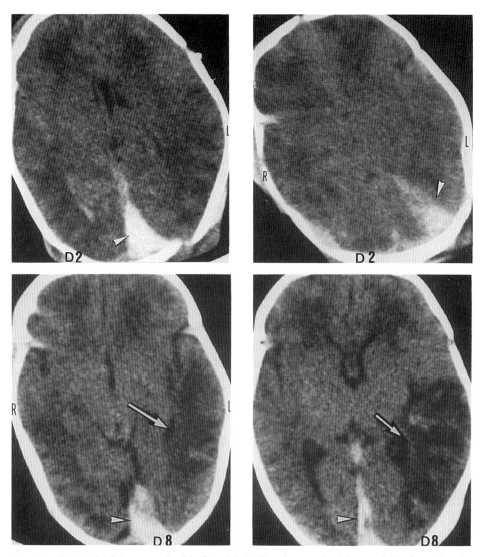

Fig. 6.36. *(Top)* Axial CT scans on day 2 in Case 6.5. *(a)* Density covering left tentorial leaflet and mesial occipital surface, compatible with basal subdural haemorrhage *(arrowheads)*. *(Bottom)* Control scans on day 8 show hypoperfusion within territory of posterior branches of middle cerebral artery *(arrows)*.

Prognosis and management
The possible sequelae of cortico-subcortical parenchymal loss have been outlined in the section on arterial infarction. A typical defect is shown in Figure 6.37, the follow-up scan at 14 months of a term infant with subgaleal bleeding and bilateral parietal fracture following vacuum delivery. This girl developed contralateral hemiplegia.

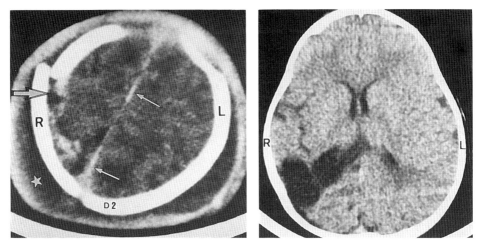

Fig. 6.37. Axial CT scan on day 2 *(left)* following difficult vacuum extraction resulting in subgaleal haemorrhage *(asterisk)*: note subdural haemorrhage *(large arrow)* and contusion under right parietal bone fracture, together with intradural haematoma *(small arrows)*. Control CT scan at 14 months *(right)* shows a triangular defect in cortical and subcortical tissue. This lesion was associated with contralateral hemiplegia.

The importance of damage to the vertebral arteries has been stressed as a possible cause of ataxic cerebral palsy, cranial nerve palsies and visual deficit (Yates 1973). One syndromic entity worth mentioning is the triad temporal lobe epilepsy, homonymous hemi- or quadranopia and enlarged occipital horn following perinatal infarction of the posterior cerebral artery territory (Remillard *et al.* 1974).

Central tentorial damage (tentorial laceration or tear, falco-tentorial injury)
Anatomical description
This section covers traumatic lesions associated with overstretching and tearing of the central tentorial fibres, mainly the 'vertical stress band' as described by Holland (1937) (Fig. 6.38), sometimes associated with falx injury in the vicinity of the inferior sagittal sinus. The tentorium can be torn across its full thickness, when the free anterior margin is almost invariably involved, or have partial superficial tears (fraying) (Pape and Wigglesworth 1979). If (i) the line of injury crosses a major vein, such as the straight sinus, vein of Galen (Fig. 6.39) or in rare cases the transverse sinus, or if (ii) even in the absence of a true tentorial laceration, a persistent tentorial sinus (or one of its tributaries) is damaged, acute and massive peritentorial bleeding will often lead to early death from both hypovolaemic shock and hypertension within the posterior fossa (Craig 1938, Pape and Wigglesworth 1979). The site of blood collection is within the middle cranial fossa (basal SDH) (Gröntoft 1953), between the bases of the cerebral hemispheres (basal interhemispheric SDH) and high up in the posterior fossa (superior posterior fossa SDH)

67

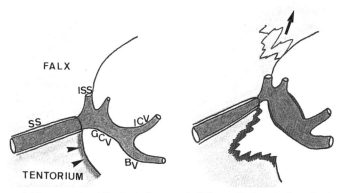

Fig. 6.38. The mesial free margin of the tentorium cerebelli bears the brunt of mechanical stress during cranial compression. The falco-tentorial junction may be lifted upwards and anteriorly, leading to tentorial tear and congestion of the great vein of Galen. (SS = straight sinus; ISS = inferior sagittal sinus; GCV = great cerebral vein; ICV = internal cerebral vein; BV = basal vein.)

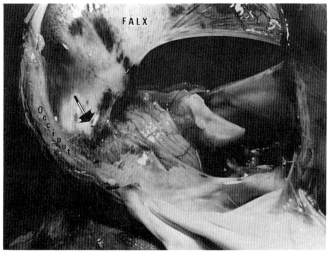

Fig. 6.39. Post-mortem view of fatal tentorial injury *(arrow)* following difficult vacuum extraction with several cup detachments. Leaflet is completely torn from free margin to skull bone revealing the cerebellum.

(Fig. 6.40). If only minor vessels (bridging veins to cerebellum and brainstem or small tentorial veins) are involved, haemorrhage can be minimal and not fatal, with signs not apparent before the second half of the first day (subacute presentation). Full thickness tears sometimes lack haemorrhage, suggesting that rupture of bridging veins in the vicinity has more clinical importance, although the injured tentorium serves as one of the hallmarks of mechanical trauma. Onset of hydrocephalus beyond the first week following posterior fossa or peritentorial

68

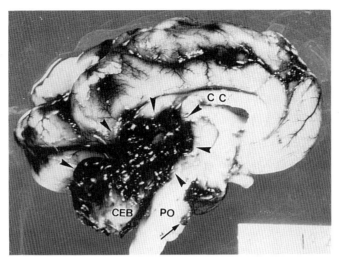

Fig. 6.40. Post-mortem view of fatal central tentorial injury following failed instrumental delivery. *Arrowheads* show haemorrhage around and above cerebellar vermis, into cisterna ambiens and in supracallosal region between both hemispheres. (CC = corpus callosum; CEB = cerebellar vermis; PO = pons.) (Courtesy Prof. J.S. Wigglesworth.)

haematoma constitutes the chronic presentation, sometimes delayed into the second month of life (French and Dublin 1977). The alleged possibility of tentorial arterial damage is not documented in neonates (Welch and Strand 1986). Unilateral tears are more common if they occur after intrauterine death (Gröntoft 1953), but may also relate to oblique distortion of the skull as, for instance, by inaccurate application of forceps blades (Pape and Wigglesworth 1979). The review by Schwartz (1964) demonstrated particular vulnerability of the transition zone between straight sinus and great cerebral vein to displacement of the falco-tentorial junction, leaving the vein of Galen kinked, distended, often thrombosed and sometimes ruptured. Rarity of the latter findings in present perinatal autopsies is partially explained by reduction of the duration of labour over the past few decades. The association between occipital osteodiastasis and tentorial changes is detailed elsewhere.

Incidence
There is doubt whether the incidence of severe tentorial damage has fallen in the latter part of this century. Already in the years 1921 to 1941 only 11 tentorial tears were discovered in a total of 602 necropsies from 38,826 term deliveries (0.3/1000) (Sulamaa and Vara 1952). The incidence of cranial birth trauma, most cases probably involving tentorial damage, was 3.1 per 1000 total births in the British Perinatal Mortality Survey of 1958 (Butler and Bonham 1963). The lowest rate was recorded in term infants (about 1/1000) and the highest in those with gestational

ages >43 weeks (40/1000). Barson (1983), reviewing records covering the period 1976 to 1981 in Manchester, England, recorded 0.96 tentorial tears per 1000 total births of all gestational ages. He documented as much as 10 per cent of tentorial trauma in perinatal deaths with gestational ages <29 weeks. At UZ Gent the incidence of *in vivo* recognized tentorial damage among liveborn infants weighing ⩾1000g at birth is around 0.8/1000. These data cannot be compared because the reporting centres differ in selection of referred cases, because the incidence of tentorial damage in survivors was never recorded before the advent of modern imaging, and because even with it some lesions will go unnoticed. In addition most authors refer to tentorial damage as a percentage of their perinatal autopsy material which is useless for comparison between centres. Personal observations over the last few years suggest that for every tentorial injury discovered at post-mortem examination, there are at least two survivors with *in vivo* suspected tentorial injury. That would suggest an incidence of between two and three major tentorial lesions per 1000 live births, possibly increasing to around 1 per cent in instrumental deliveries. These data should of course be confirmed by prospective study. In a recent prospective MRI study of neonatal intracranial pathology no attempt was made to deduce the actual incidence of tentorial damage (Keeney *et al.* 1991).

Pathogenesis
Most pathophysiological considerations, if not all, have been founded on post-mortem examination experience. In summary, several authors around the turn of the century, *e.g.* Beneke (1910) and later on Holland (1937), popularized the concept of tentorial stress during delivery. Holland pointed out the vulnerability of the vertical central tentorial fibres (Beneke's *Tentorium-strahlung der Falx)*. Overstretching of these dural structures is due to (i) excessive calvarial moulding, because of either bitemporal (Beneke) or occipito-frontal (Holland) compression, with subsequent rostral lift of the falco-tentorial junction, or (ii) forward displacement of the occipital bone as in difficult breech delivery or inaccurate application of forceps blades (Wigglesworth and Husemeyer 1977). As pointed out by many authors, the obstetric context is that of a stormy or prolonged spontaneous vaginal delivery (Beneke 1910), a difficult midpelvic or high cavity instrumental delivery (Holland 1937, Craig 1938, Kehrer 1939, Sulamaa and Vara 1952, Chiswick and James 1979) or an assisted breech delivery (Hemsath 1934, Holland 1937, Tank *et al.* 1971), the latter especially if associated with forceps extraction of the trapped aftercoming head. Caesarean section before the onset of labour can complete this list as an exceptional circumstance leading to tentorial injury. Mode of birth in relation to time of presentation in a series of 90 reported cases (see below) is shown in Figure 6.41. The general idea is that excessive skull traction results in proportionately excessive skull compression (see section on skull trauma during birth, p. 25).

In a review of *in vivo* diagnosed or suspected tentorial damage, an association

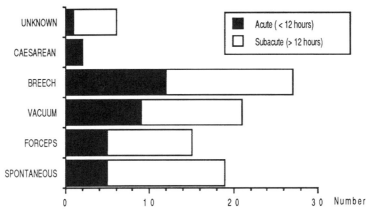

Fig. 6.41. Mode of delivery in 90 reported infants with (acute or subacute) posterior fossa subdural haemorrhage. (See Table 6.14 for source of data.)

with vacuum extraction was found in those countries where this method of delivery is popular (*e.g.* Japan, Russia, Belgium and the Scandinavian countries) (Govaert *et al.* 1990*b*). A contemporary report (Hanigan *et al.* 1990*b*) stating that vacuum delivery causes tentorial damage by direct traction on the falx is misplaced in two ways: it does not substantiate the concept of direct ventouse influence on deeper cranial structures and it omits references to several necropsy studies where the relation between vacuum delivery and tentorial injury had already been clearly established (*e.g.* Aguero and Alvarez 1962). A report by Saunders (1948) seems superficially to support this idea of direct stress because galeal traction over the anterior fontanelle in dead neonates was clearly shown to lift and stretch the falco-tentorial junction in the direction of the traction applied ('galea forceps'); it cannot be excluded that galeal traction increased the general skull compression and thus produced this sequence of events.

Clinical setting
The presenting signs and symptoms of 15 personally observed cases and 63 *in vivo* cases with suspected central tentorial tears gathered from the literature have been earlier reviewed in an attempt to propose management guidelines (Govaert *et al.* 1990*b*). The features described are essentially those of posterior fossa SDH. Two recent reports (Hanigan *et al.* 1990*b*, Huang and Shen 1991) increase to 90 the total number of clinically detailed peritentorial haemorrhages that can be evaluated here. Tables 6.14 and 6.15 show the presenting neurological syndrome as well as outcome in relation to mode of presentation and whether or not suboccipital craniotomy was performed. The arbitrary cut-off between acute and subacute presentation is made 12 hours after birth; comparison between presentation and outcome illustrates the somewhat artificial nature of this separation. The obstetric

71

TABLE 6.14

Neurological signs in 90 neonates with posterior fossa subdural haematoma*

General signs	N	(%)	Localizing signs	N	(%)
Tense fontanelle	53	(59)	Apnoea	28	(31)
Hypotonia	32	(36)	Irregular breathing		
Seizures	32	(36)	(gasping, sighing)	27	(30)
Lethargy, depressed			Opisthotonus	12	(13)
primitive reflexes	29	(32)	Skew eye deviation	11	(12)
Vomiting	15	(17)	Facial palsy	10	(11)
Irritability	13	(14)	VIth nerve palsy	4	(4)
Weak cry	11	(12)	Unequal pupils	4	(4)
High-pitched cry	11	(12)	Retroauricular haematoma	3	(3)
Hypertonia	9	(10)	IIIrd nerve palsy	1	(1)

*Data compiled from: Govaert *et al.* (1990*b*), Hanigan *et al.* (1990*b*), Huang and Shen (1991).

TABLE 6.15

Neonatal posterior fossa subdural haematoma: outcome vs. presentation and management in 90 infants*

	Craniotomy		No craniotomy	
	Acute (N=15)	Subacute (N=29)	Acute (N=19)	Subacute (N=27)
Birth asphyxia	0	2	7	3
Apnoea	5	6	11	6
Tense fontanelle	14	18	13	8
Seizures	4	7	10	11
Irregular breathing	8	7	6	5
Fixed bradycardia	4	3	3	4
Skew eye deviation	5	1	2	2
Cranial nerve palsy	5	4	5	1
Hydrocephalus				
Requiring shunt	5	9	3	2
Treated conservatively	0	0	0	3†
Fatal outcome	0	3	9	6
Apparently normal survival	10	12	8	13

*For data sources see Table 6.14.
†Serial lumbar punctures and acetazolamide.

history preceding each type is similar, as are the incidences of seizures and hydrocephalus. Probable indicators of severity are intracranial hypertension with apnoea and/or abnormal breathing patterns such as sighing and gasping, resulting in the need for ventilatory support. Cranial nerve palsies, of facial and eye musculature, seem to be more common in acutely presenting tentorial damage (Dubose Ravenel 1979, Balériaux *et al.* 1980, Serfontein *et al.* 1980, Hernansanz *et al.* 1984). Lumbar puncture theoretically endangers the infant by enhancing the risk

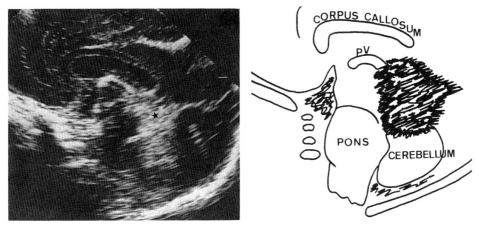

Fig. 6.42. Sagittal ultrasound scan on day 2 in Case 6.7 (see p. 76) *(asterisk* indicates haemorrhage); the corresponding structures are identified in the drawing. (PV = plexus ventriculi tertii.)

of cerebellar coning in cases of frank hypertension within the posterior fossa (Dubose Ravenel 1979).

We conclude that, apart from opisthotonus and retroauricular haematoma (Young and Zalneraitis 1980), fixed bradycardia and sighing might be somewhat indicative of severe posterior fossa haemorrhage. Neither seizures nor intracranial hypertension are obligatory. Pulmonary haemorrhage was recorded as an agonal event in lethal tentorial injury (Blank *et al.* 1978).

Radiological assessment
Several recent reports corrected the previous lack of *in vivo* descriptions of tentorial damage by means of ultrasound, CT scan and MRI (Scotti *et al.* 1981, Govaert *et al.* 1990*b*, Huang and Shen 1991, Keeney *et al.* 1991). Skull X-rays may show occipital osteodiastasis, suture diastasis around the occipital bone (see section on skull trauma during birth) or bone fractures. Ultrasound is a very reliable screening method for detection of severe falco-tentorial bleeding (Bejar *et al.* 1985), but lacks precision in delineating lesions in the posterior fossa and interhemispheric fissure. Axial incidence and scanning through the posterior fontanelle can increase the diagnostic yield. The lesion to be sought is an additional density situated on the superior part of the cerebellar vermis behind the brainstem and filling the cisterna ambiens (Fig. 6.42).

Very few reports link CT findings with post-mortem observations (Blank *et al.* 1978, Menezes *et al.* 1983). Reviews by Govaert *et al.* (1990*b*) and Huang and Shen (1991) independently arrived at remarkably similar conclusions. On CT scan tentorial damage is very likely in the presence of: (i) a pericerebellar and some-times parenchymal haemorrhagic density (Fig. 6.43*a*); (ii) marked haemorrhages on sections through the tentorial apex, around the straight sinus and behind the

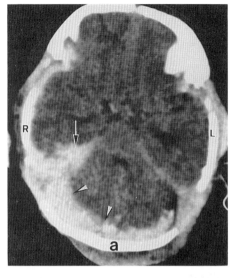

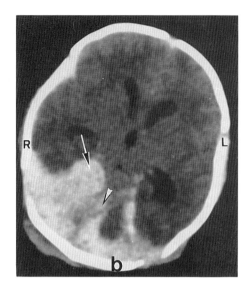

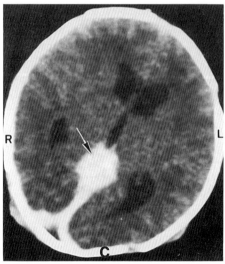

Fig. 6.43. Axial CT scans on day 2 in Case 6.7: sections from below *(a)*, at *(b)* and above *(c)* cerebellar tent. In *(a)* the *arrow* indicates basal subdural haemorrhage, the *arrowheads* show retrocerebellar posterior fossa subdural haematoma. In *(b)* the *arrowhead* indicates the straight sinus while the *arrow* points to haemorrhage of right mesial tentorial margin. In *(c)* a nodular haemorrhage extends between both hemispheres behind third ventricle *(arrow)*. Note also mild ventricular distension and anterior displacement of posterior horns of both lateral ventricles.

third ventricle, coalescing to form a somewhat triangular density with its basis against the occipital bone (Fig. 6.43*b*); or (iii) bleeding in between the posterior cerebral hemispheres (basal interhemispheric SDH) (Fig. 6.43*c*). Coronal images, either direct or by reconstruction, are most helpful in demonstrating the regional distribution of blood (Serfontein *et al.* 1980, Scotti *et al.* 1981, Rolland *et al.* 1982, Menezes *et al.* 1983, Koch *et al.* 1985, Coker *et al.* 1987, Govaert *et al.* 1990*b*). MRI, it is suggested, is even superior in delineating the precise anatomical locations of haemorrhage, in demonstrating associated parenchymal damage due to asphyxia or vascular lesions and in documenting superior sagittal sinus thrombosis (Hanigan *et al*. 1990*b*, Keeney *et al*. 1991). Minor haemorrhages, especially those which would otherwise be missed, are likely to be diagnosed by MRI, even several weeks after the acute event. Personal experience is limited because the latter method either requires adequate sedation of the infant, with its accompanying problems, or the availability of skilled staff with plenty of time just to soothe a restless baby. With MRI, although the result is clearly superior and the radiation exposure absent, further study is needed to show how much will be missed by careful ultrasound scanning and one early (in the first three days of life) CT scan.

Management and prognosis
Controversy has dominated the literature on this aspect; having had recent experience with both surgical and conservative treatment (Govaert *et al*. 1990*b*) I thus attempt here to clarify the state of the art.

Neurosurgical intervention has an invaluable place in some patients because it can correct raised ICP instantly (Gilles and Shillito 1970, Carter and Pittman 1971, Menezes *et al*. 1983). The only obvious indication is either acute hydrocephalus because of obliteration of the CSF pathways in the posterior fossa, or life-threatening brainstem compression with apnoea and/or fixed bradycardia and/or systemic hypertension and/or ocular palsies. If a neurosurgical approach is preferred the only safe method is to perform suboccipital craniotomy before ventricular drainage, because primary shunting of the supratentorial ventricles may result in acute upward herniation of the cerebellum and brainstem. Care must be taken not to injure the transverse sinus in the process of removing the postcerebellar clots and not to cause additional damage to the cerebellar hemispheres (Tanaka *et al*. 1988). The goal seems to be correction of intracranial hypertension and not removal of all posterior fossa clot. After a couple of days the collection, its volume ranging from 10 to 75mL, partially liquefies to become a genuine hygroma in the chronic stage.

Both conservative and neurosurgical treatment permit neurologically intact survival in about 50 per cent of the infants, most with comparable amounts of bleeding (Fishman *et al*. 1981, Gouyon *et al*. 1981).

Craniotomy does not prevent late-onset 'resorptive' hydrocephalus (Govaert *et al*. 1990*b*). As outlined by Tanaka *et al*. (1988), there is a biphasic ventricular dilatation after severe posterior fossa haemorrhage with an acute phase due to obstruction of CSF pathways by compression and a chronic phase due to deficient absorption or circulation of CSF. The latter is related to the amount of associated subarachnoid haemorrhage or caused by recurrent bleeding into an hygromatous collection (French and Dublin 1977). Even in late-onset hydrocephalus at the age of 6 months, after demonstration of the communicating nature of the ventricular dilatation, *e.g.* by isotope cisternography, conservative treatment with serial lumbar punctures and drugs that inhibit CSF production can be successful (Koch *et al*. 1985, Von Gontard *et al*. 1988, Govaert *et al*. 1990*b*). Immediate postsurgical problems include the formation of a CSF fistula or a pseudomeningocele (Dubose Ravenel 1979), both necessitating reintervention in some infants.

On follow-up, in addition to post-haemorrhagic hydrocephalus, one should be looking for the development of cysts in and around the cerebellum (Koch *et al.* 1985, Huang and Shen 1991), posterior fossa subdural hygroma (French and Dublin 1977, Govaert *et al.* 1990*b*, Huang and Shen 1991) (Fig. 6.44) and cystic dilatation of the retrocerebellar subarachnoid space (Adam and Greenberg 1978, Dorsic *et al.* 1983, Govaert *et al.* 1990*b*) (Fig. 6.45). The relevance of these findings is poorly understood.

Even following a very large peritentorial haemorrhage, the only sequelae can be delayed gross motor development in infancy or residual nystagmus, with apparently normal later development.

Case histories
CASE 6.7
This male child was outborn at term with six difficult vacuum tractions following a prolonged second stage (100 minutes). Apgar scores were 2 and 5 at one and five minutes; birthweight was 3700g. The infant was referred 16 hours after birth with anaemia, macrocrania, seizures, hypotonia, fever and blood-stained CSF. Rapid deterioration occurred over the next few hours, with impaired consciousness, apnoeic episodes, deep gasping and fixed bradycardia at 80 to 110 bpm. Initial ultrasound and CT scans are shown in Figures 6.42 and 6.43. Surgery was withheld because apnoeic episodes did not persist and the fontanelle was not tense. Diffuse 'epileptic' disturbances were recorded on EEG, clinical seizures being noticeable for three days. Onset of sucking and minimal spontaneous motor activity were first evident on day 5. Transient ventriculomegaly was noted on ultrasound between days 6 and 10. Complete oral feeding was achieved by day 14. A posterior fossa hygroma was seen on repeat CT scan on day 18 (Fig. 6.44). Ventriculomegaly recurred toward the end of the first month and then spontaneously regressed. Head circumference remained around the 90th centile until day 140 when acute onset of hydrocephalus caused intracranial hypertension requiring treatment. Ultrasound and isotope cisternography confirmed communication between lumbar CSF and lateral ventricles. This was managed by serial lumbar punctures (23 in all) until day 180, as well as furosemide and acetazolamide up to day 240. Mental development was apparently normal at 2 years of age; he sat alone at 7½ months and walked at 14 months; nystagmus, however, persisted.

CASE 6.8
This girl was outborn at 38 weeks with breech delivery by 'easy Bracht manoeuvre'. Apgar scores were 5 and 9 at one and five minutes: birthweight was 2300g. At the first attempt at feeding two hours after birth she was pale and lethargic with a tense fontanelle; she was referred with fixed bradycardia (90 bpm), irregular jerky vertical eye movements, anaemia, metabolic acidosis and hyperglycaemia, no reaction to painful stimuli, absent primitive reflexes and a clenched left fist. CT scans before and after surgery are shown in Figure 6.46. Emergency suboccipital craniotomy was undertaken because of evidence of brainstem compression about six hours after birth. After removal of 20mL of solid clot, immediate return to normal intracranial tension was established. Cerebellar ischaemia was suspected because of compression of the cerebellum, not from laceration (occipital osteodiastasis not recognized). An injured left transverse sinus was the probable origin of massive

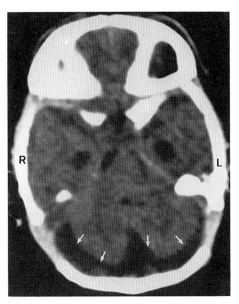 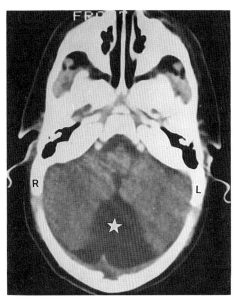

Fig. 6.44. Axial CT scan on day 18 in Case 6.7, showing posterior fossa subdural hygroma *(arrows)*.

Fig. 6.45. Axial CT scan on day 140 in Case 6.7, showing retrocerebellar CSF collection *(asterisk)*.

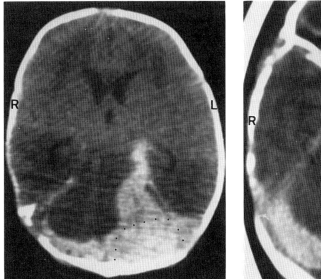 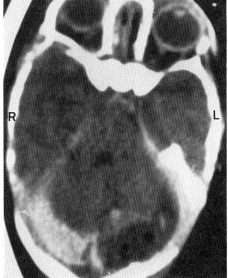

Fig. 6.46. Axial CT scans on days 1 and 5 in Case 6.8. *(Left)* Before surgery a left retrocerebellar haematoma extends to the level of the cisterna ambiens. *(Right)* Following posterior fossa craniotomy partial removal of the clot has allowed cerebellum to return to its normal position.

haemorrhage. Dural prosthetic replacement of part of the removed occipital bone was necessary. She was extubated on the fifth day, and oral feeding was started on the following day. Control CT scan documented removal of about half the postcerebellar blood clot. Complete right facial nerve paralysis was noticeable for two months. At 1 year of age she showed gross motor delay, but normal mental development.

Superficial cerebral venous thrombosis

Anatomical description

Thrombotic occlusion of major superficial veins including the superior sagittal, transverse, sigmoid and straight sinus are discussed in this section. If thrombosis involves or propagates to the great cerebral vein of Galen there is risk of deep cerebral venous thrombosis with secondary thalamo-ventricular haemorrhage and/or (in the case of thrombosis extending to the internal cerebral veins) haemorrhagic periventricular white matter infarction. In the absence of influential local factors, the most common site of origin for thrombosis within the superior sagittal sinus is the central area between both fontanelles (Fig. 6.47). Major cerebral veins empty into that region, increasing the vessel size and changing local flow patterns, their entry being in a direction opposite to bulk flow in the sinus (Byers and Hass 1933). In a milestone study of dural sinus thrombosis, Bailey and Hass (1958) outlined the preferential localization of thrombi (Table 6.16). Whatever the variable presence of collateral circulation to the middle cerebral veins or the transverse sinus, the superior sagittal sinus is the chief venous drain for the upper and mesial regions of the cerebrum. Thus, even if thrombosis is limited to the aforementioned weak spot, permanent neurological damage may result from associated infarction within the (sub)cortical cerebral parenchyma drained by unperfused cerebral veins (Byers and Hass 1933, Bailey and Hass 1958, Friede 1989). The areas involved, though often bilateral, are usually asymmetrical. Major infarctions are haemorrhagic, so-called red softening or '*ramollissement rouge*'. Unilateral isolated thrombosis of a transverse sinus is compatible with intact neurological survival (Byers and Hass 1933, Baram *et al.* 1988). Some degree of subarachnoid haemorrhage is invariably associated and may even mislead the clinician (Byers and Hass 1933, Bailey and Hass 1958, Scotti *et al.* 1974). Even minor subdural haematoma formation is not uncommon (Byers and Hass 1933, Bailey and Hass 1958, Baram *et al.* 1988). In case of associated primary or secondary disseminated intravascular coagulation, the extent of intracranial haemorrhage might become important. Post-thrombotic hydrocephalus, a rare event, can be due to deep thrombosis and subsequent intraventricular bleeding, to white matter atrophy or to deficient CSF circulation over the hemispheres and/or absorption in the major sinus (Bailey 1959).

Incidence and pathogenesis

Some data suggest that superficial intracranial venous thrombosis in the newborn infant is underdiagnosed. Within the period under study in Gent (1980–91) six cases

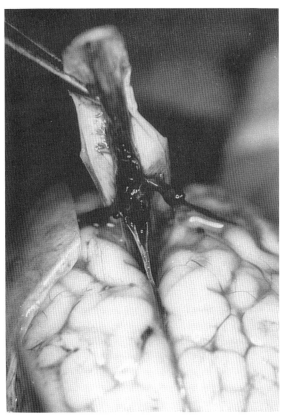

TABLE 6.16

**Site of dural sinus thrombosis in
early infancy (N=31)***

Site	N
Superior sagittal sinus	31
Lateral sinus	17
Superior cerebral veins	15
Straight sinus	10
Great vein of Galen	7
Cavernous sinus	2

*After exclusion of precipitating
focal events; data from Bailey and
Hass (1958).

Fig. 6.47. Post-mortem view showing preferential site of superior sagittal sinus thrombosis at the vertex. This boy, who died 13 days after spontaneous delivery at term, had postpartum asphyxia, barotrauma, early bronchopulmonary dysplasia and unexplained haemoperitoneum. Bridging veins are clearly thrombosed, leading to left occipital cortico-subcortical haemorrhagic infarction (not shown in this picture). (Courtesy Drs Bridger and Kirkham, Royal Sussex County Hospital, Brighton.)

were diagnosed in term babies: two are discussed in Chapter 8 (p. 139); two others were due to traumatic forward displacement of the occipital squama into the superior sagittal sinus; one was associated with congenital nephrotic syndrome (described in detail below); and one occurred in a boy with meconium aspiration syndrome, persistent pulmonary hypertension, mild bronchopulmonary dysplasia, and a limited tortuous calcification on follow-up CT scan believed to be a thrombosed superior sagittal sinus bridging vein (see Fig. 6.50, p. 85). These cases are listed, together with three recent observations from Hammersmith Hospital, in Table 6.17. There was involvement of the superior sagittal sinus in all nine cases, and five also suffered from deep thrombosis of the great cerebral vein.

Voorhies *et al.* (1984) gathered five babies with a thrombosed superior sagittal sinus from a population of 48 severely asphyxiated term infants. More recently, the

TABLE 6.17

**Superficial cerebral venous thrombosis:
details of nine patients*

Birthweight <2500g	4
Male sex	8
Mode of delivery	
Spontaneous vaginal	5
Breech	2
Vacuum	1[1]
Emergency caesarean	1[2]
Apgar score <4 @ 1 min.	2
<7 @ 5 mins	4
Cause	
Birth asphyxia	1
Birth trauma	4
Other	4[3]
Onset of symptoms: day 1	5[4]
day 2	2
Neonatal death	4
Cerebral palsy	4

*Six from UZ Gent, three from Hammersmith Hospital.
[1]After 5 minutes of second stage.
[2]Face presentation.
[3]One congenital nephrotic syndrome; one iatrogenic, due to a tight nuchal negative pressure ventilator collar; two persistent pulmonary hypertension of unknown cause.
[4]Possibly prenatal in the infant with nephrotic syndrome.

use of MRI scanning permitted recognition of subtle lesions restricted to the transverse sinus in term neonates with a paucity of clinical symptoms and in the absence of obvious precipitating factors (Baram *et al.* 1988).

Pathogenetic mechanisms recognized in the neonatal period are listed in Table 6.18. In severe birth asphyxia, infants who go on to develop intracranial venous thrombosis suffer from severe brain oedema and loss of arterial pulsation, indicating brain death (Voorhies *et al.* 1984). Birth trauma, though not getting much credit from Friede (1989), was the likely cause in a case with forward displacement of the interparietal ossicle reported by Meier (1938) and in two personal observations of forward displacement of the occipital squama tip, one following vacuum delivery of a growth retarded infant (Govaert *et al.* 1992*e*). Newton and Gooding (1975) even documented relevant forward displacement of the superior sagittal sinus in an infant lying supine with his head straight so that the occiput was against bedding. Severe dehydration has been amply documented as the only cause of thrombosis in young children with acute diarrhoea, most of them presenting with serum sodium levels >150mmol/L (Yang *et al.* 1969). Scalp

TABLE 6.18

Aetiology of superior sagittal sinus thrombosis in neonates

1. Severe birth asphyxia (Voorhies *et al.* 1984)
2. Birth trauma (Meier 1938, Govaert *et al.* 1992*e*)
3. Dehydration (primary or marantic) (Byers and Hass 1933, Bailey and Hass 1958, Yang *et al.* 1969, Patronas *et al.* 1981)
4. Infection (of the scalp; meningitis; bacteraemia) (Byers and Hass 1933, Bailey and Hass 1958)
5. Polycythaemia (cyanotic congenital heart disease; infant of diabetic mother) (Cottrill and Kaplan 1973, Schubiger *et al.* 1982)
6. Deficient anticoagulation
   —heterozygous antithrombin III deficiency (Brenner *et al.* 1988)
   —homozygous protein C (or S) deficiency (Marciniak *et al.* 1985)
   —congenital nephrotic syndrome (present study)
7. Iatrogenic
   —misplaced central venous catheter (Hurst *et al.* 1989)
   —tight nuchal ventilator collar (Govaert *et al.* 1992*a*)
   —penetrating fetal scalp electrode (Wigger 1991)

infection was formerly another cause (Byers and Hass 1933, Bailey and Hass 1958). Polycythaemia is not a prerequisite for thrombosis in cyanotic heart disease, a condition where intracranial venous thrombosis is much more common than arterial cerebral occlusion (Cottrill and Kaplan 1973). In nephrotic syndrome the frequent occurrence of both venous and arterial thromboses has been attributed to thrombocytosis, platelet hyperaggregability, elevation of factors I, V and VIII, and decrease in circulating free protein S and antithrombin III (Kanfer 1990, Parag *et al.* 1990, Lye and Tan 1991, Marsh *et al.* 1991).

Clinical setting
The major event, with acute occlusion of the superior sagittal sinus in its middle and posterior parts, presents with signs of intracranial hypertension such as vomiting, irritability and bradycardia (Byers and Hass 1933, Bailey and Hass 1958). Seizures, sometimes focal, are common, and detailed neurological examination may show focal motor deficit. High fever and opisthotonus have been mentioned regularly. Indicators of severity are eyelid and scalp vein congestion, hinting at obstruction of deep venous return. Other ophthalmological findings have been nystagmus, fundal oedema and retinal vein congestion. Progression to coma with irregular breathing is an agonal event. Disseminated intravascular coagulation can be a consequence, but is yet to be shown as one of its causes (Leissring *et al.* 1968, Govaert *et al.* 1992*e*). Limited involvement of the anterior part of the superior sagittal sinus or thrombosis of one transverse sinus is a difficult diagnosis because of the lack of neurological signs: jitteriness, irritability, mild hypertonia and focal sharp waves on EEG may be the only findings in MRI-confirmed diagnoses (Baram *et al.* 1988). In the early recovery period a wide open eye gaze is indicative of superior sagittal sinus thrombosis (personal observations).

Radiological assessment

Diagnosis used to be achieved by such means as invasive sinography, arteriography and isotope sinography, but now the CT scan has become a reliable tool (Eick *et al.* 1981, Patronas *et al.* 1981, Segall *et al.* 1982) (Fig. 6.48*a,b*). Direct signs on uncontrasted scans, often more accentuated by appropriate changes in window setting, are opacities within the major vessels. Following enhancement, filling defects produce an appearance like an 'empty triangle' or 'delta' sign. Indirect confirmation is provided by cerebral swelling, gyral enhancement, haemorrhagic conversion of infarcted tissue in typical parasagittal superior cerebral areas and collateral veins highlighting the tentorium or crossing the cerebral white matter (dilated transmedullary veins).

In infancy, ultrasound offers non-invasive diagnosis: 10MHz scanning allows recognition of the ischaemic parasagittal parenchyma and will demonstrate intravascular densities in the superior sagittal sinus under either fontanelle (Govaert *et al.* 1992*e*) (Fig. 6.48*c,d*). With luck, even partial thrombosis can be visualized. Differentiation of brain damage in superior sagittal sinus thrombosis has to be made from parasagittal cerebral injury in arterial border zones: both present as hyperdense ultrasound and hypodense CT areas near the sinus, but the asphyxial context and bilaterality will point to the latter diagnosis (Huang *et al.* 1987).

Colour Doppler flow imaging might show absent flow in a completely occluded vessel and its subsequent recanalization (Fig. 6.48*e*). Several authors have pointed to the superiority of MRI to make this diagnosis in the newborn infant: in the acute stage an absence of flow void will mark the occluded sinus, whereas after a few days and up to at least 4 weeks of age thrombi will be hyperintense on T1 and T2 images due to the presence of methaemoglobin (McMurdo *et al.* 1986, Baram *et al.* 1988, Hurst *et al.* 1989, Draaisma *et al.* 1991). In the sagittal plane, supracerebellar location of a posterior fossa SDH will be differentiated from venous thrombosis by the presence or absence of proximity to the posterior cerebellar vermis (Keeney *et al.* 1991). Easy accessibility and increased use of the latter technique might make intracranial venous thrombosis in the perinatal period sufficiently well known that it will no longer be an '*histoire à éclipses*'—a story with periods in which acquired knowledge seems to be forgotten and in constant need of rediscovery.

Case histories

CASE 6.9

This firstborn boy was delivered at term after an uneventful pregnancy, presenting with the occiput anterior. The first stage of labour took five hours; five minutes after the onset of expulsive efforts fetal bradycardia prompted vacuum delivery. His Apgar scores were 7 and 8 at one and five minutes. Birthweight was 1970g, crown–heel length 46cm and head circumference 32cm. 14 hours after birth he was described as moaning, looking pale and jaundiced. On referral, head movement seemed painful, and his cry was high pitched. A boggy feeling at the back of the head suggested subgaleal bleeding confined to occipital and nuchal areas. The head circumference had increased to 33.5cm. Signs of intracranial hypertension were absent. Eye movements had a full range but the irides were blood-

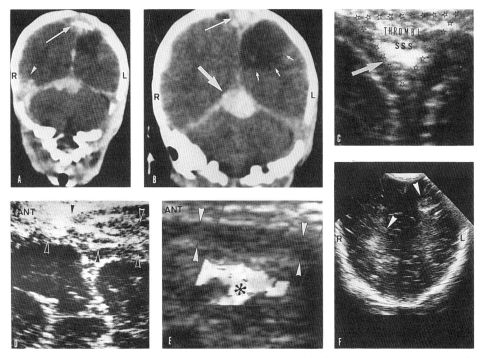

Fig. 6.48. Imaging results in Case 6.9 within the first three days of life (except *E*, taken in second week). *(A)* Coronal CT scan demonstrating basal subdural haemorrhage *(arrowhead)* and forward displacement of tip of occipital bone *(arrow)*. *(B)* Coronal CT scan documenting central tentorial haematoma and/or dilated great cerebral vein *(large arrow)*, clot within superior sagittal sinus *(arrow)* and low attenuation of ischaemic parietal parenchyma on left *(small arrows)*. *(C)* Coronal and *(D)* sagittal ultrasound scan showing thrombi within superior sagittal sinus. *(E)* Sagittal ultrasound scan with colour Doppler flow imaging, indicating presence of flow *(asterisk)* in cortical vessels and flow void *(between arrowheads)* in superior sagittal sinus. *(F)* Coronal ultrasound scan demonstrating asymmetrical echodense ischaemic parenchyma in both occipital lobes *(arrowheads)*.

stained. No seizures were recorded. Investigations revealed anaemia and disseminated intravascular coagulation. There was no diastasis of the main sutures on lateral skull X-ray. High frequency ultrasound scanning demonstrated cerebral parenchymal densities in the occipital periventricular and subcortical area on both sides (Fig. 6.48*f*) and suggested a haemorrhagic lesion in the quadrigeminal cistern riding on the cerebellar vermis. The superior sagittal sinus was filled with high density reflections, and on colour Doppler flow imaging was shown to be void of blood circulation (Fig. 6.48*e*). Additional features on CT scan were the suspected forward displacement of the tip of the occipital squama, haemorrhage within the falx and a right basal convexity SDH (Fig. 6.48*a,b*). The hyperdense zones on ultrasound were hypodense on uncontrasted CT scan, indicating their ischaemic nature. This boy recovered with minimal motor disability involving the right hand evident at 1 year of age.

CASE 6.10
This boy was born vaginally at 38 weeks of gestation. There had been meconium staining of

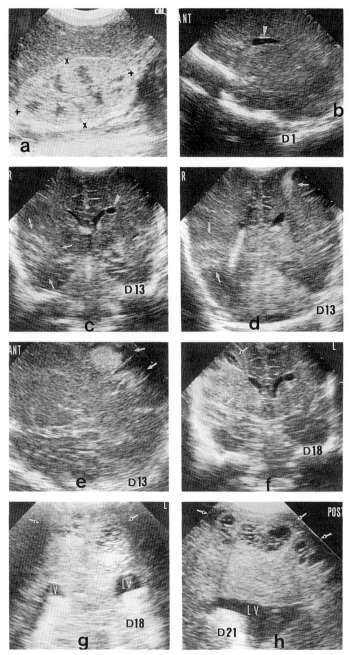

Fig. 6.49. Ultrasonographic findings in Case 6.10. Hyperdense renal parenchyma *(a)*, associated with congenital nephrotic syndrome and left frontal paraventricular cyst *(arrowhead)* on day 1 *(b)*. Asymmetrical parenchymal densities *(arrows)* on day 13 are shown in frontal coronal *(c)*, occipital coronal *(d)* and left parasagittal *(e)* views. These developed cystic necrosis *(dotted arrows)* on day 21 *(f,g,h)*. (LV = lateral ventricle.)

84

the liquor. He was referred because of birth asphyxia. Apgar scores were 3 and 4 at one and five minutes. His birthweight was 2710g; the placenta weighed 1370g. He presented with a left pneumothorax and mild hydrops. His neonatal course was complicated, and final diagnoses included: left renal vein thrombosis, congenital nephrotic syndrome of the Finnish type, enteritis and retinitis associated with *Candida glabrata* infection. Seizures were probably due to partial thrombosis of the superior sagittal sinus (Fig. 6.49). He developed spastic quadriplegia and severe mental impairment and died at the age of 2 years. Consent for post-mortem examination was refused.

Management and prognosis
Apart from obvious symptomatic and aetiological treatment such as correction of secondary haemostatic problems, sufficient hydration seems to be the only recommended measure. Antithrombotic drugs, of theoretical benefit, have not yet been used in the neonatal period because of the fear of increasing haemorrhagic conversion of ischaemic territories. Depending on the extent of parenchymal damage, contralateral neurological deficit is to be expected (Bailey 1959). The important representation of hand function in the paracentral supero-lateral cortex explains how mild spasticity of one hand could be the only sequela in the Case 6.9 outlined above. From adult experience it can be envisaged that superior sagittal sinus thrombosis could trigger the emergence of dural arterio-venous fistulae (Graeb and Dolman 1986). Neonatal thrombosis of the superior sagittal sinus has been mentioned as one of the causes of minimal brain damage and even 'schizophrenic' behaviour (Towbin 1971). Minimal venous thrombosis may leave no recognizable neurological deficit (Fig. 6.50).

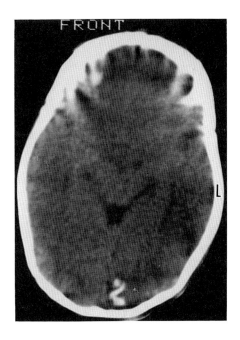

Fig. 6.50. Follow-up axial CT scan at 2 months in term delivered boy with persistent pulmonary hypertension of unknown cause: note (unsuspected) undulating dense structure in left occipital area, suggestive of calcified old thrombus in a bridging vein. At age 2 years this boy was developing within normal limits.

7
INSTRUMENTAL DELIVERY: THE OBSTETRIC PERSPECTIVE

Paul Defoort

Introduction

The nightmare of obstructed labour has haunted mankind throughout history. Despite the occasional heterodox viewpoint like that of Gebbie (1981) who holds that pelvic dystocia is but a recent by-product of urban society, the evidence is that throughout the world and in the most remote and primitive societies, customs and practices—varying from rituals to gross physical interference—testify of preoccupation with the problem of non-progress in childbirth (Speert 1973). In Europe, from the time of the Renaissance onward, surgeons and male accoucheurs in the chauvinistic spirit of their age, began to express their concern and irritation at the ingrained practice of midwives to simply amputate the prolapsed presenting part, even when this was by no means a mechanical solution to cases of obstructed labour. However, they themselves had nothing to offer at the time but feto-destructive procedures (Thiery, personal communication).

A solution to this problem compatible with survival of the child is a relatively recent acquisition in human history, the forceps coming into general use in the 18th century. It soon became apparent, however, that not just survival but also the quality of life could be affected by the obstetrician's acts. In 1862, Little presented convincing evidence of the relationship between birth events and neurological sequelae. His concepts led directly to the work of Waitz (1931), Schwartz (1961), Courville (1971) and others who in this century studied the relationship between fetal brain trauma and (mechanical) events during birth.

As a result, the obstetrician nowadays hardly needs convincing of the dangers of birth for the infant. The consciousness of the obstetric community is expressed in timeless maxims like, 'For the child, the act of being born possibly carries the biggest risk to which it will ever be exposed in its lifetime' (Holm 1982), or 'No amount of prenatal care can compensate for poor care at the time of delivery' (Miller 1935).

This awareness, however, is subject to many shifts of emphasis and can lead to different responses. While at first the main preoccupation was with the danger of mechanical trauma, soon enough the risk of 'asphyxia' or hypoxia was brought to the fore. As hypoxia was *inter alia* associated with labour 'stress' and duration, this engendered the tendency to keep the second stage of labour as short as possible by the practice of 'prophylactic forceps' (De Lee 1921, De Rom and De Rom 1954).

This practice was, if anything, extended when the Malmström vacuum extractor became available, allowing great flexibility in the application of vaginal instrumental delivery.

Recent views on perinatal brain damage have tended to give more importance to fetal events such as growth retardation, where the decisive insult may have taken place before birth (Rosen and Hobel 1986, Perkins 1987). This has focused the attention of the obstetrician on fetal surveillance and the prevention of fetal damage and coined the image of the obstetrician as the 'antenatal paediatrician'. Management of the second stage of labour, once the whole *raison d'être* and substance of the specialty, is now more or less taken for granted and no longer the centre of attention of many practitioners. At the cost of caesarean section rates soaring at 25 to 30 per cent in some countries, there remain practically no problems to be resolved by instrumental delivery (Plauché 1992*a*, Yeomans and Hawkins 1992).

With all this, it should be recognized that obstetric management of the second stage has not been subjected to definitive scientific investigation. While nowadays direct mechanical trauma to the term baby presenting by the head may be a distinctly rare event, the benefit of the generally accepted obstetric practice of hastening delivery after a certain time in the second stage had elapsed, is not proven (Cohen 1977, Sleep *et al*. 1989). In this light, even a small additional risk due to elective instrumental delivery is not to be accepted lightly. Indeed, this thought may rightly 'provide a basis for reconsidering some area of current obstetric practice' (Wigglesworth 1984). In this overview I will re-evaluate the obstetric arguments for cutting short the second stage in the normal case, and the possible risk of instrumental delivery with the emphasis on vacuum extraction. Only the case of the normal singleton at term, presenting by the head, will be considered.

Perinatal risk and the duration of the second stage of labour
During the second stage of labour the child survives in peculiar circumstances. In most cases the presenting part is no longer surrounded by amniotic fluid. It passes through the birth canal, which demands a change both in attitude (flexion, rotation) and in shape (moulding). Under increasing pressure from the vis a tergo, when the woman starts bearing down, the head stretches the perineum. This leads to augmenting mechanical pressure on the brain and its blood vessels. At the same time, bearing down during contractions possibly diminishes placental blood flow, while the umbilical cord may be locally compressed between the fetal parts and the soft tissue of the birth canal. These factors all combine to induce in the baby a degree of acidosis, which can become more threatening when metabolic acidosis exists from exhaustion in the mother. This interplay of mechanical and biochemical factors makes the second stage a stressful period for the unborn child. A moot point is whether a physiological limit to the duration of this period can be proposed.

Such a limit could be defined in two ways. Either it can be viewed as a function of the duration of the mechanical expulsion process, or it can be posed in terms of the maximum duration of the birth process before manifest effects on the unborn baby become apparent. The two limits are not necessarily the same. Indeed, the natural history of obstructed labour would suggest that a baby can still be expelled long after it has succumbed in the process. It is evident that delimiting the 'physiological' duration of the second stage of labour in terms of fetal effects is, for the obstetrician as for the neonatologist, a more realistic concept than finding a time limit for the mechanical expulsion process.

Probability of delivery and duration of the second stage

Approximately 77 per cent of all parturients are delivered within one hour in the second stage, and 92 per cent within two hours. Means of 50 to 57 minutes for primiparae and 15 to 20 minutes for multiparae are quoted (Hellman and Prystowski 1952, Friedman and Kroll 1969, Friedman 1978). The probability of delivery as a function of the prior duration of the second stage has been calculated by statistical survival analysis (Kadar *et al.* 1986). According to these data, the probability of delivery attains its maximum after 68.5 minutes. A 10 years increase in maternal age reduces this by 60 per cent. The probability is halved when birthweight exceeds 3000g. Between two and three hours in the second stage, a cumulative increase of 10 to 15 per cent in spontaneous deliveries is to be expected. Past the third hour, a similar cumulative increase is achieved only by a further three hours waiting. A non-interventionist* attitude toward the second stage ('open-ended approach') would allow an increase of 41 to 62 per cent in spontaneous deliveries. However, the supplementary waiting time would be least beneficial to those women who for several reasons have the least chance of spontaneous delivery. For the majority of primiparous women the limit of an efficient second stage is three hours. The additional time needed to increase the number of spontaneous deliveries by 40 to 60 per cent ranges from 30 minutes to many hours, depending on certain determining population features. Thus, a 23-year-old woman who has not given birth after three hours still has a one in three chance to do so within six hours, and a two in three chance if the baby weighs <3000g. For a woman of 35 years with a child >3000g, the chance of a spontaneous delivery after a six hour second stage is virtually non-existent. It should be noted that these figures are exemplary and are not generally applicable.

Factors which, together with time spent in the second stage, determine the probability of delivery are: parity (in which being nulliparous or not is predominant, subsequent birth order having less importance); birthweight; duration of pregnancy, and weight gain during pregnancy, which correlate positively with the duration of the birth process; and body length, which correlates

*The term 'non-intervention' is here used in a pragmatic sense, and should not be taken to imply the dogma of the 18th century school of Denman, who carried the attitude of not interfering with the birth process to extreme limits. (The 'non-interventionist' school was discredited when Princess Charlotte and her child both died after prolonged labour managed following strictly non-interventionist principles.)

negatively. Occipito-posterior presentation of the fetal head increases the duration of pregnancy only in nulliparous women (Nesheim 1988).

These factors may also increase the duration of the deceleration phase of the first stage (Nesheim 1988). Prolongation of this phase is strongly predictive of an unfavourable progression in the second stage (Friedman 1967, Davidson *et al.* 1976). When the time span to progress from 7 to 10cm dilatation exceeds two hours, spontaneous delivery ensues in only 5 per cent. When this interval is three hours or more, spontaneous delivery no longer occurs (Davidson *et al.* 1976).

It follows that there are limits to sensible non-intervention in the management of the second stage. The effect of the determining factors is that the longer the second stage is protracted, the more the chance that the parturient will prove able to achieve birth spontaneously recedes.

Fetal oxygenation and the duration of the second stage

From the point of view of fetal well-being also, the time spent in the second stage is to be limited (Jeffcoate 1950, Hellman and Prystowski 1952). The deleterious effects of prolongation of the second stage can be due to interference with fetal oxygenation (acidosis) and to mechanical effects on the fetal head (moulding, pathological moulding). Katz *et al.* (1987) found that the mean pH of umbilical artery blood exceeds 7.31 when the second stage takes less than 15 minutes, but falls to 7.25 when 30 minutes are exceeded. A significant increase in excess lactate is seen in nulliparous and multiparous women. A prolonged expulsion can make the moderate respiratory acidosis in the fetus, that normally resolves rapidly after birth, evolve into a potentially dangerous metabolic acidosis.

The limits to a safe duration of the second stage are not clearly defined. For some authors 30 to 45 minutes is the advisable limit (Roemer *et al.* 1976, Katz *et al.* 1987), while for others it may be prolonged up to 180 minutes without untoward effects (Cohen 1977). Nelson and Ellenberg (1988) claim that the duration and severity of asphyxia required to produce damage in the child are extreme, and very uncommon in developed countries. However, this claim is mainly based on Apgar scores, though it is in accordance with the outcome of asphyxia experimentally induced in rhesus monkeys (Myers 1977). In fact, the correlation between the increased risk for an untoward fetal outcome and the duration of the second, and also the first, stage cannot be considered as proven (Dale and Stanley 1980, Sleep *et al.* 1989).

The period of risk is seemingly not the whole of the second stage but only the perineal phase, being the interval between the presentation of the head at the pelvic floor and the completion of birth, or the duration of perineal 'bulging' (Wood *et al.* 1973*b*). The duration of the phase of active bearing down has a three to seven times increased influence on fetal acid-base parameters compared to the whole duration of the second stage (Beard and Morris 1965, Roemer *et al.* 1976, Piquard *et al.* 1989). When cord compression occurs this influence is 25 times higher (Roemer *et al.* 1976).

Significant lowering of the pH in the umbilical artery and vein and an increase of the base deficit by 6mmol/L are already apparent when the interval between presentation at the perineum and birth exceeds 200 seconds. Electively shortening this phase of the second stage by outlet vacuum or forceps extraction improves the outcome in terms of pH (+0.3), without, however, bettering the outcome in terms of Apgar scores (Wood 1973a).

When only the pH in the umbilical artery is considered, the duration of the second stage, in the absence of cord complications, may go up to 93 minutes, and with the cord coiled around the neck up to 63 minutes, before the pH is down to 7.20. Taking into account statistical exceptions to the general trend, a limit of 45 minutes is advisable (Roemer et al. 1976). When monitoring, and in the presence of a normal heart frequency registration, an expectant attitude may be sustained longer. Accepting these principles in lieu of the 20 or 30 minutes rule may reduce the number of instrumental deliveries by 35 per cent in nulliparous and 9 per cent in multiparous women, over the whole of the duration of the second stage, and by 4.5 and 1.2 per cent, respectively, for the expulsion phase.

Not all authors however, would accept this optimistic view. Amiel-Tison et al. (1988) stressed that pressure on the skull may effect the cerebro-vascular circulation so as to cause hypoxaemia, even in conditions which some authors would still consider to be normal, i.e. early decelerations. They also emphasized that, as pressure on the presenting part remains high even between contractions, 'prolongation of labour may be deleterious, even if the contractions are spaced relatively far apart'. They recommend no further procrastination at full dilatation, and 'protecting the fetal head from the pressure of the soft tissues by appropriate instruments, including forceps or ventouse', thus re-establishing for physiological considerations the prophylactic forceps concept of the 1920s (Amiel-Tison et al. 1988).

Mechanical stress on the skull in the second stage
The influence of the forces of labour on the presenting fetal head is complex. The compression forces are absorbed and diverted through adaptation in shape of the skull (moulding) and displacement of the child (progression through the birth canal). Their physiological effect on the fetus is further determined by secondary, mainly vascular, reactions, and sometimes compounded by acidosis.

The pressure increase from the contractions, when estimated in the equatorial plane of the skull, is two to four times the intra-amniotic pressure (Schwarcz et al. 1970, Mann et al. 1972, Eskes et al. 1975, Amiel-Tison et al. 1988, Svenningsen 1989). The increase in intracranial pressure lags from 0.54 to 0.58 seconds behind the increase in intra-amniotic pressure, which is indicative of the dependence of the pressure increase on counterpressure from the surrounding tissue (Eskes et al. 1975). Pressure is highest in the equatorial plane of the skull, where it can reach up to 7.4kg in total (Mann et al. 1972). Lindgren (1960, 1973, 1981) made a detailed study of the forces acting on the presenting fetal head, and brought to attention the friction forces between the head and the maternal soft tissues. Lindgren calculated a resulting pressure of 210mmHg at the equatorial plane of the head, and of 35mmHg at the apex (about 6cm lower) for an intra-amniotic pressure of 60mmHg. The friction coefficient between the head and the cervix is about 0.20. Pressure reaches its maximum during the latter phase of cervical dilatation (engagement in the uterus) and again when the head is on the pelvic floor. The summation of the expulsion forces while bearing down (contraction pressure and abdominal pressure) on one side, and the resistance from the cervix and subsequently the pelvic floor on the other, integrated in time, were described as the 'fetal head compression pressure' (FHCP) by Svenningsen (1989).

Unequal resistance of the bony skull to this force leads to deformation of the skull (moulding) which calls for adaptation of the internal structures, especially the falx and tentorium cerebri and their vessels, the elasticity of which is not unlimited. This deformation is to a certain extent an adaptation mechanism whereby the FHCP does not get locally excessive. On the other hand, a threshold can be reached beyond which deformation no longer plays the role of 'pressure distributor' and becomes in itself deleterious.

Earlier obstetric thinking accepted a unidirectional model for the deformation of the fetal head (Moloy 1942, Schwartz 1961, Courville 1971). It has now become clear that the deformation of the head of the neonate 'does not tell the whole story of what shapes the head took during the intrapartum period' (Kriewall and McPherson 1981). Dynamic studies of moulding during labour gave a different picture (Rydberg 1954, Borell and Fernström 1958, Lindgren 1960, Schwarcz *et al.* 1970, Kriewall and McPherson 1981, Svenningsen 1989). During birth the head goes through at least three phases of compression and decompression (Lindgren 1981), in which even in the normal pelvis excessive moulding and pressure can develop. One factor in this is the duration of deformation in one direction. Of prime importance is the realization that there are no natural regulatory mechanisms to protect the fetus from excessive FHCP and its sequelae. The intracranial circulation has few autoregulatory mechanisms and depends upon intracranial pressure. Fetal heart rate changes by intrauterine pressure are due to imbalance between sympathetic and parasympathetic (vagal) nervous systems. With severe increase in head compression and decrease in cerebral perfusion, brain oedema may ensure resulting in an even greater increase in intracranial pressure, and a simple reflex bradycardia may become a bradycardia due to a combination of increased intracranial pressure and fetal hypoxia (Amiel-Tison *et al.* 1988). This complex interaction of mechanical stress with haemodynamic and even metabolic repercussions, prevents the simple and direct correlation of the condition of the individual neonate with the FHCP (Svenningsen 1989). There is, however, the indication that precisely because of these interactions, compression of short duration is in any case better tolerated than a longer expulsion stage. Obstetric intervention, by limiting the duration of this stage, can obviate the lack of a natural feedback mechanism and thus safeguard the fetus.

Instrumental delivery

Rationale

The relationship between duration of the expulsion stage and fetal outcome in terms of acidosis, and the analysis of mechanical forces during spontaneous delivery, both indicate that the duration of the second stage might better be limited. In a number of cases, where arrest of labour and/or fetal distress occurs, this is mandatory. In other cases, where there is no individual urgency, the obstetrician may feel that as a general rule it is better to cut short the second stage after a given time. In these cases, the procedure may be considered elective. In any case, the obstetrician will have to weigh benefit against possible harm. Just as s/he may be considered the only 'safety mechanism' at the disposal of the fetus against untoward developments in labour, s/he is also the only one in a position to judge the optimum force to exert on the baby during extraction. As Courville (1971) has pointed out, s/he must therefore assume the responsibility—not to be taken lightly—for any breakdown in procedure that would bring about physical birth injury.

Vacuum and forceps

Two extraction instruments are available in modern obstetrics: forceps, and the Malmström cup vacuum extractor and its derivatives.

Both instruments have their merits and demerits. Preferential use of one or the other may be individually determined, but generally speaking the vacuum extractor has found wide acceptance in continental Europe and met with much diffidence in the USA (Plauché 1992*b*). In Flanders, from 1987 to 1991, vacuum extraction was used in 12.9 per cent of registered singleton births, and forceps in 1.7 per cent (with a rate of 10.9 per cent for caesarean sections) (SPE 1992).

Forceps have a number of disadvantages, which may be part of the reason why the search for an alternative instrument has never altogether ceased.
• Application of forceps requires accessory space in the birth canal, which creates further difficulty in a borderline pelvis.
• The head can be compressed excessively between the blades of the forceps.
• The head cannot rotate spontaneously during forceps extraction. It is bound to follow the rotation applied by the obstetrician. This in turn requires an accurate diagnosis of position prior to application. There is evidence that a correct estimation of position is achieved in at best 60 to 70 per cent of cases.
• Finally, it is generally recommended that forceps should only be applied after analgesia/anaesthesia.

The disadvantages of the vacuum extractor are more insidious. When in 1953 Malmström introduced the flanged cup which made effective traction possible, enthusiasm for this easily applied instrument led to a number of over-enthusiastic applications—extraction from a high station or with incomplete dilatation ('assisting dilatation'), or even application to guide the breech—that on closer consideration have been abandoned (Malmström 1957, Sjösted 1967, Chalmers

92

1971). They may account for a number of traumatic cases.

The degree of experience vacuum requires is also sometimes underestimated especially in difficult cases when progress of the head has to be judged carefully. Here Courville's heeding takes on its most fulsome meaning. As a rule, it is mandatory to desist after three to five tractions when there is no clear evidence of progress. It has repeatedly been stated that vacuum extraction is not indicated when fetal distress occurs, because of the time it takes to build up the vacuum. In fact, Malmström's original recommendation to build up the vacuum step by step needs no adhering to (Nyirjesy *et al.* 1963, Bird 1982, Thiery 1985), and vacuum extraction, not requiring additional analgesia, is at least as quick as forceps in cases of fetal distress (Vacca and Keirse 1989).

Vacuum extraction should not be done in breech or face presentation, and will often fail in a dead fetus, where a proper caput does not build up.

Occasionally, cases are mentioned where a forceps delivery has been achieved after failed vacuum extraction. In these cases, one of two situations applies: either the neonate is traumatized, because the forceps extraction will have been achieved by too tight a grip or excess pulling force, in a borderline pelvis; or the baby will be perfect, in which case the vacuum extraction was bungled in the first place. There is *no* third explanation.

This author feels that every obstetrician should stick to the instrument s/he is experienced and feels confident with. There is no occasion where vacuum can be used but not forceps, equally vice versa. There are cases that should be treated vaginally with whichever instrument the operator adheres to, and cases where s/he should desist from vaginal delivery. A case an experienced vacuum operator cannot conclude successfully must be one of borderline disproportion, because in a case of manifest disproportion, trial of vacuum should not have begun. There is in my experience no case where a vacuum extraction, if indicated, cannot be properly handled by the application of the original Malmström No. 5 cup, despite the fact that other sizes of this cup have been made available, as well as other cups (*e.g.* Bird, O'Neill, Saling) designed for various specific applications. Plastic cups of different shapes have been marketed, more, one suspects, for consumer than for sound technical reasons. Most have bell-shapes from the pre-Malmström era, rendering their efficiency doubtful (Thiery 1985). While of plastic, they are neither handy nor vagina-friendly to apply. In fact, their designers seem mostly to have forgotten that when they are to be applied, the head has still a vagina around it.

The forces of vacuum extraction
The clue to the Malmström cup's efficiency is that, through the vacuum, subcutaneous oedema of the scalp forms a 'caput succedaneum artificiale', 'cup caput' or 'chignon', filling the cup. The cup then grips this caput like hand with inward-curved fingers, and traction is applied to the skin and transmitted to the fixed skin layer at the base of the neck, and not to the fetal skull (Malmström 1957, Donald 1972). In contrast to the forceps, the application of the instrument in itself

causes no increase of pressure on the head. Compression is caused only by the progress of the head through the birth canal, and in principle equals the force needed to overcome the resistance of the vagina and pelvic floor to progression, in other words the force to be achieved in spontaneous labour.

Rosa (1955) calculated that the intracranial pressure for a traction of 10kg at $0.5kg/cm^2$ on the Malmström No. 5 cup rated $75g/cm^2$. For a corresponding traction force to be achieved with forceps, compression forces would be almost 20 times higher ($1400g/cm^2$) at the tips and higher still in the concavity between the blades. Mishell and Kelly (1962) also found that compression was less with vacuum extraction than with forceps, but other authors have found contradictory results. During spontaneous vertex delivery the average compression force on the head varies, according to parity and position of the head, from $1.9kg/cm^2/s$, to $29kg/cm^2/s$ as against $4.6kg/cm^2/s$ for vacuum extraction and 3.0 to $4.4kg/cm^2/s$ for a number of forceps types (Thiery 1985). Moolgaoker *et al.* (1979) found greater divergences, but vacuum extraction in the hands of these authors required a longer time and the obstetric background of their cases may not be strictly comparable (Thiery 1985). When a negative pressure of $0.5kg/cm^2$ is applied to the Malmström No. 5 cup, the maximal traction that can be applied before the cup comes off is 14.8kg. Doubling the negative pressure allows for a traction force of 29.8kg to be applied (Rosa 1955). In traction experiments with a dead neonate, Donald (1972) found the cup came loose at a traction force of 23lbs (10.5kg). This was much less than the pulling force possible with forceps, and Donald considered this an important element of safety of the vacuum extractor. As it is, in a living fetus, which can build up an effective cup caput, higher pulling forces can presumably be achieved. Mostly a vacuum of 0.8 to $0.9kg/cm^2$ is built up in practice. Available equipment for the most part allows a negative pressure of $1kg/cm^2$. According to Bird (1982), such pressure can be applied without harm.

Clinical measurements (Mishell and Kelly 1962, Saling and Hartung 1973, Saling *et al.* 1973, Thiery *et al.* 1973, Moolgaoker *et al.* 1979) show that a pulling force of 20kg can be surpassed in vacuum extraction, and this is significantly more than the 15kg expelling force that is achieved during spontaneous birth. The actual extent of the forces is dependent on several factors:
• vacuum level and the size of the suction cup;
• cervical dilatation: as the friction between fetal head and uterine tissue is considerable (Lindgren 1973, 1981), incomplete dilatation increases proportionately the force to be applied;
• vis a tergo: a cooperative patient diminishes the actual pulling force to be applied;
• birthweight: the force exerted over the whole of the second stage (force–time integral, FTI) is doubled when the birthweight for a midpelvic extraction lies between 2500 and 2900g or above 3700g (Saling and Hartung 1973). This accords well with the known influence of birthweight on spontaneous labour (Kadar *et al.* 1986, Nesheim 1988);

• position of the head: mean FTI, compression and traction forces decline by a factor of four from the pelvic inlet to the outlet (Saling and Hartung 1973, Moolgaoker *et al.* 1979);

• attitude of the head: the degree of flexion is all important, as birth with a certain degree of deflexion considerably heightens the force to be applied (Bird 1976) and also predisposes to undue deformation of the skull and elongation of the falx.

The cup has therefore to be be applied on the 'flexion point' of the head. This is located on the sagittal suture, 3cm frontally from the posterior fontanelle (flexing, median application) (Bird 1976, Vacca and Keirse 1989). With a strongly moulded or deflected head or in the presence of oblique presentation of the head (asynclitism), this eventually requires manual correction prior to extraction.

A further word of caution when comparing instrumentally assisted delivery to spontaneous delivery is due. It may not be sufficient simply to compare quantitative estimation of compression forces in instrumental and spontaneous delivery. Kriewall and McPherson (1981) have pointed out that the skull is designed to resist compression forces and can to a degree cope with them by redistributing them to certain stress-absorbing structures and by adaptation of shape, but that the same does not apply to traction forces. They thus expressly contradict the contention of Kelly (1963) that the maximum amount of safe forceps pull equals the amount of pressure on the head during spontaneous delivery in the primigravida. The same would, of course, apply for vacuum. Kriewall and McPherson's work implies that the structure of the fetal head may be relatively resistant to compression forces, but not so to pulling forces. In cases of cephalopelvic disproportion and muscular spasm of the lower uterine segment, the applied loads are increased and the pressure distribution altered, so that the risk in these cases is the greater, as it is in the softer preterm head.

Direct mechanical trauma was seen as the main cause of intracranial trauma at the beginning of the century (Amiel-Tison *et al.* 1988, Brand and Saling 1988). It may now have dwindled to 1 or 2 per cent or even 1 or 2 per mille of the total incidence of birth trauma (Wigglesworth 1984, Alberman 1988, Geirsson 1988, Nelson and Ellenberg 1988). Taylor *et al.* (1985) even found no link between cerebral palsy and instrumental delivery. But even discounting the lurid casuistics of trauma through glaring misuse of the instrument, there is no room for complacency, and the notion of this totally avoidable damage should be present in the mind of the obstetrician deciding upon an instrumental delivery.

When judging the risks of instrumental delivery, care should be taken to separate the part played by the instrument from that of the circumstances leading up to its use. One illustrative example is to be found with forceps application: mid-forceps application is now considered unsafe and is no longer recommended, whereas outlet forceps is a safe procedure. One would surmise from this that inlet forceps should be even more dangerous, but Brand and Saling (1988) actually found it to be safer than mid-forceps, because inlet forceps implied a number of elective procedures, while mid-forceps implied a number of therapeutic procedures in malrotation and prolonged labour. Wigglesworth (1988) is of the opinion that trying to disentangle the roles of mechanical trauma and obstetric circumstances may well prove impossible.

While vacuum extraction does not allow 'crushing' the head as a misapplied forceps might conceivably do, the relatively easy high application of the instrument might engender higher pulling forces than are warranted, while sudden pressure changes by cup detachment are also a cause for concern. The last event should be prevented by proper technique (three-finger grip and avoiding tangential traction). Retinal haemorrhages, which are also seen after spontaneous delivery, have been much discussed, but it now seems established that they are not due to vacuum extraction as such but to the conditions of use (nulliparity, large baby, prolonged second stage—Tranou-Sphalangakou 1968, Van Zundert *et al.* 1986) and also that they are not related to intracranial haemorrhage (von Barsewisch 1979).

Cup caput is due to the working mechanism of the instrument and is not to be seen as a trauma (Thiery 1985). Together with superficial scalp abrasion, however, it seems to account for the abandonment of the vacuum extractor for consumer reasons in the United States (Plauché 1992*b*). The fear that profuse bleeding may be caused by applying the cup over a scalp electrode or the microblood sampling puncture (after proper compression for a few moments) is not upheld by the facts.

In fetuses with bleeding tendency (Bird 1982) there is an increased risk of subcutaneous ecchymosis (cup haematoma) or subgaleal haematoma, which may result in serious and possibly life-threatening bleeding (Plauché 1979). Cephalhaematoma, the accumulation of blood between the cranial bone and pericranium which occurs in 0.4 to 2.5 per cent of spontaneous deliveries, is seen more often after high or prolonged vacuum extraction especially when complicated by cup detachment. While rare and mostly of little clinical importance, skull fractures after vacuum extraction (Sjösted 1967) may illustrate the point concerning fetal skull resistance made by Kriewall and McPherson. Intracranial haemorrhage (ICH) is the most serious hazard, though seemingly rare in vacuum extraction. Here especially, the part of the instrumental delivery, and factors leading up to it (prolonged delivery, hypoxia), are difficult to distinguish from each other. Cranial injury related to vacuum delivery is discussed in Chapter 6.

Conclusion

There are many serious arguments indicating that a prolonged second stage is inefficient as well as in the end deleterious for the child. It is also clear that in many cases a longer limit to the duration can be adhered to than is generally the case, and that it is not so much the whole of the second stage as the perineal phase that is better cut short. In these cases the dictum applies: 'Elective termination of labour because an arbitrary period of time has elapsed in the second stage is clearly not warranted' (Cohen 1977).

An expectant attitude may be adapted when the following conditions apply: term labour, normal fetal heart rate, and a cooperative and comfortable parturient, for whom the first stage progressed normally. There must be no cephalopelvic disproportion, in which case caesarean section is indicated. Refraining from a number of elective instrumental deliveries will create for some women the additional satisfaction to have given birth to their baby 'all by themselves'. Indeed, many women experience instrumental delivery as a disappointment or a personal failure.

The obstetrician should stick to the instrument with which s/he has a thorough experience. By definition, a correct instrumental delivery should imply no additional risk to the child (Thiery 1985; Vacca and Keirse 1989; Plauché 1992a,b; Yeomans and Hawkins 1992).

The Committee on Obstetrics of the American College of Obstetrics and Gynecology (1988) declared that there was no difference in perinatal outcome when forceps deliveries were compared to similar spontaneous deliveries. There is certainly even less reason to consider vacuum extraction, with correct median-flexing application, as hazardous.

By all means, proper obstetric judgement of all factors involved is the unborn child's only way to safety. Whenever the obstetrician decides upon instrumental vaginal delivery, s/he must remember that s/he will be the only one, in Courville's words, to judge properly, and be responsible for, the further course of events.

REFERENCES

American College of Obstetrics and Gynecology Committee on Obstetrics (1988) *Obstetric Forceps.* Washington DC: ACOG (Publication No. 59).

Alberman, E. (1988) 'Epidemiology and causative factors.' *Baillière's Clinical Obstetrics and Gynaecology*, **2**, 9–19.

Amiel-Tison, C., Sureau, C., Shnider, S.M. (1988) 'Cerebral handicap in full-term neonates related to the mechanical forces of labour.' *Baillières Clinical Obstetrics and Gynaecology*, **2**, 145–165.

Beard, R.W., Morris, E.D. (1965) 'Foetal and maternal acid–base balance during normal labour.' *Journal of Obstetrics and Gynaecology of the British Commonwealth*, **72**, 496–506.

Bird, G.C. (1976) 'The importance of flexion in vacuum extraction delivery.' *British Journal of Obstetrics and Gynaecology*, **83**, 194–200.

—— (1982) 'The use of the vacuum extractor.' *Clinical Obstetrics and Gynecology*, **9**, 641–661.

Borell, U., Fernström, J. (1958) 'Die Umformung des kindlichen Kopfes während normaler Entbindungen in regelrechter Hinterhauptslage.' *Geburtshilfe und Frauenheilkunde*, **18**, 1156–1160.

Brand, M. Saling, E. (1988) 'Obstetrical factors and intracranial haemorrhage.' *In*: Kubli, F., Patel, N., Schmidt, W., Linderkamp, O. (Eds) *Perinatal Events and Brain Damage in Surviving Children.* Berlin: Springer-Verlag, pp. 216–227.

Chalmers, J.A. (1971) *The Ventouse: the Obstetric Vacuum Extractor.* London: Lloyd-Luke.

Cohen, W.R. (1977) 'Influence of the duration of second stage labor on perinatal outcome and puerperal morbidity.' *Obstetrics and Gynecology*, **49**, 266–269.

Courville, C.B. (1971) *Birth and Brain Damage: an Investigation into the Problems of Antenatal and Paranatal Anoxia and Allied Disorders and their Relation to the many Lesion-complexes Residual Thereto.* Pasadena, CA: Courville.

Dale, A., Stanley, F.J. (1980) 'An epidemiological study of cerebral palsy in Western Australia, 1956–1975. II. Spastic cerebral palsy and perinatal factors.' *Developmental Medicine and Child Neurology*, **22**, 13–25.

Davidson, A.C., Weaver, J.B., Davies, P., Pearson, J.F. (1976) 'The relation between ease of forceps delivery and speed of cervical dilatation.' *British Journal of Obstetrics and Gynaecology*, **83**, 279–283.

De Lee, J.B. (1921) 'The prophylactic forceps operation.' *American Journal of Obstetrics and Gynecology*, **1**, 34–44.

De Rom, F.M., De Rom, R.M. (1954) 'Le rôle du forceps prophylactique dans la protection de l'enfant au cours de l'accouchement chez les primipares.' *In: La Prophylaxie en Gynécologie et Obstétrique.* Geneva: Librairie de l'Université Georg, pp. 1226–1230.

Donald, I. (1972) *Practical Obstetric Problems.* London: Lloyd-Luke.

Eskes, T.K.A.B., Martinez, A., de Haan, J., Briët, J.W., Jongsma, H.W. (1975) 'Pressure on the hydrocephalic fetal head during the first stage of labor.' *European Journal of Obstetrics and Gynecology and Reproductive Biology*, **4**, 171–176.

Friedman, E.A. (1967) *Labor: Clinical Evaluation and Management.* New York: Appleton Century Crofts.

—— (1978) *Labor: Clinical Evaluation and Management. 2nd Edn.* New York: Appleton Century Crofts.

—— Kroll, B.H. (1969) 'Computer analysis of labour progression.' *Journal of Obstetrics and Gynaecology of the British Commonwealth*, **76**, 1075-1079.

Gebbie, D.A.M. (1981) *Reproductive Anthropology—Descent Through Woman.* Chichester: J. Wiley.

Geirsson, R.T. (1988) 'Birth trauma and brain damage.' *Baillière's Clinical Obstetrics and Gynaecology*, **2**, 195–212.

Hellman, L.M., Prystowski, H. (1952) The duration of the second stage of labor.' *American Journal of Obstetrics and Gynecology*, **63**, 1233–1239.

Holm, J.P. (1982) *Epidural Anaesthesia in Risk Birth.* (Thesis, University of Groningen.)

Jeffcoate, T.N.A. (1950) 'Delay in the second stage of labour.' *British Medical Journal*, **1**, 1359–1362.

Kadar, N., Cruddas, M., Campbell, S. (1986) 'Estimating the probability of spontaneous delivery conditional on time spent in the second stage.' *British Journal of Obstetrics and Gynaecology*, **93**, 568–576.

Katz, M., Lunenfeld, E., Meizner, J., Bashan, N., Gross, I. (1987) 'The effect of the duration of the second stage of labour on the acid-base status of the fetus.' *British Journal of Obstetrics and Gynaecology*, **94**, 425–430.

Kelly, J.V. (1963) 'Compression of the fetal brain.' *American Journal of Obstetrics and Gynecology*, **85**, 687–694.

Kriewall, T.J., McPherson, G.K. (1981) 'Effects of uterine contractility on the fetal cranium. Perspectives from the past, present and future.' *In*: Milunsky, A., Friedman, E.A., Gluck, L. (Eds) *Advances in Perinatal Medicine. Vol. I.* New York: Plenum, pp. 295–356.

Lindgren, L. (1960) 'The causes of fetal head moulding in labour.' *Acta Obstetricia et Gynecologica Scandinavica*, **39**, 46–62.

—— (1973) 'Biodynamics of the cervix during pregnancy and labour.' *In*: Blandau, R.J., Moghissi, K. (Eds) *The Biology of the Cervix.* Chicago: University of Chicago Press, pp. 385–413.

—— (1981) 'Effects of pressure gradient on the fetal cranium.' *In*: Milunsky, A., Friedman, E.A., Gluck, L. (Eds) *Advances in Perinatal Medicine. Vol. I.* New York: Plenum, pp. 375–428.

Little, W.J. (1862) 'On the influence of abnormal parturitions, difficult labours, premature birth, and asphyxia neonatorum, on the mental and physical condition of the child, especially in relation to deformities.' *Transactions of the London Obstetrical Society*, **3**, 293–344.

Malmström, T. (1957) 'The vacuum extractor (an obstetrical instrument) and the parturiometer (a tocographic device).' *Acta Obstetricia et Gynecologica Scandinavica*, **36**, Suppl. 3.

Mann, L.L., Carmichael, A., Duchin, S. (1972) 'The effect of head compression on FHR, brain metabolism and function.' *Obstetrics and Gynecology*, **39**, 721–725.

Miller, N.F. (1935) *Quoted in:* Hayashi, R.H. (1992) 'Foreword.' *Clinical Obstetrics and Gynecology*, **35**, 443.

Mishell, D., Kelly, J.V. (1962) 'The obstetrical forceps and the vacuum extractor: an assessment of their compressive force.' *Obstetrics and Gynecology*, **19**, 204–206.

Moloy, H.C. (1942) 'Studies of fetal head molding during labor.' *American Journal of Obstetrics and Gynecology*, **44**, 762–772.

Moolgaoker, A.S., Ahamed, S.O.S., Payne, P.R. (1979) 'A comparison of different methods of instrumental delivery based on electronic measurements of compression and traction.' *Obstetrics and Gynecology,* **54**, 299–309.

Myers, R.E. (1977) 'Experimental models of perinatal brain damage: relevance to human pathology.' *In*: Gluck, L. (Ed.) *Intrauterine Asphyxia and the Developing Fetal Brain.* Chicago: Year Book Medical, pp. 37–97.

Nelson, K.B., Ellenberg, J.H. (1988) 'Intrapartum events and cerebral palsy'. *In*: Kubli, F., Patel, N., Schmidt, W., Linderkamp, O. (Eds) *Perinatal Events and Brain Damage in Surviving Children.* Berlin: Springer-Verlag, pp. 139–148.

Nesheim, B.J. (1988) 'Duration of labour: an analysis of influencing factors.' *Acta Obstetricia et Gynecologica Scandinavica,* **67**, 121–124.

Nyirjesy, I., Hawks, B.L., Falls, H.C., Munsat, T.L., Pierce, W.E. (1963) 'A comparative study of the vacuum extractor and forceps.' *American Journal of Obstetrics and Gynecology,* **85**, 1071–1082.

Perkins, R.P. (1987) 'Perspectives on perinatal brain damage.' *Obstetrics and Gynecology,* **69**, 807–819.

Piquard, F., Schaefer, A., Hsiung, R., Dellenbach, P., Haberey, P. (1989) 'Are there two biological parts in the second stage of labor?' *Acta Obstetricia et Gynecologica Scandinavica,* **68**, 713–718.

Plauché, W.C. (1979) 'Fetal cranial injuries related to delivery with the Malmström vacuum extractor.' *Obstetrics and Gynecology,* **53**, 750–757.

—— (1992*a*) 'Forceps delivery.' *In*: Plauché, W.C., Morrison, J.C., O'Sullivan, M.J. (Eds) *Surgical Obstetrics.* Philadelphia: W.B. Saunders, pp. 265–279.

—— (1992*b*) 'Vacuum extraction.' *In*: Plauché, W.C., Morrison, J.C., O'Sullivan, M.J. (Eds) *Surgical Obstetrics.* Philadelphia: W.B. Saunders, pp. 281–296.

Roemer, V.M., Harms, K., Buess, H., Horvath, T.J. (1976) 'Response of fetal acid–base balance to duration of second stage of labour.' *International Journal of Gynaecology and Obstetrics,* **14**, 455–471.

Rosa, P. (1955) 'Défense de l'extraction par ventouse.' *Bulletin de la Société Royale Belge de Gynécologie et d'Obstétrique,* **26**, 142–148.

Rosen, M.G., Hobel, C.J. (1986) 'Prenatal and perinatal factors associated with brain disorders.' *Obstetrics and Gynecology,* **68**, 416–421.

Rydberg, E. (1954) *The Mechanism of Labor.* Springfield, IL: C.C. Thomas.

Saling, E., Hartung, M. (1973) 'Analyses of tractive forces during application of vacuum extraction.' *Journal of Perinatal Medicine,* **1**, 245–251.

—— Blücher, U., Sander, H. (1973) 'Equipment for the recording of traction power in vacuum extractions.' *Journal of Perinatal Medicine,* **1**, 142–144.

Schwarcz, R.L., Strada-Saenz, G., Althabe, O. (1970) 'Compression received by the head of the human fetus during labor.' *In*: Angle, R.C., Bering, E.A. (Eds) *Physical Trauma as an Etiological Agent in Mental Retardation.* Washington, DC: US Department of Health, Education and Welfare, pp. 133–141.

Schwartz, P. (1969) *Birth Injuries of the Newborn.* Basel: Karger.

Sjösted, J.E. (1967) *The Vacuum Extractor and Forceps in Obstetrics. A Clinical Study.* (Thesis, University of Helsinki.)

Sleep, J., Robert, J., Chalmers, I. (1989) 'Care during the second stage of labour.' *In*: Enkins, M., Chalmers, I., Keirse, M.J.N.C. (Eds) *Effective Care in Pregnancy and Childbirth, Vol. 2.* Oxford: Oxford University Press, pp. 1129–1144.

Speert, H. (1973) *Iconographia Gyniatrica. A Pictorial History of Gynecology and Obstetrics.* Philadelphia: F.A. Davis.

SPE (1992) *Evaluatie van de perinatale Activiteiten in Vlaanderen, 1987–1991.* Brussels: Studiecentrum Perinatale Epidemiologie.

Svenningsen, L. (1989) *Measurement of the Forces During Spontaneous Delivery and under Vacuum Extraction. Their Relevance for the Clinical Condition of the Newborn.* (Thesis, University of Oslo.)

Taylor, D.J., Howie, P.W., Davidson, J., Davidson, D., Drillien, C.M. (1985) 'Do pregnancy complications contribute to neurodevelopmental disability?' *Lancet,* **1**, 713–716.

Thiery, M. (1985) 'Obstetric vacuum extraction.' *In*: Wynn, R.M. (Eds) *Obstetrics and Gynecology Annual, Vol. 14.* Norwalk, CN: Appleton Century Crofts, pp. 73–111.

—— Van Kets, H., Derom, R. (1973) 'Recording of tractive power in vacuum extractions.' *Journal of Perinatal Medicine,* **1**, 291–292. *(Letter.)*

Tranou-Sphalangakou, L. (1968) *About Retinal Haemorrhages in the Newborn.* (Thesis, University of Athens.)

99

Vacca, A., Keirse, M.J.N.C. (1989) 'Instrumental vaginal delivery.' *In*: Enkins, M., Chalmers, I., Keirse, M.J.N.C. (Eds) *Effective Care in Pregnancy and Childbirth. Vol. 2.* Oxford: Oxford University Press, pp. 1216–1233.

Van Zundert, A., Jansen, J., Vaes, L., Soetens, M., De Vel, M., Van der Aa, P. (1986) 'Extradural analgesia and retinal haemorrhages in the newborn.' *British Journal of Anaesthesiology*, **58**, 1017–1021.

von Barsewisch, B. (1979) *Perinatal Retinal Haemorrhages. Morphology, Aetiology and Significance.* Berlin: Springer-Verlag.

Waitz, R. (1931) *Les Lésions Cérébro-méningées à la Naissance.* Paris: Doin.

Wigglesworth, J.S. (1984) *Perinatal Pathology.* Philadelphia: W.B. Saunders.

—— (1988) 'Trauma and the developing brain.' *In*: Kubli, F., Patel, N., Schmidt, W., Linderkamp, O. (Eds) *Perinatal Events and Brain Damage in Surviving Children.* Berlin: Springer-Verlag, pp. 64–69.

Wood, C., Ng, K.H., Hounslow, D., Benning, H. (1973*a*) 'Time—an important variable in normal delivery.' *Journal of Obstetrics and Gynaecology of the British Commonwealth*, **80**, 285–288.

—— —— —— —— (1973*b*) 'The influence of differences of birth times upon fetal condition in normal deliveries.' *Journal of Obstetrics and Gynaecology of the British Commonwealth*, **80**, 289–294.

Yeomans, E.R., Hawkins, G.D.V. (1992) 'Operative vaginal delivery in the 1990s.' *Clinical Obstetrics and Gynecology*, **35**, 487–493.

8
DEEP HAEMORRHAGE

Neonatal subarachnoid haematoma (focal subarachnoid bleeding)
Anatomical description
Some newborn infants develop large extravasations of blood within the pial–arachnoid membranes, usually restricted to one side of the cerebrum (Chessells and Wigglesworth 1970, Larroche 1977). The term 'haematoma' is preferred because of the volume of the collection, sometimes up to a few centimeters in thickness, and because of its firmness due to clotting (Fig. 8.1). Blood may spread along the subjacent sulci and fissures thus penetrating deep into the parenchyma. It is therefore not surprising to find subsequent necrosis of the related cerebral (sub)-cortex, possibly also due to associated uncal herniation and systemic vascular changes. A predilection for the base of the temporal lobe and temporo-parietal convexity is not readily explicable.

Incidence
Its relative scarcity is clearly shown by its absence from a series of *in vivo* diagnosed intracranial haemorrhages at or near term (Flodmark *et al.* 1980*b*, Guekos-Thöni *et al.* 1980, Leblanc and O'Gorman 1980, Ludwig *et al.* 1980, Brockerhoff *et al.* 1981, Fenichel *et al.* 1984, Pierre-Kahn *et al.* 1985, Welch and Strand 1986, Romodanov and Brodsky 1987, Sachs *et al.* 1987, Oelberg *et al.* 1988).

On the other hand, Chessells and Wigglesworth (1970) documented the lesion in five neonatal autopsies (one term and four preterm infants) in one centre during an eight month period. Two prenatal cases were also observed within the 1980s Hammersmith series (unpublished data). Larroche (1977) gathered 60 instances out of 2000 stillbirths and neonatal deaths (3 per cent). The virtual absence from reports on living newborn infants, in contrast to post-mortem data, suggests the high potential of this lesion to cause neonatal death. Within the UZ Gent material there were no instances among term infants, but three cases were documented in big preterm infants (gestational ages 32–36 weeks) between 1989 and 1991, two of which were fatal.

Pathogenesis
The event is clearly of venous or capillary origin, as its distribution is not related to arterial regions (Larroche 1977). The most likely cause is haemostatic failure (Chessells and Wigglesworth 1970). The intermediary mechanism is disseminated intravascular consumption of platelets and coagulation factors. This type of 'secondary haemorrhagic disease' can be related to (i) profound hypothermia in slightly preterm infants, (ii) asphyxia, and (iii) severe rhesus iso-immunization;

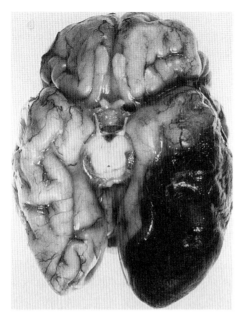

Fig. 8.1. Post-mortem view of temporal lobe subarachnoid haematoma. (Courtesy Prof. J.S. Wigglesworth, Hammersmith Hospital.)

however, in my experience the usual underlying disease is bacterial sepsis. Against this background it is not surprising to find disseminated fibrin thrombi within several visceral microvessels (Chessells and Wigglesworth 1970). Barson (1990) reviewed perinatal infections evidenced at autopsy and listed subarachnoid haematoma as an indirect indicator of septicaemia, together with disseminated abscess formation, purulent vasculitis, the presence of intravascular bacteria and evidence of fibrin formation within small vessels. He registered 27 instances (22.3 per cent) in 42 necropsies with evidence of disseminated intravascular coagulation (DIC) from a series of 121 bacteraemic stillbirths, neonatal and postnatal deaths with positive post-mortem heart blood culture, as compared with 17 instances (2.2 per cent) in 32 necropsies with evidence of DIC from a series of 781 culture-negative dead infants. His findings confirm the non-specific link between bacteraemia, intravascular consumption of coagulation factors and subarachnoid haematoma. Typical subarachnoid haematoma has also been reported in association with hereditary clotting disturbance, *e.g.* haemophilia (Yoffe and Buchanan 1988). A similar lesion has also been reported in association with congenital toxoplasmosis and calcifying brain damage (Dische and Gooch 1981).

Of two prenatal cases observed recently at Hammersmith Hospital, one was associated with chronic fetal anaemia and non-immune hydrops ending in subacute multi-organ failure, while the other had alloimmune thrombocytopenia due to human platelet antigen 1 (HPA1) incompatibility as the underlying disorder. Association in the latter infant with minor subpial bleeds and the finding with reticulin staining of a limiting membrane and some molecular layer remnant on the

102

surface of the suspected subarachnoid haematoma suggest that differentiation between subarachnoid and pial haematoma cannot be made with the naked eye and may even require special histological techniques. This could help explain why, in spite of the association with DIC, most of the haematomas are solid; that is, cerebral thromboplastic material may give local assistance in the process of clotting. The presence of clot accounts for the obvious hyperdensity of the haematoma on ultrasound scan.

Although put forward as an alternative, there is little evidence that trauma is responsible (Larroche 1977). A recent observation at Hammersmith Hospital concerned a male infant with extensive subgaleal bleeding, bilateral tentorial fraying, left parietal and frontal bone fractures and fatal hypovolaemic shock after failed vacuum extraction at 34 weeks of gestation: the extensive, more diffuse subarachnoid haemorrhage in this infant was probably secondary to consumption of platelets and factors in the subgaleal space, preventing clotting underneath the arachnoid membrane.

More nodular but extensive subarachnoid bleeds have been observed in neonates with ruptured intracranial vascular anomalies such as arterio-venous angioma, aneurysm of the great vein of Galen and arterial 'berry' aneurysm.

Clinical setting
The context is that of a seriously ill neonate with anaemia, an abnormal bleeding tendency, intracranial hypertension and seizures. The three preterm infants cared for at UZ Gent (see above) were all born by spontaneous vaginal delivery without birth asphyxia; all developed septic shock with metabolic acidosis between the first and 14th days of life.

Details of the associated haemostatic profile are provided by Chessells and Wigglesworth (1970): these document the characteristic features of DIC in clear-cut cases.

Radiological assessment
One typical case, diagnosed *in vivo* by ultrasound scan, is described in the literature (Larroche 1992): the ultrasound appearance is similar to that observed in one of the UZ Gent cases (Fig. 8.2). Differentiation from subdural bleeding is not difficult by the use of CT scan (Fig. 8.3) (Govaert *et al.* 1992*b*). The images are that of an extracerebral density indenting sulci and fissures (bilateral in only 3/33 cases reviewed by Larroche, on the left in 22). All the haemorrhages described by Chessells and Wigglesworth were located on the right. They are usually found beneath and around the base of the temporal lobe.

Management
Treatment is that of DIC, whatever its origin, though any initiating factors such as infection or severe metabolic acidosis must also have prompt attention. The management of severe DIC not surprisingly lacks controlled studies and is not

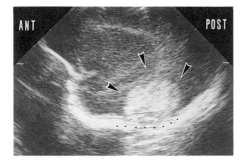

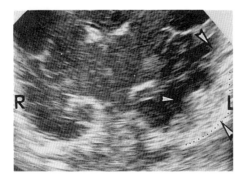

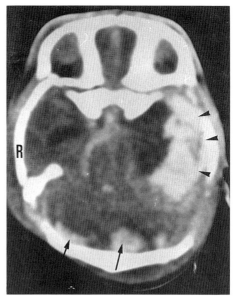

Fig. 8.2. Left parasagittal *(top)* and coronal *(bottom)* ultrasound scans demonstrating temporal density *(arrowheads)* resting on underlying bones *(dotted line)* and invading cerebral sulci.

Fig. 8.3. Axial CT scan: left temporal lobe is hypodense in its medial aspect and replaced by haematoma in its lateral aspect *(arrowheads)*. There is further haemorrhage in or on top of the cerebellum *(arrows)*.

generally agreed. It may include exchange transfusion with fresh citrate phosphate dextrose blood, platelet concentrate, fresh frozen plasma and cryoprecipitate. Personal experience with preterm infants suggests a desperately downhill course in cases with severe intracranial hypertension, despite emergency neurosurgical treatment. On the other hand, presentation with seizures and a midline shift is compatible with survival and limited neurological impairment.

Subpial haemorrhage
Anatomical description
This type of bleeding is found immediately below the pial membrane, which remains intact. Mingling of erythrocytes and CSF does not take place because the haemorrhage is retained within the brain tissue of the molecular or external granular layer of the cerebrum and cerebellum respectively. In most cases subpial haemorrhages symmetrically cover part of the parieto-temporal cerebral cortex or the cerebellum. Larger haemorrhages penetrate into the brain substance along the blood vessels. At post-mortem examination they remain on the brain surface once the arachnoid membrane has been gently peeled away. Accurate histological

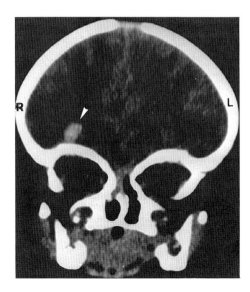

Fig. 8.4. Coronal CT scan on day 50 showing right frontal subpial haemorrhage *(arrowhead)* in girl who died as a consequence of pituitary agenesis.

description of their subpial nature can be achieved with reticulin staining to show the intact covering pial membrane (Friede 1972).

Incidence and pathogenesis
Minor lesions (a few millimeters thick) have not been demonstrated in life through the intact skull. A moderately large pial bleed is shown in Figure 8.4, the CT image of a term infant who died in the second month of life due to pituitary agenesis and after a course complicated by bacteraemia and respiratory insufficiency. Pathological descriptions are limited to a couple of reports, the only comprehensive ones by Friede (1972, 1989). He mentions eight neonatal cases in 230 detailed studies of newborn and older infant brains. Gröntoft (1953) gathered 12 pial bleeds in a careful study of 86 meningeal haemorrhages from 319 autopsies on stillbirths and neonatal deaths. Friede suggests a common pathogenesis with subarachnoid haemorrhage, because of its association with low birthweight and respiratory distress. Nevertheless the rather constant topographical characteristics, namely distribution on the temporal lobe surface and identical subpial level in different haemorrhages, suggest a local factor. Hypothetically, glial necrosis and oedema of the superficial layer could induce subsequent tractional damage to the small vessels under the pial membrane. In association with haemostatic disorders major haemorrhages have been recognized by the use of CT and MRI (Kuhn *et al.* 1992) (see sections on subarachnoid haematoma and cerebellar haemorrhage).

Prognosis
Subpial blood clots do not benefit from the washing effect of neighbouring CSF

105

bulk flow and resorption may thus be difficult. This has led to the as yet unsubstantiated suggestion that they might play a role in the genesis of superficial brain siderosis (Friede 1972): this may result when ferritin is biosynthesized by glial cells in response to prolonged contact with haemoglobin iron.

Haemorrhagic encephalopathy
This section relates to disseminated petechial intraparenchymal cerebral haemorrhage around the small vessels of the CNS. This is caused either by agonal diapedesis (Cammermeyer 1953), or in the case of severe venous congestion by capillary wall rupture (Pape and Wigglesworth 1979). Microscopically one finds extravasated blood around small veins and capillaries without signs of inflammation (Craig 1938, Larroche 1977). Since before the advent of neonatal intensive care, pathologists had been concerned about the presence of such lesions in 'vital centres' of the brainstem, debating whether they were the cause or consequence of neonatal respiratory distress (Hirvensalo 1949, Morison 1963).

The relevance of these lesions is ill-defined, mainly because the only information about them comes from necropsy findings and also because in most cases they are unimpressive and overshadowed by other problems. Craig (1938), in a study of 126 neonatal intracranial haemorrhages, recorded six instances of numerous but limited areas of bleeding throughout the cerebrum and, to a lesser extent, in the cerebellum and brainstem. Prolonged labour ending in difficult delivery aided by forceps was the presumed cause in these patients, who presented with a congested brain of uniformly red to purple appearance.

Another definite cause was illustrated by Larroche (1977) in describing widespread purpura of the cerebral cortex, subcortical white matter, thalamus and basal ganglia in infants with immune fetal hydrops. As the probable common denominator is severe venous congestion, it is not surprising to recognize such lesions in situations with agonal hypervolaemia such as that seen in the recipient twin in feto-fetal transfusion or in abruptio placentae.

Although Craig (1938) gave a detailed account of the torpid clinical evolution in his patients who were described as having a typical expression of fear, these observations date from an era of contemplative neonatal medicine. It is likely that those infants, in whom the contribution of birth asphyxia is not clearly delineated, would nowadays survive. As the haemorrhages are too small to be detected by ultrasound or CT scan, one will have to await reports using other brain scanning methods before describing the clinical findings typical of severe cerebral venous congestion in the absence of asphyxia.

Lobar parenchymal haemorrhage
As in the adult, on rare occasions a perinatal brain haemorrhage will lodge inside one cerebral lobe, as if it originated in its white matter. If the cortex above it is not affected these lesions are either primary haematomas or lacunar infarctions with secondary haemorrhagic transformation. In association with extensive (grade III)

intraventricular haemorrhage they can be periventricular venous infarctions. Their striking asymmetry suggests that local factors, such as trauma or vascular lesion, are generative. The absence of data on this event in the term newborn infant is so striking that a subdivision similar to the adult counterpart is worth making.

Frontal lobe haemorrhage

ANATOMICAL DESCRIPTION

Recent CT studies of living term neonates with seizures suggest the existence of a separate clinical entity associating unexplained unilateral frontal parenchymal haemorrhage with conspicuous extracerebral bleeding either between the lobe and the falx or in the sylvian fissure (Chaplin *et al.* 1979, Blanc *et al.* 1982, Bergman *et al.* 1985, Pierre-Kahn *et al.* 1985, Welch and Strand 1986, Hayashi *et al.* 1987). All case histories lack evidence of intraventricular haemorrhage. The associated extracerebral bleeding was either subdural or subarachnoid (Hayashi *et al.* 1987) in location.

INCIDENCE AND PATHOGENESIS

Though not reported in sufficient detail, two such haemorrhages were found in a recent prospective MRI study of 100 high-risk newborn infants (Keeney *et al.* 1991), and a further two were noted in 25 traumatic parturitional haemorrhages collected by Welch and Strand (1986).

Seven cases from the literature for whom sufficient clinical and descriptive details are given are summarized in Table 8.1. These case histories share the absence of a definite aetiology such as mechanical birth trauma (except possibly for case 1), birth asphyxia, or a disturbed clotting mechanism (except for case 3 where DIC was recorded, probably secondary to the initial bleeding and to intrauterine growth retardation).

Hayashi *et al.* (1987) put forward interfrontal bone displacement as the causal factor in cases 6 and 7, based on neurosurgical findings of parenchymal 'contusion'. Although this is an attractive hypothesis, against it are the excellent status of all infants at birth, the absence of moulding or calvarial damage worthy of note on postnatal clinical examination, and the non-existence of available evidence that this type of displacement can induce direct parenchymal destruction. Arterio-venous malformation and angioma have been excluded by angiography (Hayashi *et al.* 1987). Future investigation, either by MRI or at post-mortem examination, will have to focus on aetiology.

CLINICAL SETTING

As indicated in Table 8.1, one possible presentation is with contralateral focal clonic seizures and hemiparalysis (cases 1 and 2). If very large, the haemorrhage causes anaemia and a tense fontanelle. These two infants remained remarkably alert and able to feed normally in between the convulsions, and seizure control was reported to be easy (Chaplin *et al.* 1979). Lumbar CSF was haemorrhagic.

TABLE 8.1
Unilateral frontal intracerebral haemorrhage at term in seven infants*

	1	2	3	4	5	6	7
Sex	F	M	?	M	?	F	F
Birthweight (g)	3840	3400	1950	3950	3200	2750	3720
Gestational age (wks)	42	42	39	42	37	40	38
Mode of delivery							
Spontaneous vaginal				+		+	+
Forceps	+[1]	+					
Caesarean			+		+		
Apgar score @ 1 min.	8	8	5	10	8	9	9
@ 5 mins	9	9	9	10	9	9	10
Event–symptoms interval	36h	13h	?	<1d	<1d	2d	2d
Focal seizures	R	L	?	?	—	R	R
Hemiparesis	+	+	?	—	—	—	—
Intracranial hypertension	—	—	?	+	—	+	+
Side of bleeding	L	R	R	L	L	L	L
Associated extracerebral haematoma							
Interhemispheric	—	+	+	+	—	+	—
In sylvian fissure	—	—	—	—	+	—	+
Midline shift	—	+	—	+	—	+	+
Craniotomy	—	—	—	+	—	+	+
Apparently normal at 1 year	+	+	—	+	+	?	?

*Cases 1,2—Chaplin *et al.* (1979); case 3—Blanc *et al.* (1982): case 4—Pierre-Khan *et al.* (1985); case 5—Bergman *et al.* (1985); cases 6, 7—Hayashi *et al.* (1987).
[1]Prolonged labour.

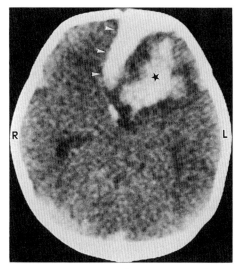

Fig. 8.5. Axial CT scan (Table 8.1, case 6): left frontal lobe haematoma *(asterisk)* accompanied by interhemispheric extracerebral bleeding *(arrowheads)*. (Hayashi *et al.* 1987, by permission.)

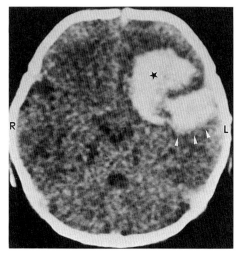

Fig. 8.6. Axial CT scan (Table 8.1, case 7): left frontal lobe haematoma *(asterisk)* accompanied by extracerebral bleeding in sylvian fissure *(arrowheads)*. (Hayashi *et al.* 1987, by permission.)

X-ray and ultrasound findings were not considered striking in the reports mentioned. On CT scan the lesion presents as an irregular density within the frontal white matter, sparing the cerebral cortex but sometimes surrounded by hypoperfused non-haemorrhagic white matter (Figs 8.5, 8.6). Sparing of a rim of cortex renders haemorrhagic infarction of the anterior cerebral artery an unlikely diagnosis. Frank haematoma within a large infarction could mimic these images (Inoue *et al*. 1980). As already explained, an extensive extracerebral haemorrhage is associated in most cases, either between the frontal lobe and the falx or within the sylvian fissure. Although impossible to be certain on CT scan alone, the location and surgical findings in cases 6 and 7 suggest a subarachnoid origin. In an infant not included in the table (because clinical details were insufficient) an appearance suggestive of an extracerebral haemorrhage between mesial frontal lobe and falx, either subarachnoid or pial, was the only finding on CT scan on the third day after severe birth asphyxia at term (Magilner and Wertheimer 1980): this infant presented with clonic seizures, aspiration pneumonia, bilateral retinal haemorrhages and evidence of DIC. The child's neurological status at the age of 11 months was considered normal. If sizeable, the combined lesion displaces the falx and shifts the midline. Angiography defines the normality of the main related vessels (Hayashi *et al*. 1987).

The presence of severe intracranial hypertension will indicate the need for surgical decompression (Pierre-Kahn *et al*. 1985, Hayashi *et al*. 1987). Despite the obvious sequela of a triangular brain defect, with its base facing the frontal bone, most children have been reported to recover completely without residual cerebral palsy. Post-haemorrhagic hydrocephalus has not been mentioned. The shape of the brain defect must not be mistaken for regional atrophy following arterial cerebral infarction.

Temporal lobe haemorrhage

A clear-cut example of this type of bleeding is depicted by Slovis *et al*. (1984). A term baby, birthweight 3402g, was delivered vaginally after prolonged labour. The Apgar scores, despite meconium staining of the liquor, were 8 at one and five minutes. The neonatal course was complicated by hypoglycaemia, hypocalcaemia and polycythaemia. Seizures prompted CNS investigations on day 4: CT scan appearances suggested haemorrhage involving the entire right temporal lobe. Ten days later the lobe had become cystic. Hyperviscosity—the mother had diabetes mellitus—was the mechanism proposed by the authors.

Though similar in appearance on CT scan, an infant described by Fouché *et al*. (1982) probably suffered from left subarachnoid haematoma and not lobar parenchymal haemorrhage, as the clinical context was one of DIC with congenital toxoplasmosis. Post-mortem details were not recorded.

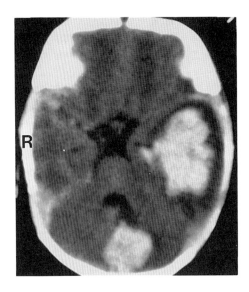

Fig. 8.7. Axial CT scan on day 6 in Case 8.1, showing large left temporal haemorrhage surrounded by hypodense parenchyma, and similar lesion in left cerebellar hemisphere near midline.

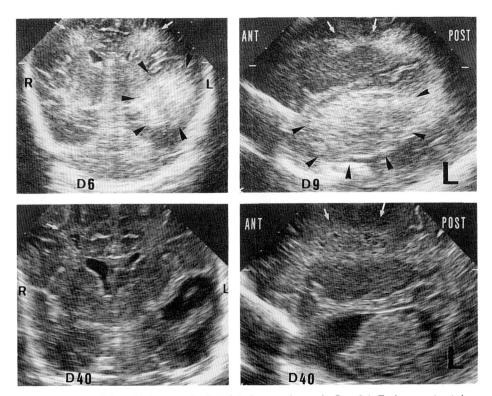

Fig. 8.8. Coronal *(left)* and left parasagittal *(right)* ultrasound scans in Case 8.1. Early scans *(top)* show hyperdensity within left temporal lobe *(arrowheads)* and periventricular white matter *(arrows)*. On late scans *(bottom)* cystic changes are visible in both areas of injury.

110

In an article on primary cerebral bleeding at term, Bergman *et al.* (1985) reported a macrosomic neonate without birth asphyxia who presented at two hours with apnoea, tonic seizures and a left VIth nerve palsy; CT scan, not shown in the paper, was said to document left temporal cerebral haemorrhage.

Baumann *et al.* (1987) described left temporal lobe haematoma in a thrombocytopenic newborn infant with subsequent contralateral hemiparesis and hemianopia. They considered partial infarction of the area perfused by the middle cerebral artery to be the primary event.

CASE 8.1
This firstborn infant was shown by ultrasound to be behind in growth from about the 29th week of gestation onwards. Oligohydramnios was added to this finding later on. Delivery was normal at 37 weeks of gestation (first stage two hours, second stage 10 minutes), though the liquor was meconium stained. Her birthweight was 2100g; Apgar scores were 4 and 8 at one and five minutes. She presented with minimal respiratory distress and hypoglycaemia. Her platelet count fell to 22×10^9/L on day 3, when her gastric residue became bloodstained. Feto-maternal incompatibility for platelet surface antigen HPA1 was subsequently shown without demonstration of specific platelet antibodies. The platelet count started to rise following intravenous immunoglobulin treatment, the first normal count being achieved on day 9. On day 6 she was referred with generalized oedema, a tense fontanelle, irritability and a paretic right arm. There were no petechiae or bruises. The initial coagulation screen suggested DIC. CT scan findings (Fig. 8.7), in addition to suggesting a large left temporal lobe haematoma, were also compatible with haemorrhage into the parenchyma of the right occipital lobe and into the left cerebellar hemisphere. The evolution of the brain lesions on ultrasound is shown in Figure 8.8: parietal cystic periventricular leukomalacia developed together with cavitary changes in preceding haematomas. An acute cholestatic episode on day 21 finally led to surgical exploration of the abdomen the following week, after exclusion of hilar angioma on aortography. The proximal bile ducts were obviously dilated because of a hilar scarring process around the main duct; histological examination excluded malignancy and confirmed the surgeon's diagnosis of previous haemorrhage by showing fibrous tissue with siderophages. At 2 years of age this child has spastic diplegia, squints and has horizontal nystagmus. The final neurological diagnosis was: multiple parenchymal haemorrhages in a growth retarded infant with thrombocytopenia of uncertain cause. Investigations for congenital infection had proved negative. The temporal and cerebellar location of haematomas, together with the presence of additional (cystic) parietal leukomalacia, militate against a diagnosis of ischaemic white matter disease as a primary event.

Lobar temporal haematoma due to venous ischaemia, haemorrhagic diathesis or other causes has to be differentiated from subarachnoid haematoma and basal subdural haemorrhage with underlying cerebral contusion or arterial infarction (see Chapter 6). The outcome of infants with cystic necrosis of one temporal lobe is not well described.

Parietal lobe haemorrhage
A search for clear-cut primary parietal bleeding, appearing as a rounded mass on scans and without the cortical involvement and anatomical distribution of arterial infarction, has not been very rewarding.

Fenichel *et al.* (1984) reported two male infants, both born normally, one at and one post-term. One presented with apnoea and multifocal seizures at 24 hours, the other with focal facial twitching on day 7. The corresponding scans were described but not shown. Both infants ended up with cerebral palsy and mental retardation.

Bergman *et al.* (1985) described a macrosomic neonate, birthweight 5000g, with bilateral intraventricular and right parieto-temporal cerebral haemorrhage at the end of the first month of life. This infant of a mother with gestational diabetes mellitus presented with diarrhoea, fever and seizures on day 27. As her haemoglobin level was 18g/dL the suggested cause of this event was hyperviscosity with deep venous thrombosis, but this was impossible to confirm as no imaging studies were available. A case history, documented by Cartwright *et al.* (1979) concerned a term male infant with seizures, pallor and intracranial hypertension on the second day after difficult rotational forceps delivery. His birthweight was 3120g; Apgar scores were 8 and 9 at one and five minutes. His CSF was uniformly blood-stained. CT scan indicated a right posterior parietal haematoma with midline shift. He developed contralateral hemiparesis.

CASE 8.2
This second-born child presented with fetal distress, heralded by meconium staining of the liquor and loss of beat-to-beat variation on cardiotocogram for 30 minutes before delivery. He was born normally, at term, after a short second stage. His Apgar score was 3 at one and three minutes; birthweight was 2100g. Before referral he became hypothermic (34°C) and hypoglycaemic. His respiratory difficulties were thought to result from meconium inhalation and persistent pulmonary hypertension, with an additional left pneumothorax. Haemoglobin on the first day was 14g/dL. The platelet count fell to 61×10^9/L on day 6. CT scans are shown in Figure 8.9. Association of the parietal bleeding with a major intraventricular haemorrhage suggested an anatomical diagnosis of periventricular venous haemorrhagic infarction. The sparing of adjacent cortex was striking and excluded complete arterial stroke. An ipsilateral vitreal haemorrhage accompanied the cerebral lesion. The child developed post-haemorrhagic hydrocephalus but escaped shunting after stabilization with serial lumbar punctures and diuretics. At seven months he was generally developmentally retarded, with global hypotonia rather than spasticity.

These few observations show the need for further study into the nature of lobar parietal or occipital haematoma. Differentiation must be made if possible between primary white matter damage, venous infarction associated with ventricular bleeding, arterial stroke and contusion.

Capsular haemorrhage
Limited nodular parenchymal haemorrhage within the internal capsule has been reported in at least one term infant presenting with tonic seizures on the second day of life following normal delivery without birth asphyxia (Fenichel *et al.* 1984). Attenuation was recorded on ipsilateral EEG tracings. Contralateral hemiplegia was later evident.

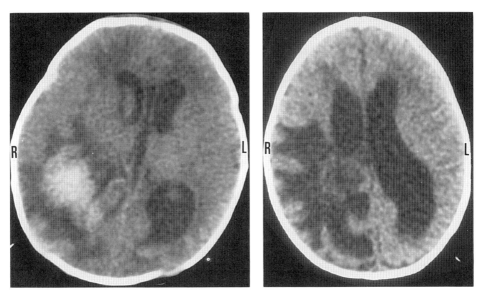

Fig. 8.9. Axial CT scans on days 12 *(left)* and 60 *(right)* in Case 8.2: early lesion is a mainly parietal haemorrhage related to left ventricle trigone and surrounding white matter, together with ipsilateral grade III intraventricular haemorrhage. On follow-up there is clear hypodensity of white matter, sparing adjacent cortex.

Case history

CASE 8.3

This boy was born normally at 37 weeks gestation. The cord was tight around his neck, and he looked pale. Apgar scores were 5 and 7 at one and five minutes; umbilical artery pH was 7.1; birthweight 2800g. At 1 hour the P_aco_2 was normal, pH was 7.17 and base deficit 14mmol/L. Short-lived respiratory distress was observed, thought to be due to initial pulmonary hypertension. A Kleihauer test on day 3 was negative, and the haemoglobin dropped to 10g/dL. A platelet count on day 6 was 51×10^9/L. On day 7 a septic screen was performed after routine testing showed raised serum C-reactive protein: this proved negative, but he was given antimicrobial therapy. On day 8 clonic movements of all four limbs were noted. Examination of the CSF excluded meningitis. Echographic scans and MRI on day 18 were compatible with a well-delineated small left capsular haemorrhage (Figs 8.10, 8.11). The cause was felt to be either a limited deep venous thrombosis possibly associated with incipient but promptly treated infection, or a haemorrhagic embolic infarct. Follow-up at 4 months showed no evidence of contralateral hemiplegia.

These isolated reports do not clarify the basic mechanisms of capsular haemorrhage. Limited infarction (or haemorrhage) of the internal capsule in older children has been shown to cause isolated motor cerebral palsy (Okuno *et al*. 1980). Even with current techniques, differentiating between lacunar and striatocapsular lesions, as in the adult, is still not routinely done in the newborn infant (Bladin and Berkovic 1984). During neonatal ECMO (extracorporeal membrane oxygenation),

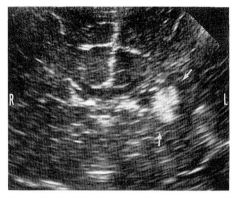

Fig. 8.10. Detail of coronal ultrasound scan of Case 8.3 on day 18, showing nodular density *(arrows)* within anterior limb of left internal capsule between head of caudate and putamen.

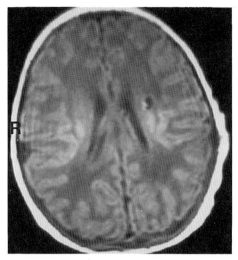

Fig. 8.11. Axial T1-weighted MRI in Case 8.3 on day 18: note hypointense nodular lesion with isodense mesial margin (suggestive of subacute haemorrhage because of central hyperintensity on T2-weighted image).

bilateral multifocal small haemorrhages, similar to the one described in Case 8.3 are not uncommon findings.

Haemorrhagic white matter necrosis
Anatomical description
The evolution and natural history of leukomalacia are presented in Figure 8.12.

Necrotic white matter can be haemorrhagic because of the venous nature of the infarct (Pape and Wigglesworth 1979, Takashima *et al.* 1986, Gould *et al.* 1987, Haddad *et al.* 1992). This variant of haemorrhagic leukomalacia ought to be exceptional at term, as its mechanism is compression of medullary veins by a large germinal matrix bleeding. Areas of ischaemia can also suffer from secondary haemorrhagic conversion. The latter can be triggered by clotting failure (Armstrong and Norman 1974). In term infants white matter injury is usually part of a lesional complex affecting cerebral (sub)cortex (Leech and Alvord 1974, Larroche 1977, De Vries *et al.* 1988*b*, Dambska *et al.* 1989), basal ganglia (Armstrong and Norman 1974, Rushton *et al.* 1985, Armstrong *et al.* 1987, De Vries *et al.* 1988*b*) and/or brainstem structures. Total ischaemia, with loss of glia and neuropil (De Girolami *et al.* 1984), results in colliquative necrosis extending into the gyral white matter core (Dambska *et al.* 1989). The pathologically well-defined entities of linear leukomalacia (Leech and Alvord 1974, Rodriguez *et al.* 1990) and telencephalic leuko-encephalopathy (Gilles and Murphy 1969) are still obscure from the clinical point of view.

114

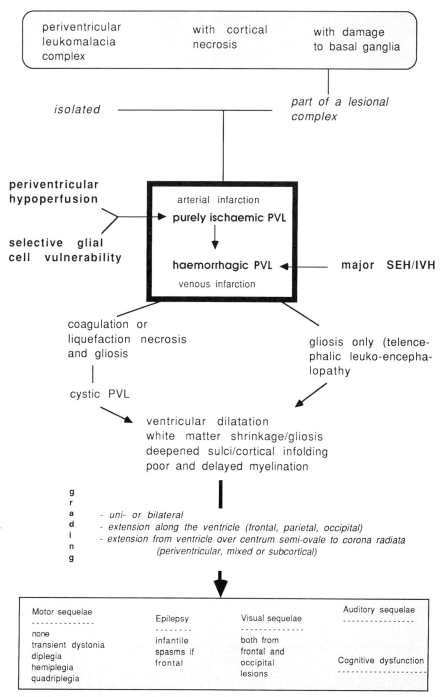

Fig. 8.12. The evolution and natural history of periventricular leukomalacia (PVL). (SEH = subependymal haemorrhage, IVH = intraventricular haemorrhage.)

Pathogenesis
Reviewing the literature describing pathological findings reveals that about one fifth of leukomalacias, irrespective of gestational age, are haemorrhagic. At term, leukomalacia has been recorded in infants with intrauterine growth retardation, sepsis and/or meningitis, congenital heart disease, respiratory difficulties and hypoglycaemia (Larroche 1977). The common denominator seems to be hypotension (Pape and Wigglesworth 1979, Ment *et al.* 1985, Kopelman 1990). This could explain alleged associations with early onset group B streptococcal bacteraemia (Faix and Donn 1985, Colan 1986, Takashima *et al.* 1987) or hypoplastic left heart syndrome (Armstrong and Norman 1974, Glauser *et al.* 1990).

The arterial border zone hypothesis (De Reuck *et al.* 1972, Takashima and Tanaka 1978), still the most attractive pathogenetic mechanism, has been challenged and expanded by documentation of vessel immaturity (Kuban and Gilles 1985), pressure passivity of cerebral circulation during hypotension (Volpe 1990) and specific vulnerability of glial cells to circulating endotoxins (Gilles *et al.* 1977, Ando *et al.* 1988).

Radiological assessment and relation to prognosis
Sonographic detection of intraparenchymal echodensities should raise suspicion about underlying leukomalacia. Symmetrical soft and radiating densities in frontal and occipito-parietal regions can be normal features up to two months post term (peritrigonal blush) (Laub and Ingrisch 1986, Hope *et al.* 1988). Pathological densities are more irregular and often asymmetrical or unilateral. Though most examiners will suspect a density to be pathological because of its abnormal brightness, comparison with the echodense aspect of the choroid plexus can be tricky (Carson *et al.* 1990).

Histopathological correlates can be: (i) coagulation necrosis (Dolfin *et al.* 1984, Nwaesi *et al.* 1984); (ii) spongiosis with gliosis and microcalcification (Trounce *et al.* 1985); (iii) haemorrhagic leukomalacia (Fig. 8.13) (McMenamin *et al.* 1984, Rushton *et al.* 1985, Trounce *et al.* 1986, De Vries *et al.* 1988*b*, Schellinger *et al.* 1988); (iv) necrosis as part of an arterial infarct; or (v) simple venous congestion (Trounce *et al.* 1986). In the rare event of a perinatal leukodystrophy, white matter hyperechogenicities persist for weeks without cavitation or ventricular dilatation. Within dystrophic areas, focal hyperdensities may indicate calcification.

Prolongation of these flares or echodensities beyond the first couple of weeks is considered abnormal. Even in the absence of an intermediate cystic stage, they can precede definite motor impairment (Appleton *et al.* 1990). The cystic intermediate (Fig. 8.14) is an absolute indicator of subsequent cerebral palsy, the degree correlating with the anatomical grading of damage (Guzzetta *et al.* 1986, Trounce *et al.* 1986, De Vries 1987, Monset-Couchard *et al.* 1988, Zorzi *et al.* 1988). Disappearance of flares without residual ventriculomegaly indicates intact survival of the involved white matter (Stewart *et al.* 1987).

CT scanning has a place in the differentiation between purely ischaemic and

116

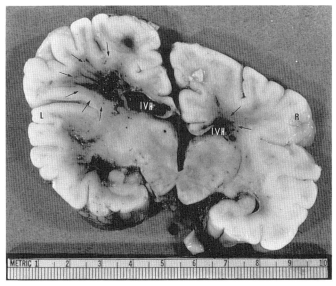

Fig. 8.13. Post-mortem appearance of brain of term infant with seizures, bacteraemia and diffuse intravascular coagulation who died on day 4: note symmetrical haemorrhagic periventricular white matter damage *(arrows)*, most marked on left, and associated intraventricular bleeding (IVH). (Armstrong and Norman 1974, by permission.)

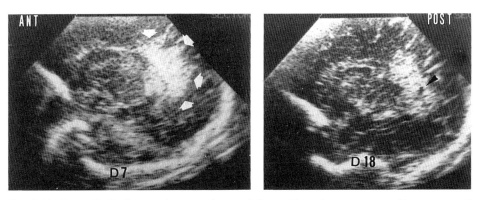

Fig. 8.14. Parasagittal ultrasound scans of term infant with early onset group B streptococcal bacteraemia, hypotension and persistent fetal circulation, showing hyperdense periventricular white matter in left trigonal area on day 7 *(arrows)*, and early cystic changes on day 18 *(arrowhead)*. (Faix and Donn 1985, by permission.)

haemorrhagic white matter damage within the neonatal period (Fig. 8.15). MRI has already been shown to be superior in the definition of the later stages of white matter damage (Dubowitz *et al.* 1985, Keeney *et al.* 1991).

Fast magnetic imaging as well as objective measurement of echodensity will provide easy estimation of the intensity of leukomalacia in the near future.

117

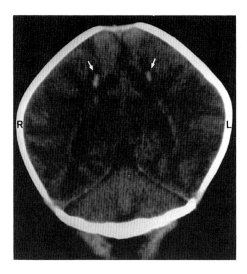

Fig. 8.15. Post-mortem coronal CT scan on day 50 in infant who died as a consequence of pituitary agenesis: *arrows* indicate symmetrical haemor- rhagic periventricular leukomalacia.

Haemorrhagic arterial cerebral infarction
Anatomical description and natural course
Extravasation of erythrocytes into a cerebral arterial infarct to the extent that it produces macroscopically visible bleeding, would qualify the infarction as haemorrhagic. In the series of reports referred to below, one term neonatal cerebral stroke in five appears to be affected by this phenomenon. Borderzone (watershed) and lacunar infarcts are not discussed because of an intriguing lack of documentation in this age group. For similar reasons I will not expand on cerebellar infarctions, which have not so far, to my knowledge, been described in the living newborn infant (Fischer *et al.* 1972, Aoki *et al.* 1986, Rosman *et al.* 1992).

Although extrapolation is not entirely justified, some patterns of evolution emerge from a wealth of adult human and experimental data (Laurent *et al.* 1976, Inoue *et al.* 1980, De Girolami *et al.* 1984, Saku *et al.* 1990, Macfarlane *et al.* 1991, Garcia 1992). One should however not take for granted the existence in the newborn infant of the proposed sequence: ischaemia → reactive hyperaemia → no reflow → luxury perfusion.

The evolutionary staging of an infarct from CT and histological findings is summarized in Table 8.2 (for a review, see Raybaud *et al.* 1985). Cytotoxic oedema increases the water content from 30 minutes to a few hours after the onset of arterial occlusion. From about six hours to six days vasogenic oedema and coagulation necrosis supervene. The basis for this event is thought to be reperfusion of a pressure-passive vascular bed through the recanalized artery or via existing anastomoses. Disruption of the endothelial blood–brain barrier has been documented, although the involved region is not enhanced by contrast. By 24 hours post-insult most arterial infarcts in the term newborn brain are detectable because

118

TABLE 8.2

Stages in the evolution of an arterial cerebral infarct

Timing	Pathology	Uncontrasted CT scan	Contrast enhancement	Mass effect
30 mins–hrs	Cytotoxic oedema	Normal or early reactive hyperaemia	—	—
6 hrs–6 days	Vasogenic oedema	Hypodense grey and white matter or haemorrhagic due to reactive hyperaemia	—	+
3 days–4 wks	Organization, breakdown	Differential hypodensity (white > grey matter), delayed hyperaemia due to neovascularization	+	—
>4 wks	Residual atrophy	Cortico-subcortical triangular defect	—	—

of obvious hypodensity on uncontrasted CT scan (Fujimoto *et al.* 1992). A mass effect is encountered in a minority (three out of 15 instances studied by Fujimoto *et al.*). Throughout the late neonatal period the infarct will then organize, involving gliosis, breakdown of myelin, microcyst formation and neovascularization. Vascular reaction is most marked in, but not confined to, grey matter. Petechial haemorrhages, appearing from three to six days post-insult in the cortex and basal ganglia, are found in 90 per cent of all infarcts at nine to 14 days. On CT, gyriform brightness of the cortex can be a transient marker of these changes (Close and Carty 1991). Contrast will mainly enhance grey matter, whereas white matter will remain relatively hypodense. If curvilinear haemorrhages are clearly visible on uncontrasted scans, the infarct is termed 'haemorrhagic'. Neovascularization is not a prerequisite for haemorrhagic conversion. Within hours of infarction early cortical haemorrhage can be caused by a rise in systemic tension opening leptomeningeal anastomotic vessels. In adults migration of the embolus renders most embolic strokes haemorrhagic within hours to a few days (Olsen and Lassen 1984, Okada *et al.* 1989). Ongoing partial perfusion of the penumbra is an alternative mode of haemorrhagic necrosis. Post-infarct hyperperfusion has been recently reviewed by Macfarlane *et al.* (1991). Variables to be considered are the control of flow to healthy surrounding tissue, systemic blood pressure, seizure activity, arterial O_2 and CO_2 levels, haemoglobin level and affinity for oxygen, as well as drug effects (Jones *et al.* 1988, Del Toro *et al.* 1991, Pryds 1991). Frank haematoma in an infarct presents as a high density mass in the central white matter of the ischaemic territory. Experimental work suggests that it is merely an exaggerated form of haemorrhagic infarction, to be differentiated from a venous infarct. Haemorrhagic diathesis might promote both haemorrhagic conversion and haematoma formation.

From the second month onwards complete infarction of a major arterial region will leave a cortico-subcortical triangular void area of tissue loss, based against the skull bone. Infarctions close to the site of occlusion or centrally in the arterial territory may spare cortical grey matter.

Incidence

Barmada *et al.* (1979) calculated a prevalence rate for arterial infarctions of 17 per cent among autopsied term neonates. Ment *et al.* (1984) isolated 10 term infants with arterial cerebral ischaemia, of prenatal origin in two, from a population of 882 admissions of any gestational age. Clancy *et al.* (1985) described seizure activity in 11 term infants observed during a two-year period in three affiliated intensive care nurseries. In a cohort of 50 term neonates with seizures, Levy *et al.* (1985) found seven instances of arterial cerebral stroke. Nine of 19 term infants with persistent fetal circulation studied by Klesh *et al.* (1987) were affected by arterial stroke. Taylor *et al.* (1989) reported four haemorrhagic infarcts in a series of 17 neonatal deaths following ECMO.

In a well-defined Swedish region around Göteborg, 0.44 children per 1000 aged between 6 and 15 years were born at term and later fulfilled the criteria for a diagnosis of congenital hemiplegia (Uvebrant 1988); as 20 per cent of their CT scans revealed cortico-subcortical cavitation, one can cautiously estimate the incidence of arterial cerebral stroke in term neonates to be around one in 10,000 children, including cases of possible prenatal origin.

Aetiology

A total of 81 term newborn infants with sufficient published detail of their histories and in whom differentiation between plain ischaemic and haemorrhagic stroke could be made were collated from the literature (Gross 1945; Barmada *et al.* 1979; Billard *et al.* 1982; Hill *et al.* 1983; Mannino and Trauner 1983; Mantovani and Gerber 1984; Ment *et al.* 1984, 1987; Clancy *et al.* 1985; Levy *et al.* 1985; Klesh *et al.* 1987; Roodhooft *et al.* 1987; Hernanz-Schulman *et al.* 1988; Raine *et al.* 1989; Taylor *et al.* 1989; Fujimoto *et al.* 1992). Clinical details of these 81 cases are given in Table 8.3, while the arteries involved are shown in Figure 8.16. Except for ECMO and haemorrhagic diathesis there are currently no events known with a predisposition to haemorrhagic conversion. This conversion was recorded in 14 of the 79 infants with middle cerebral artery infarctions (18 per cent), and in two of the 19 infants in the anterior plus posterior group. Whether or not the extent of tissue damage plays a role in the phenomenon is not known. The comparatively greater frequency of left middle cerebral artery infarction is striking. Hypothetical explanations are preferential direction of emboli and proximity of the open ductus arteriosus and its flow changes near the left carotid and vertebral arteries (Mannino and Trauner 1984).

The recognized causes of neonatal cerebral stroke are gathered in Table 8.4 (reviews by Pavlakis *et al.* 1991, Allan and Riviello 1992). The most likely

TABLE 8.3
**Neonatal arterial cerebral infarction: review of 81
reported cases***

	Ischaemic (N=66)	Haemorrhagic (N=15)
Birthweight >4000g	9	2
Event–diagnosis interval		
Range (days)	1–90	1–30
1–3 days	34	9
4–7 days	10	3
≥8 days	12	3
Birth asphyxia	22	3
Birth trauma	8	0
Haemorrhagic diathesis	0	3[1]
Bacteraemia/meningitis	3	0
Hypertension	2	0
Polycythaemia	3	1
Embolism/PPHN[2]	3/6	4/0

*See text for references.
[1]Three ECMO-treated infants.
[2]Evidence of embolism in other organs, on angiography or
at necropsy; PPHN (persistent pulmonary hypertension of
the newborn) is included in this group because of the
presence of direct connection from venous return to brain
arteries.

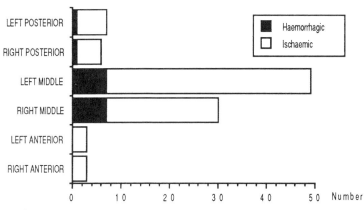

Fig. 8.16. Arteries involved in 81 term infants with cerebral stroke. (See text for source references.)

intermediate stage between hyperviscosity and brain damage is venous thrombosis.
Iatrogenic stroke was documented in an infant with thrombosis around the tip of an
umbilical venous catheter (Ruff *et al.* 1979) and in others where flushing of a
partially occluded temporal artery catheter led to ipsilateral middle cerebral artery
infarction (Prian *et al.* 1978, Simmons *et al.* 1978). Embolic haemorrhagic infarction

TABLE 8.4
Aetiology of neonatal arterial stroke

1. Embolism
   —from the ductus arteriosus (Gross 1945, Knowlson and Marsden 1978)
   —from the heart (Terplan 1973)
   —through the heart
     ■ from the placenta (Ment *et al*. 1984, Chandra *et al*. 1990)
     ■ from systemic veins (Ruff *et al*. 1979)
   —during ECMO (Taylor *et al*. 1989)
   —from a temporal artery catheter (Prian *et al*. 1978, Simmons *et al*. 1978)

2. Vasculitis (meningitis)
   —bacterial (Headings and Glasgow 1977, Snyder *et al*. 1981, Taft *et al*. 1986, Ben-Ami *et al*. 1990)
   —viral (Roden *et al*. 1975)

3. Bacteraemia and intravascular coagulation (Barmada *et al*. 1979, Hill *et al*. 1983)

4. Polycythaemia (Amit and Camfield 1980, Miller *et al*. 1981)

5. Birth asphyxia (Cocker *et al*. 1965, Barmada *et al*. 1979, Magilner and Wertheimer 1980, Babcock and Ball 1983, Hill *et al*. 1983, Martin *et al*. 1983, Voorhies *et al*. 1984, Clancy *et al*. 1985, Levy *et al*. 1985, Sran and Baumann 1988)

6. Postnatal asphyxia (Clancy *et al*. 1985)

7. Birth trauma (see Chapter 3)

8. Hypertension (Hill *et al*. 1983, Clancy *et al*. 1985)

9. Severe respiratory distress (Mannino and Trauner 1983, Klesh *et al*. 1987)

10. Maternal cocaine abuse (Chasnoff *et al*. 1986)

of the right frontal lobe has been associated with dilatation and thrombosis of a persistent ductus arteriosus (Gross 1945). Its occurrence against a background of birth asphyxia is well documented (Cocker *et al*. 1965, Magilner *et al*. 1980, Babcock and Ball 1983, Martin *et al*. 1983, Voorhies *et al*. 1984).

Elusiveness of a clear-cut aetiology has been emphasized by several authors (Mantovani and Gerber 1984, Levy *et al*. 1985, Roodhooft *et al*. 1987, Raine *et al*. 1989).

Clinical setting
Arterial stroke classically presents with contralateral seizures (Mannino and Trauner 1984, Mantovani and Gerber 1984, Clancy *et al*. 1985, Fujimoto *et al*. 1992). Where there is associated generalized ischaemic brain damage, these specific alarm signals may be lacking (Aso *et al*. 1990). Amidst various necropsy confirmed types of anoxic–ischaemic brain injury, stroke does seem to correlate best with electrical seizures (Aso *et al*. 1990). Middle (complete or partial) and posterior cerebral artery involvement has been found in infants with seizures on one side of the body, whereas anterior cerebral artery occlusion can present with arm and face

twitching (Billard *et al.* 1982). Twitching of a leg was mentioned in an infant with anterior middle cerebral artery stroke (Billard *et al.* 1982). Generalized seizures from the onset have also been reported (Levy *et al.* 1985, Roodhooft *et al.* 1987). EEG-confirmed clinical seizures carry more weight in predicting residual epilepsy (Allan and Riviello 1992). Most authors have reported no difficulty in controlling the fits (Fujimoto *et al.* 1992), a feature ascribed to their cortical origin (Camfield and Camfield 1987). Subtle seizures reported in middle cerebral artery infarction, rarely as an isolated phenomenon, include: blinking of the eyes, staring, eye fluttering, vertical nystagmus, hiccups, chewing, sucking, and thumb adduction (Mantovani and Gerber 1984, Levy *et al.* 1985, Klesh *et al.* 1987, Raine *et al.* 1989). Other authors have referred to apnoeic spells or cyanotic attacks (Miller *et al.* 1981, Hill *et al.* 1983, Mantovani and Gerber 1984, Raine *et al.* 1989, Fujimoto *et al.* 1992). Between fits most children seemed to be alert and could be fed normally. Others were lethargic and did not suck well (Levy *et al.* 1985, Roodhooft *et al.* 1987).

One term infant presented with temperature instability (Roodhooft *et al.* 1987), another died unexpectedly, late in the neonatal period (Gross 1945). A few authors have reported concomitant acute pallor and loss of pulse in a limb due to arterial embolism or spasm (Asindi *et al.* 1988, Raine *et al.* 1989, Gudinchet *et al.* 1991).

Radiological assessment
Radionuclide brain scanning at about one week after the acute event used to be the, relatively reliable, method for differentiating between normal brain, diffuse encephalopathy and focal infarction. In a series of 85 asphyxiated term neonates, 68 presenting with fits, eight had the 'middle cerebral artery' pattern of isotope uptake (O'Brien *et al.* 1979, Mantovani and Gerber 1984).

Ultrasound has now become the initial detection method (Hill *et al.* 1983, Mannino and Trauner 1984, Fischer *et al.* 1988, Hernanz-Schulman *et al.* 1988). Due to coagulation necrosis, irregular hyperdensity is present throughout the affected area after 24 hours. Vessel pulsations are absent within, and may be increased around, the infarct. Effacement of sulci explains the lack of gyral definition. A dense head of caudate may be striking within the first 24 hours (Fischer *et al.* 1988). There is no objective proof of an increase in echodensity following haemorrhagic conversion.

Demonstrative CT pictures are presented in the Hammersmith atlas of acquired perinatal brain damage (De Vries *et al.* 1990). Figure 8.17 shows a typical haemorrhagic and an ischaemic infarct in the same patient (Roodhooft *et al.* 1987). Frank haematoma into an infarct was suspected in a patient reported by Klesh *et al.* (1987) (Fig. 8.18). Calcified remnants can be found on follow-up (Gudinchet *et al.* 1991, Fujimoto *et al.* 1992).

MRI imaging may greatly improve our knowledge of the exact anatomical description and natural course of these lesions (Baumann *et al.* 1987).

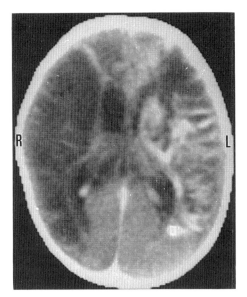 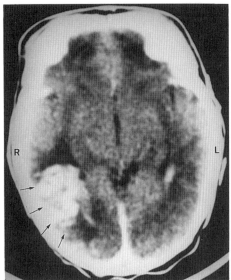

Fig. 8.17. Axial CT scan with contrast enhancement on day 7 in term infant with unexplained bilateral complete middle cerebral artery infarction: right side is purely ischaemic, whereas on left gyriform contrast enhancement is seen (together with haemorrhagic conversion on uncontrasted CT scan). (Roodhoft *et al.* 1987, by permission.)

Fig. 8.18. Axial CT scan on day 6 in macrosomic post-term infant with fetal distress, birth asphyxia and seizures: note large haemorrhagic density involving white and cortical grey matter *(arrows)* in posterior perfusion area of right middle cerebral artery, compatible with haematoma into an infarct. (Klesh *et al.* 1987, by permission.)

For ready interpretation the main arterial regions are depicted in Figure 8.19. Smaller lacunar and capsular ('super' or 'giant' lacunar) infarctions have been well defined in older children (Brückmann *et al.* 1989, Kappelle *et al.* 1989) and adults (Bogousslavsky 1992). They comprise capsulo-putamino-caudate (lateral lenticulo-striate branches of the middle cerebral artery), capsulo-pallidal (perforating branches of the anterior choroidal artery) and capsulo-caudate (medial lenticulo-striate branches from the anterior cerebral artery or Heubner's artery) infarction. The haemorrhagic infarct reported by Levene (1988) in an asphyxiated term infant could be of the capsulo-pallidal variety.

Management
Aetiological treatment is mandatory. At present systemic heparinization and vasodilator therapy find only anecdotal support (Raine *et al.* 1989). Thrombolysis and anti-thrombotic drugs are expected to increase the risk of haemorrhagic conversion. The benefit (better perfusion of penumbral areas with a chance of recovery) or disadvantage (additional necrosis and a bigger mass effect) of such treatment is still unclear, even in the adult (Garcia 1992).

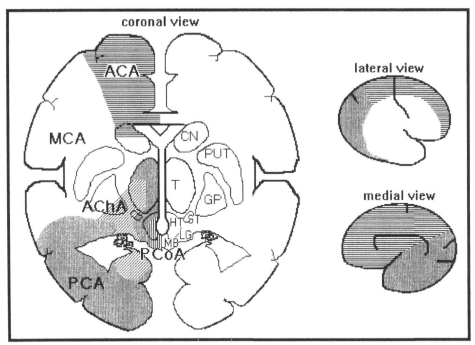

Fig. 8.19. Regional arterial perfusion of the brain summarized in a coronal section (ACA = anterior cerebral artery; MCA = middle cerebral artery; PCA = posterior cerebral artery; PCoA = posterior communicating artery; AChA = anterior choroidal artery; CN = caudate nucleus; PUT = putamen; GP = globus pallidus; THAL = thalamus; HT = hypothalamus; ST = subthalamic nucleus; MB = mammillary bodies; LG = lateral geniculate). *Inset:* lateral and mesial cerebral surfaces.

Prognosis

Table 8.5 presents data from a series of reports on neonatal stroke with absence of birth asphyxia, clear delineation of the artery involved, and evidence of cortico-subcortical tissue loss on follow-up of at least six months (Miller *et al*. 1981, Billard *et al*. 1982, Mantovani and Gerber 1984, Ment *et al*. 1984, Clancy *et al*. 1985, Levy *et al*. 1985, Trauner and Mannino 1986, Roodhooft *et al*. 1987, Sran and Baumann 1988, Raine *et al*. 1989, De Vries *et al*. 1990, Fujimoto *et al*. 1992).

Apparently normal neurological outcome has been reported repeatedly: this may be because of underperfusion of an area rather than necrosis or ischaemia, only partial involvement of an arterial territory, or plasticity of remaining healthy tissue (Varga-Khadem *et al*. 1985, Fujimoto *et al*. 1992). Personal observation suggests that normal development is compatible with the presence of hyperecho-genicity in an arterial region, shown to the hyperdense on CT scan.

The extent of infarction does influence the outcome. Complete infarction within the region of the middle cerebral artery invariably causes contralateral hemiplegia. This can be partial following infarction of the anterior cerebral artery

TABLE 8.5

Outcome in 16 term neonates with arterial cerebral infarction*

Artery	N	Neonatal seizures	Residual epilepsy	Spastic hemiplegia	Cognitive dysfunction
Anterior	2	2	0	2[1]	1
Posterior	3	2	0[2]	0	0
Middle					
Anterior	5	4	1	1	3[3]
Posterior	2	2	0	0	0
Complete	4	4	0	4	?

*See text for source references.
[1]One with complete hemisyndrome, one with spastic leg only.
[2]There is evidence that temporal lobe epilepsy and homonymous hemi-anopia can follow perinatal infarct within the region of this artery (see Chapter 6).
[3]Mental dysfunction was mild.

and discrete or absent following partial infarction of the middle cerebral artery.

Middle cerebral artery infarction is not a prerequisite for lesions of the cortico-spinal tract: fibres of this tract can be affected within the territory of the anterior cerebral artery at cortical level, of the posterior cerebral artery at peduncular level, and of the anterior choroidal artery as it irrigates the internal capsule (Fujimoto *et al.* 1992). Children with congenital hemiplegia and cortico-subcortical cavitation (as opposed to those with normal scans or unilateral ventriculomegaly) usually have more severe hemiplegia (Kotlarek *et al.* 1981, Molteni *et al.* 1987). Involvement of the upper limb, with prounounced astereognosis, is quite typical (Molteni *et al.* 1987, Uvebrant 1988).

Language deficits, even if only subtle, are invariably detected in the case of middle cerebral artery infarction (Varga-Khadem *et al.* 1985).

Residual epilepsy is documented in around 60 per cent of cases (Kotlarek *et al.* 1981, Uvebrant 1988). Temporal lobe epilepsy can be a sequel of infarction within the territory of the posterior cerebral artery (Remillard *et al.* 1974).

Mild mental impairment (IQ 75–90) affects about half of the infants.

Intraventricular haemorrhage (IVH)
Anatomical description
Bleeding into the supratentorial ventricle is not exceptional in term neonates. For practical reasons, in the following section this group of disease entities will be subdivided according to their presentation on brain imaging pictures (Table 8.6). Fourth ventricle bleeding is discussed together with parenchymal cerebellar haemorrhage.

Incidence
Isolated subependymal haemorrhage in the caudo-thalamic groove is surprisingly

TABLE 8.6

Types of intraventricular haemorrhage (IVH) at term

1. *Pure* IVH

2. IVH *associated with subdural/subarachnoid haematoma:* may be due to birth trauma, to haemorrhagic diathesis or to rupture of an intraventricular clot through the occipito-temporal cerebral substance with secondary basal subdural haematoma formation and a relatively small residual ventricular coagulum

3. IVH *associated with primary thalamic or thalamo-ventricular haemorrhage,* the most likely cause of which is deep venous thrombosis

4. *Primary cerebral* IVH with secondary intraventricular bleeding

5. Ventricular flooding in the case of *vascular brain malformation or tumour*

TABLE 8.7

Intraventricular haemorrhage at term (UZ Gent 1980–91)

	Trauma*	Isolated asphyxia	Haemorrh. diathesis	Bacteraemia +meningitis	Other	Total
Pure IVH	1	2	1[1]	1	5	9
IVH+ subdural haem.	3	0	0	0	0	3
IVH+ thalamic haem.	1	0	0	1	0	2
IVH+ cerebral haem.	1	1	0	1	1	4
Total	6	3	1	2	6	18

*Two spontaneous vaginal deliveries, one breech, three instrumental; four also had birth asphyxia.
[1]Likely cause was maternal salicylate ingestion.

frequent in healthy term infants: an incidence of 3.7 per cent (19/505) has been found within the first three days of life (Hayden *et al.* 1985). Of those 19 cases, 14 were bilateral, with four on the left and one on the right. At least one was prenatal in origin judging by its central cystic regression. In the absence of post-mortem confirmation, this incidence may be an overestimate because simple congestion or gliosis of the germinal area might look like haemorrhage on an ultrasound scan. There were no obvious risk factors in obstetric histories or the immediate neonatal period to account for these lesions. These findings show the possibility of germinal matrix injury around term. The location infero-lateral to the foramen of Monro would be in accord with the proposed caudo-rostral regression of the germinal matrix (Hambleton and Wigglesworth 1976).

During the study period from 1980 to 1991 at UZ Gent 18 neonates presented with IVH not related to preterm birth: Table 8.7 attempts to organize this material from both the anatomical and aetiological points of view. This section will concentrate on pure IVH and its causes.

Various sources point to an incidence of IVH of at least one in 10,000 infants liveborn at or near term, whether derived from autopsy studies (Butler and

Alberman 1969, Wigglesworth *et al.* 1976) or from a population of living neonates (Sachs *et al.* 1987). In a recent centre-based study an incidence of 3.6 per 10,000 live term births was recorded (Jocelyn and Casiro 1992). Towards 36 weeks of gestation the incidence may rise to about 1/1000 (Wigglesworth *et al.* 1976). Average neonatal intensive care units ought to diagnose it at least once a year (Nanba *et al.* 1984). In necropsies of term infants the range of incidence is from 2 to 25 per cent. Larroche (1984) reported 15 instances in over 500 autopsies of term infants (stillbirths, neo- and postnatal deaths): the source was vascular malformation in five, unknown in four, choroid plexus haemorrhage in three, deep venous thrombosis in two and matrix haemorrhage in one. Focusing on clinical signs, higher incidences have been found: 7.8 per cent in a prospective study of neonates with 'some neurological sign' (Ludwig *et al.* 1980), 13 per cent following birth asphyxia with hypoxic–ischaemic encephalopathy (Fitzhardinge *et al.* 1981) and 10 per cent in persistent pulmonary hypertension of the newborn (Oelberg *et al.* 1988). Ludwig *et al.* (1980) found no evidence of IVH in 33 control CT scans of asymptomatic children.

Pathogenesis and aetiology
Associated factors in a series of 53 term infants with IVH diagnosed *in vivo* by cranial ultrasound or CT scan, comprising nine personal cases from UZ Gent and 44 from the literature (Cartwright *et al.* 1979, Chaplin *et al.* 1979, Palma *et al.* 1979, Flodmark *et al.* 1980*b*, Guekos-Thöni *et al.* 1980, Mitchell and O'Tuama 1980, Blanc *et al.* 1982, Scher *et al.* 1982, Fenichel *et al.* 1984, Nanba *et al.* 1984, Bergman *et al.* 1985, Oelberg *et al.* 1988, Keeney *et al.* 1991, Jocelyn and Casiro 1992), are listed in Table 8.8.

Data from these cases and from two important necropsy surveys (Donat *et al.* 1978, Lacey and Terplan 1982) suggest that the bleeding in pure IVH originates from the choroid plexus in about 80 per cent of term infants. In contrast, the germinal matrix is accepted as the source of bleeding in about the same proportion or more of preterm infants with IVH. However, just as stromal choroid plexus haemorrhage has occurred in a small number of preterm infants, so haemorrhage originating in residual germinal matrix (almost always near the caudo-thalamic groove) has occurred in term babies. For these few it seems likely that the sequence of events will be similar to that now generally accepted for most preterm infants: acute arterial hyperperfusion of a maximally dilated immature germinal matrix vascular rete, primed by preceding hypoxia and sustained by a scanty stroma with increased fibrinolytic capacity (Pape and Wigglesworth 1989). A possible association with bolus infusions of sodium bicarbonate suggests the causal importance of sudden systemic volaemic changes, if not of osmolality changes (Simmons *et al.* 1974, Hambleton and Wigglesworth 1976).

'Venous' hypotheses invoking such mechanisms as prolonged congestion (Sänger 1924, Hausbrandt and Meier 1936, De Courten and Rabinowicz 1981), rupture of the internal cerebral vein and a stasis-promoting acute angle between the

TABLE 8.8

Aetiology of *in vivo* diagnosed pure intraventricular haemorrhage
at term (N=53)*

Traumatic delivery (with asphyxia)	11 (2)
Isolated birth asphyxia	4
Severe respiratory distress ± pulmonary hypertension	3
Haemorrhagic diathesis[1]	2
Other	
▪ Dehydration (Mitchell and O'Tuama 1980)	1
▪ Toxaemia (Bergman *et al.* 1985)	2
▪ Cardiac arrest (Mitchell and O'Tuama 1980)	1
▪ Hypertension (Guekos-Thöni *et al.* 1980)	1
▪ Fluid overload with hyponatraemia[2]	1
Unknown	27
Parenchymal extension	10
Neonatal death	4
Post-haemorrhagic hydrocephalus	14

*See text for references.

[1]One due to maternal salicylate ingestion (personal observation); one due to disseminated intravascular coagulation associated with congenital cytomegalovirus infection (Cartwright *et al.* 1979).

[2]Personal case: female 37 weeks gestation, (out)born by emergency caesarean section because of fresh meconium staining of the liquor. Birthweight 2950g; Apgar scores 1 and 10 at one and ten minutes. Seizures on day 2; serum Na 122mmol/L, Ca 1.5mmol/L; left grade III IVH, right grade II; post-haemorrhagic hydrocephalus, treated conservatively with serial lumbar punctures and acetazolamide–furosemide; hemiplegic cerebral palsy.

internal cerebral and thalamo-striate veins (Larroche 1977) are not completely forgotten, though in general have been superceded by the 'arterial' concept. Indeed, in selected situations they may still be contributory; a possible example has been reported by Wehberg *et al.* (1992), who suggested that a probable acute rise in central venous pressure caused IVH in an otherwise healthy term baby at 13 days of life after his 3-year-old brother knelt on his abdomen while climbing over him onto a bed. Deep cerebral venous thrombosis, blamed for the majority of IVHs in preterm infants by some authors in the past (Towbin 1969), is an exceptional cause of ventricular haemorrhage that merits separate description because of its specific association with haemorrhage into thalamus or caudate nucleus (see below).

The patterns of causation of haemorrhage into the choroid plexus stroma are less well documented but probably not dissimilar: (i) venous congestion (difficult delivery, birth asphyxia), (ii) systemic, arterial factors, (iii) vulnerable vascular fine structure. Older studies suggested prolonged difficult labour could lead to venous congestion and ultimate rupture of small vessels in the mature infant's choroid tissue (Donat *et al.* 1978, Lacey and Terplan 1982). Some support for this hypothesis can still be found in the rare occurrence of genuine traumatic subdural haematoma associated with IVH (Ponté *et al.* 1971; Blank *et al.* 1978; Flodmark *et al.* 1980*a,b*; Fishman *et al.* 1981; Scotti *et al.* 1981; Koch *et al.* 1985). Although limited in number and depth of observation, these case histories seem to suggest that venous congestion, more likely than arterial hyperperfusion in the context of birth trauma, can contribute to germinal matrix or choroid plexus bleeding, leading to mild IVH at term. Meningeal venous congestion was present in 26 of the 32 post-mortem cases reviewed by Lacey and Terplan (1982). The suggested causal role played by birth trauma is further supported in a description of pure IVH at term presenting with seizures, usually on the second day, after mechanically difficult delivery (Fenichel *et al.* 1984, Nanba *et al.* 1984).

Donat *et al.* (1978) introduced the concept that postnatal respiratory distress, hypoxia, acidosis and bradycardia can lead to IVH in some term babies. This is analogous to the well-known link between IVH and hyaline membrane disease in the preterm infant. There is some experimental evidence to suggest that the choroid plexus, after regression of the vulnerable germinal matrix, may be next in line to suffer from systemic haemodynamic changes. Choroid tissue, as examined by radioactively labelled microspheres, was by far the best perfused organ in a study of cerebral blood flow to fetal and newborn lamb brainstem, cerebellum, cerebral cortex, cerebral white matter, caudate nucleus and choroid plexus (Szymonowicz *et al.* 1988). Though losing 50 per cent of its vascularity from preterm fetal to neonatal age, the choroid plexus blood flow was still found to be four times superior to the next best perfused, the caudate nucleus, in neonatal lamb brains. The same researchers showed isolated reduction of regional blood flow to the choroid tissue following haemorrhagic hypotension in the neonatal lambs, in contrast to an increase in flow to the other regions (Szymonowicz *et al.* 1990). This selective vulnerability seemed to decrease from the fetal to the neonatal period. Another experimental set-up, using the same investigative method in acutely asphyxiated neonatal piglets, demonstrated a redistribution of blood flow during the event with relative overperfusion of the brainstem and reduction of flow to cerebral white matter, grey matter and choroid plexus, the latter possibly due to some sympathetic nervous influence (Coplerud *et al.* 1989). Upon recovery there was a uniform slight increase of blood flow to most brain parts. The nervous tools for modulation of vascular tone in choroid plexus vessels have been illustrated both for ortho- and parasympathetic nervous elements (Lindvall *et al.* 1977).

Further evidence for systemic 'arterial' factors in the generation of choroid plexus haemorrhage can be found in clinical observations. Maki and Shirai (1975), describing angiographic findings in six term infants with IVH, documented increased uptake and retention of contrast in the choroid plexus well into the venous phase. They further demonstrated early filling of the internal cerebral veins. The latter phenomenon, though normal for the neonatal period, does seem to militate against venous congestion as a primary event in these infants, of whom five had birth asphyxia and two were delivered by the breech. Arterial hypertension and postnatal fluid overload were thought to be the causal mechanism in two term babies with pure IVH (Guekos-Thöni *et al.* 1980, personal observation). Arterial

TABLE 8.9

Clinical features of pure intraventricular haemorrhage (IVH) in 58 term infants*

	IVH grade**		
	II (N=27)	III (N=21)	IV (N=10)
Signs and symptoms	22	15	6
Intracranial hypertension	3	3	2
Focal seizures[1]	7	2	0
Generalized seizures	3	9	4
Irritability/jitteriness	9	2	2
Lethargy	2	3	0
Fever	3	0	2
Apnoea	1	3	1
Outcome			
Neonatal death	0	2	2
Shunted hydrocephalus[2]	2	8	7
Cerebral palsy	4	4	5

*See text for references.
**Grade II = mild IVH; grade III = severe IVH + ventricular dilatation; grade IV = III + parenchymal 'extension'.
[1]Significantly more frequent in mild vs. severe IVH (χ^2, $p<0.05$).
[2]Significantly more frequent in severe vs. mild IVH (χ^2, $p<0.05$).

hypertension proximal to an interrupted aortic arch has been considered responsible for hyperdensity of the choroid plexus on CT scan in two neonates (Rand *et al.* 1990). The observation was strengthened by post-mortem findings of normal choroid plexus tissue in one of these infants who died at 3 months (CT performed at 4 weeks), thereby differentiating the striking findings of hyper-perfusion from haemorrhage, haemangioma, calcification or tumour.

The fine structure of the choroid plexus vasculature has hardly been studied in the perinatal period. In adults there seems to be a rich arterial anastomotic network between the feeding branches of the anterior and posterior choroidal arteries facing the occipital horn (Fujii *et al.* 1980). Typical for choroid plexus capillaries is the presence of vascular glomeruli, the importance of which as fragile sites has yet to be determined (Williams 1989). In the same way, gap junctions in choroid plexus capillary endothelium, unlike tight junctions elsewhere in the brain, have been proposed as a vulnerable site (Armstrong *et al.* 1980). Thus it would not be surprising to find IVH as a complication of haemorrhagic diathesis.

Clinical setting
While the tortured facial expressions, rigidity, clenched fists and piercing, shrill cries described so vividly by Craig (1938) are happily rarely seen now in term infants, more subtle signs of neurological abnormality are not often described in detail, perhaps because the observation and treatment of preterm infants has become such a priority in neonatal units. Table 8.9 summarizes clinical findings of

pure IVH as reported in a limited number of previous reports (Cartwright *et al.* 1979, Chaplin *et al.* 1979, Palma *et al.* 1979, Guekos-Thöni *et al.* 1980, Mitchell and O'Tuama 1980, Blanc *et al.* 1982, Scher *et al.* 1982, Fenichel *et al.* 1984, Nanba *et al.* 1984, Bergman *et al.* 1985). Presentation on the first day of life was recorded in half the cases where IVH was associated with trauma and in only a quarter of those with unknown aetiology. Some less commonly reported presenting signs have been vomiting (2/43), a high and shrill cry (5/43) and opisthotonus (3/43). Fever was a common sign in a recent series (47 per cent), where unfortunately the clinical findings were not matched with the grading of severity (Jocelyn and Casiro 1992). Seizures were reported to be easy to control in some neonates (Chaplin *et al.* 1979). If associated with birth trauma, recognizable convulsions usually started on the second day of life (Fenichel *et al.* 1984). In the series reported by Ludwig *et al.* (1980) none of the infants with IVH at term was asymptomatic. Hypotonia and a disproportionately tight popliteal angle for gestational age are additional signs (Dubowitz *et al.* 1981). Both thrombocytopenia during the acute stage (in assocation with persistent pulmonary hypertension) and thrombocytosis on recovery have been linked with IVH at term (Palma *et al.* 1979).

Two EEG patterns associated with term IVH are worth noting: focal ipsilateral epileptic activity (Scher *et al.* 1982), and the burst suppression type with subsequent normal outcome (Fenichel *et al.* 1984).

Radiological assessment and relation to prognosis
Shortly after the introduction of CT scanning in the management of sick preterm infants, the importance of grading IVH received appropriate attention, as did its link to immediate and long-term outcome (Papile *et al.* 1978, Krishnamoorthy *et al.* 1979, Volpe 1981). Though this link may not exist as clearly in the term neonate (see Table 8.8), no other subdivisions seem necessary. As referred to above, uncontrasted CT scans can allow recognition of posterior IVH around the glomus of the choroid plexus (Nanba *et al.* 1984). Some impairment in astroglial development and myelination is to be expected, even following isolated germinal matrix injury (Evrard *et al.* 1992). In a minority of mentally retarded children (6/299), subependymal germinolysis was the only recognized macroscopic brain finding in a study by Shaw (1987). It is important to realize that subependymal germinal matrix cysts acquired after birth can be due to haemorrhage as well as ischaemia without prior bleeding (Takashima *et al.* 1984). Certainly grade IV haemorrhage carries a gloomy prognosis (Jocelyn and Casiro 1992) (Fig. 8.20).

A warning has been given against overdiagnosis of choroid plexus haemorrhage by the use of ultrasound (Hope *et al.* 1988). The irregularity of density and variable bulk of the healthy plexus defies accurate recognition of haemorrhage. Even asymmetrical hyperdensity can be due to dissipation of clot from the ventricle into the choroid crypts. Venous congestion has been recognized as a cause of false-positive diagnosis in preterm infants (Szymonowicz *et al.* 1984). In children on ECMO, development of massive IVH may be more abrupt than usual but, despite

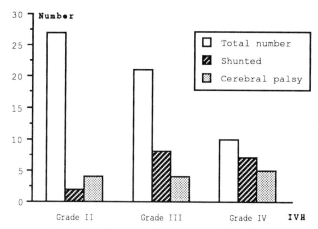

Fig. 8.20. Term intraventricular haemorrhage: grading vs. prognosis in 58 term neonates. (See Table 8.9 for grading; see text for references.)

its extent, difficult to recognize at first because of the hypodensity due to systemic anticoagulation (Bowerman *et al.* 1985). Ultrasound does remain important for follow-up of ventricle size after the acute event. Axial images are especially useful for measurement of third ventricle width and to follow the glial reaction at the ependymal lining (Gaissie *et al.* 1990).

Case history

CASE 8.4

This firstborn girl was delivered normally at 37 weeks of gestation. Mild ventricular dilatation had been recognized on ultrasound at 32 weeks. She weighed 2650g and had Apgar scores of 9 at one and five minutes. On the second day she was referred with severe respiratory distress and oedema. Our tentative diagnosis was transient tachypnoea exacerbated by fluid overload. Haematocrit on admission was 25 per cent. She was suffering from left grade III IVH and was in addition found to have complete agenesis of the corpus callosum and hypothyroidism with an ectopic sublingual thyroid gland remnant (Fig. 8.21). Left white matter hyperdensities were suggestive of periventricular leukomalacia. Post-haemorrhagic ventricular dilatation, reaching a maximum third ventricle width of 9mm, resolved spontaneously within the first month. At 6 months a mild right hemiplegia was present.

Management

Treatment of post-haemorrhagic hydrocephalus is beyond the scope of this section. There is insufficient evidence in favour of early surgical clot removal, but this viewpoint may be altered in the near future (Ritschl and Auer 1987). Attempts at prophylaxis of post-haemorrhagic hydrocephalus by intraventricular application of thrombolytic drugs deserve close attention (Whitelaw *et al.* 1992). Some prognostic considerations have been discussed above and were reviewed by Jocelyn and Casiro (1992).

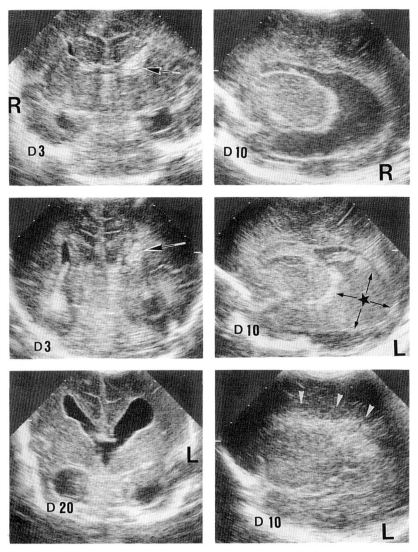

Fig. 8.21. Coronal *(left)* and parasagittal *(right)* ultrasound scans in Case 8.4: *arrows* show left intraventricular clot, while *arrowheads* indicate periventricular hyperdensity of white matter. Marked ventricular dilatation regressed spontaneously.

Primary thalamo-ventricular haemorrhage (primary thalamic bleeding, deep cerebral venous thrombosis)

Anatomical description

Several reports have described unilateral thalamic haemorrhage in term or near-term neonates as a separate entity. It usually presents after the third day of life, not infrequently well into the late neonatal period (Burger *et al.* 1978, Palma *et al.*

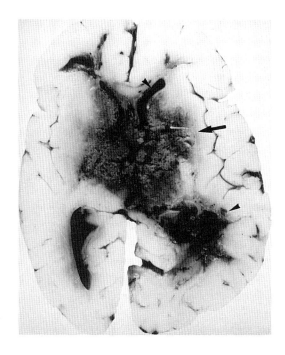

Fig. 8.22. Axial post-mortem aspect of deep cerebral venous thrombosis: *arrow* indicates red softening within thalamus, globus pallidus and part of striatum; *arrowheads* show associated intraventricular haemorrhage. (Courtesy Prof. J.S. Wigglesworth, Hammersmith Hospital.)

1979, Mitchell and O'Tuama 1980, Trounce *et al.* 1985, Montoya *et al.* 1987, Hurst *et al.* 1989, Roland *et al.* 1990). Personal observations and scrutiny of the literature link this 'new syndrome' to thrombosis of the internal cerebral vein(s) (Govaert *et al.* 1992*a*). With modern imaging techniques the salient features would be unilateral or clearly asymmetrical and irregular haemorrhagic infarction of the thalamus, associated with a variable degree of ipsilateral intraventricular bleeding. Additional structures involved are (i) the head of the caudate nucleus, (ii) the periventricular white matter of frontal, parietal and mesial occipital lobes sparing only a rim of subcortical white matter of about 2cm, and (iii) the corpus callosum. Thalamic necrosis can be complete or focal, near the upper midline in the latter instance. The ventricular haemorrhage originates from ruptured subependymal or choroid plexus vessels (Mitchell and O'Tuama 1980).

As long ago as 1936, Ehlers and Courville reviewed the available literature on thrombosis of the deep cerebral veins in early childhood and established this sequence of events: thrombosis of the internal cerebral vein → choroid plexus bleed and possibly IVH → thalamic haemorrhage. Following initial congestion, most marked in the choroid plexus, there is a phase of brain oedema (less pronounced when dehydration is the primary cause) and subsequent red or pale softening. The red softening is due to venous haemorrhagic infarction with bleeding throughout the affected region or most pronounced around its margins (Fig. 8.22). Thrombosed veins, with possibly simultaneous involvement of several vessels, stand out as black cords in the parenchyma or protrude from the ventricle walls.

135

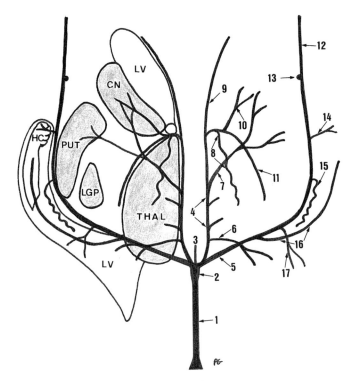

Fig. 8.23. Venous trees stemming from straight sinus, draining deep cerebral grey matter.
(1) Straight sinus; (2) great cerebral vein; (3) posterior vein of corpus callosum; (4) internal cerebral vein; (5) basal vein; (6) medial atrial vein; (7) direct lateral vein; (8) superior choroidal vein; (9) septal vein; (10) caudal vein; (11) terminal vein (thalamostriate vein); (12) anterior cerebral vein; (13) middle cerebral vein; (14) hippocampal vein; (15) inferior choroidal vein; (16) hippocampal venous complex; (17) lateral atrial vein.
(CN = caudate nucleus; LV = lateral ventricle; PUT = putamen; LGP = lateral global pallidus; THAL = thalamus; HC = hippocampus.)

Subarachnoid haemorrhage is an additional finding where thrombosis also involves superficial venous channels. If the basal vein is occluded, either directly or as a corollary to thrombosis of the great vein of Galen, variable softening of the globus pallidus and infero-lateral thalamus complete the picture. Figure 8.23 shows the related structures and vessels, and outlines the separate venous drainage of the thalamus and head of caudate nucleus, thus explaining their differential involvement (Stein and Rosenbaum 1974, Larroche 1977, Pape and Wigglesworth 1979). The importance of anastomoses in deviating blood from the affected side to the superficial dural vessels or the unaffected contralateral internal venous system has not been commented on so far.

Recently, isolated thalamic haemorrhage was singled out as a novel entity in preterm and term neonates (De Vries *et al.* 1992). In the absence of MRI findings compatible with associated IVH and major venous thrombosis, De Vries *et al.*

TABLE 8.10

Causes of neonatal thrombosis of the internal cerebral vein
and/or its tributaries

1. All instances of superficial dural sinus thrombosis with
   extension into straight sinus and cerebral vein of Galen
2. Prolonged venous congestion (as in difficult delivery)
3. Leptomeningitis and ventriculitis
4. Hyperviscosity (cyanotic heart disease, polycythaemia)
5. Severe birth asphyxia
6. Deficient anticoagulation (*e.g.* antithrombin III deficiency)
7. Extensive unruptured germinal layer haemorrhage
8. Vascular malformation

suggested it should be separated from thalamo-ventricular haemorrhage as described here. The term infant in their study was growth retarded (2200g at 38 weeks gestation) and had presented with fetal distress leading to emergency caesarean section. Roving eye movements were thought to be abnormal on day 3. A right thalamic lesion was shown to be haemorrhagic by MRI, but was not recognized on CT scan. This boy sat alone at 9 months and had minimal contralateral hypertonia. Limited venous thrombosis or lacunar arterial infarction are the likely causes of such a lesion.

Incidence
This event is rare. I have collected 23 cases from the more recent literature (Burger *et al.* 1978, Palma *et al.* 1979, Mitchell and O'Tuama 1980, Trounce *et al.* 1985, Hurst *et al.* 1989, Roland *et al.* 1990) and added three personal observations, not including the cases detailed by Ehlers and Courville (1936) and some others with insufficient clinical data (Flodmark *et al.* 1980*b*). Within the material studied at UZ Gent there were 19 cases of IVH unrelated to preterm birth, three of them primary thalamo-ventricular. Considering an incidence of about one IVH in 10,000 term livebirths, neonatal internal cerebral vein thrombosis probably affects around 1 in 50,000 term neonates. Underreporting and lack of accurate diagnosis may make this an underestimate. This could explain why Roland *et al.* (1990) found 12 of 19 term IVHs to be of this variety, although the actual incidence in their experience was in the same range (12 in *ca.*270,000 deliveries).

Pathogenesis
Although associated asphyxia and haemorrhagic diathesis (Palma *et al.* 1979) may alter the extent of parenchymal injury, thrombosis of the internal cerebral vein or tributaries is the causal mechanism. Several disease states have been known to induce this event (Table 8.10). A significant proportion of cases will result from superficial dural sinus thrombosis, and the reader is referred to the relevant section in Chapter 6 (pp. 78–85). The concept of venous stasis during delivery has been elaborated repeatedly by German pathologists (Sänger 1924, Schwartz 1964).

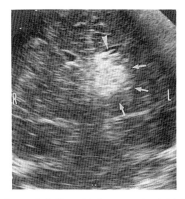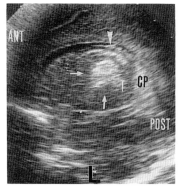

Fig. 8.24. Coronal *(left)* and left parasagittal *(right)* ultrasound scans in term neonate with group B streptococcal bacteraemia and meningitis: note minor left intraventricular haemorrhage *(arrowheads)* and unilateral left thalamic density *(arrows)*. (T = thalamus; CP = choroid plexus.)

During prolonged labour, moulding will lead to intracranial hypertension and venous compression with subsequent kinking at the junction between the great cerebral vein and straight sinus. The unusual anatomical transition from thin-walled great cerebral vein with vasa vasorum to rigid intradural straight sinus is a predisposing factor (Ruchoux *et al.* 1987). Following rupture of the membranes, the pressure release on the presenting part was also hypothesized to favour stasis in the deep venous drainage system (Schwartz 1964). These authors emphasized difficult delivery as a cause of impaired deep venous circulation.

Leptomeningeal, cortical or ependymal thrombophlebitis has been considered responsible for damage to cerebral cortex, periventricular white matter or basal ganglia in neonatal bacterial meningitis (Friede 1973). Ependymal vein occlusion was demonstrated in 5/29 cases reported by Berman and Banker (1966). Multiloculated white matter cysts, obliterating the midline structures and often communicating with a distorted loculated ventricle cavity, may be the end result (Friede 1973). The absence of purulent exudate covering these cavities, as opposed to the heavy coating found in the ventricles, supports a vascular pathogenesis for the white matter necrosis (Buchan and Alvord 1969). Focal phlebitis of a branch of the internal cerebral vein—probably the thalamo-striate vein—was the presumed cause of a primary thalamic haemorrhage in an infant with early onset group B streptococcal meningitis (personal case; Fig. 8.24). A similar observation has been made by De Vries *et al.* (1988*a*) in a preterm infant with *Listeria* meningitis. Even in the absence of obvious ventriculitis, exudative changes may affect the great vein of Galen and its tributaries within the ambient cistern, leading to phlebitis and thrombosis (Friede 1989).

Cottrill and Kaplan (1973) found cerebral venous thromboses, both superficial and deep, to be the most common CNS lesions in children dying with cyanotic congenital heart disease. They postulated that increased blood viscosity may be a contributory factor. However, it was not clear how many, if any, of the 29 patients they described were newborn infants. Minor unilateral venous infarction might be expected with hyperviscosity and could present with, for example, temporal lobe haemorrhage, as described in the polycythaemic term baby of a diabetic mother (Slovis *et al.* 1984); this infant's blood viscosity unfortunately was not recorded. Severe cardiorespiratory distress, as in pneumonia with hypotension and dehydration, can predispose to isolated deep cerebral venous thrombosis (Burger *et al.* 1978), although once again propagation from a thrombosed dural sinus is more common in this situation (see section on superficial venous thrombosis, Chapter 6). Heterozygosity for antithrombin III deficiency in association with misplacement of a subclavian venous catheter up into the jugular vein was the cause of a deep thrombosis within the vein of Galen and right internal cerebral vein of a term infant with myocardial infarction (Peeters *et al.* 1993).

In the 26 cases mentioned above, the aetiological breakdown was as follows: birth trauma (four), birth asphyxia (four), dehydration (three), polycythaemia (one), bacteraemia (four), meningitis (one) and jugular vein compression (one) (the latter two both personal cases). For the remaining eight, no obvious cause was reported. In one patient seen at UZ Gent the interval between difficult breech delivery with manual freeing of a locked chin and seizures as the presenting sign of superficial and deep cerebro-venous thrombosis was six days, suggesting a two-stage process assuming mechanical trauma was a contributory factor (Figs 8.25, 8.26).

Clinical setting
Seizures and irritability are the most striking presenting signs (Table 8.11), often surprising because of an uneventful interval between birth and thrombosis (Fig. 8.27) (Burger *et al.* 1978, Palma *et al.* 1979, Mitchell and O'Tuama 1980, Trounce *et al.* 1985, Hurst *et al.* 1989, Roland *et al.* 1990, Govaert *et al.* 1992a). The significance of delay in relation to this diagnostic entity within the range of intracranial haemorrhages was slightly overemphasized by Roland *et al.* (1990) because pure IVH shows the same bifid presentation (Cartwright *et al.* 1979, Chaplin *et al.* 1979, Palma *et al.* 1979, Guekos-Thöni *et al.* 1980, Flodmark *et al.* 1980b, Mitchell and O'Tuama 1980, Blanc *et al.* 1982, Scher *et al.* 1982, Fenichel *et al.* 1984, Nanba *et al.* 1984, Bergman *et al.* 1985, Oelberg *et al.* 1988, Keeney *et al.* 1991, Jocelyn and Casiro 1992). In addition, three well-documented instances of early thalamo-ventricular haemorrhage are on record. Of the 26 cases mentioned, 18 were male. The mean birthweight was 3078g. Special attention was paid by Trounce *et al.* (1985) and Montoya *et al.* (1987) to the eye signs, attributed in part to damage of the fronto-mesencephalic optic pathway crossing the subthalamic region: vertical upward gaze palsy, deviation of the eyes toward the lesion, ipsilateral saccadic paresis and a flat visual evoked response. These do not seem to be pathognomonic (Roland *et al.* 1990). If the extent of vessel and brain involved is great, secondary DIC may complicate the biological findings (Govaert *et al.* 1992a).

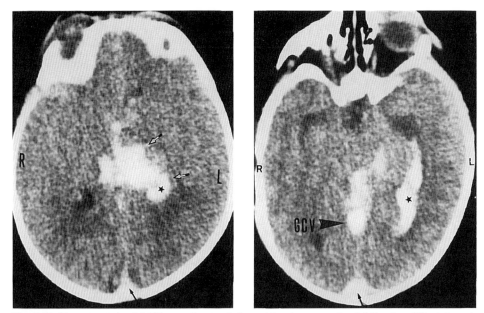

Fig. 8.25. Uncontrasted axial CT scans in term infant with seizures on day 6 following difficult breech delivery, showing spontaneous density of superior sagittal sinus *(black arrow)* and great cerebral vein (GCV), left thalamic density crossing midline *(white arrows)* and left intraventricular haemorrhage *(asterisk)*.

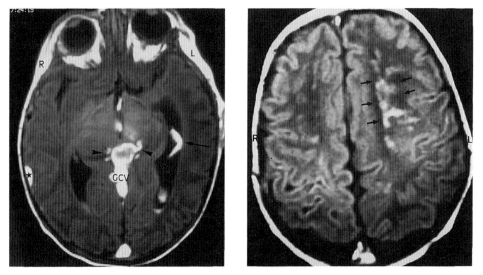

Fig. 8.26. T1-weighted MRI scan in term infant with seizures on day 7 following difficult breech delivery. *(a)* Coronal section: *arrowheads* point to thrombosed tributaries of great cerebral vein (GCV), *arrow* to thrombosed choroidal vein within left lateral ventricle; *asterisk* shows thrombosis of right anastomosing vein of Labbé. *(b)* Associated white matter injury in left corona radiata *(arrows)*.

140

TABLE 8.11

Clinical features and outcome in 29 term infants with primary thalamo-ventricular haemorrhage*

Signs and symptoms		*Outcome*	
Irritability	11	Neonatal death	3
Seizures—focal	8	Apparently normal survival	6
—generalized	10	Hydrocephalus requiring shunt	12
Intracranial hypertension	8	Cerebral palsy	13
Opisthotonus	6		
Lethargy	5		
High-pitched cry	3		
Contralateral hemiparesis	3		
Eye signs			
'Setting sun'	5		
Saccadic paresis	3		
Nystagmus	1		

*See text for references.

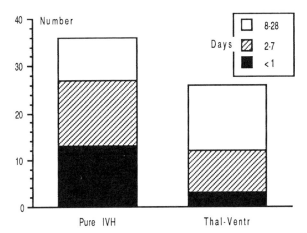

Fig. 8.27. Interval to symptoms in 36 term infants with pure intraventricular haemorrhage (Cartwright *et al.* 1979, Chaplin *et al.* 1979, Palma *et al.* 1979, Guekos-Thöni *et al.* 1980, Mitchell and O'Tuama 1980, Blanc *et al.* 1982, Scher *et al.* 1982, Fenichel *et al.* 1984, Bergman *et al.* 1985) and in 26 infants with thalamo-ventricular haemorrhage (see text for references.)

Radiological assessment

In a limited number of observations failure of direct angiography to visualize the deep cerebral veins suggested associated venous occlusion (Johnsen *et al.* 1973, Mitchell and O'Tuama 1980, Trounce *et al.* 1985, Roland *et al.* 1990). Recently MRI has provided easy diagnosis of the presumably primary thrombosis of (tributaries of) the great cerebral vein (Fig. 8.26) (Hurst *et al.* 1989, Govaert *et al.* 1992*a*). Even minor vessels, like the anastomotic vein of Labbé, can be shown to contain thrombi by this technique, and associated white matter softening is equally

TABLE 8.12

Site of lesion in 12 term infants with thalamo-ventricular haemorrhage*

Site of lesion	N (R/L/B)**
IVH grade II	10 (3/5/1)
IVH grade III	7 (2/3/1)
IVH grade IV	2 (2/0/0)
Opacified great cerebral vein	9
Opacified sagittal sinus	8
Head of caudate nucleus	12 (0/4/4)
Thalamus—focal	5 (3/2/0)
—complete	8 (2/4/1)
Globus pallidus	1 (1/0/0)

*Cases from: Burger *et al.* (1978), Palma *et al.* (1979), Mitchell and O'Tuama (1980), Trounce *et al.* (1985), Hurst *et al.* (1989), Roland *et al.* (1990), Govaert *et al.* (1992*a*).
**R/L/B = right/left/bilateral.

recognizable. Before this, several reports had commented on the diagnosis with ultrasound (Trounce *et al.* 1985) and CT scanning (Fig. 8.25). The results of a survey of 12 well-illustrated cases are summarized in Table 8.12. For recognition of the sonographic landmarks, the reader is referred to an excellent description by Naidich (1986). Thalamic haemorrhage is irregular and asymmetrical or unilateral, and in some minor thromboses is limited to the medial aspect of the organ. Thalamic involvement, in my opinion, is obligatory. Venous infarction in the head of the caudate nucleus may not be readily differentiated from subependymal haemorrhage or grade III IVH. This structure does not seem to be involved constantly, understandable because of its different venous drainage. Extension of the venous infarct into the globus pallidus is rare and attests to the severity of damage by possible involvement of the basal vein in addition to the internal cerebral vein, a feature yet to be demonstrated in the perinatal context. Most patients seem to have major IVH, grade II being restricted to only 4/12. Spontaneous opacification of the great cerebral vein and superior sagittal sinus is very common but not often quoted as being recognized.

Management and prognosis
There is no established immediate surgical or medical treatment method. Post-haemorrhagic hydrocephalus is a common sequela due to the high incidence of extensive ventricular bleeding or possibly due to associated superficial venous thrombosis. It complicates recovery in about half of the survivors (see Table 8.11), in contrast to about one in four of surviving term infants with pure IVH. No detailed studies of developmental follow-up are available. A minority of infants, those with limited thalamic involvement and without hydrocephalus or white

142

matter softening, may actually turn out to be 'neurologically intact' (Govaert *et al.* 1992*a*). Others will suffer from epilepsy, mental retardation and (usually hemiplegic or diplegic) cerebral palsy. Persistence of abnormal eye signs was reported by Mitchell and O'Tuama (1980) in an infant with hypometropic saccadic eye movements still present at the age of 5 months, and one of the UZ Gent patients still had contralateral internal ophthalmoplegia at 2 months.

Ischaemia and haemorrhage of deep cerebral grey matter
Pathological description
Following neonatal asphyxia several patterns of 'focal neuronal injury' have been recognized. Status marmoratus is the term commonly used to refer to residual damage within deep cerebral grey matter. The 'marbled' state of diencephalic structures has been appreciated for some time (Norman 1947, Malamud 1950). The term is derived from the macroscopic finding of white streaks and whorls replacing parts of the head of the caudate nucleus, anterior dorsal putamen and dorsal thalamus (Carpenter 1950, Malamud 1950, Sylvester 1960, Schneider *et al.* 1975, Leech and Alvord 1977, Jellinger 1986*a*, Friede 1989, Hayashi *et al.* 1991). Debate about histological changes within affected areas was settled by Friede and Schachenmayr (1977), who described early alterations as erratic, but microscopically normal, myelination within astroglial scars devoid of neurons or containing only remnant encrusted nerve cells (*e.g.* in the thalamus). Contrary to previous suggestions (Bignami and Ralston 1968, Borit and Herndon 1970), myelination of astroglial fibres and hypermyelination are not seen. The asphyxial scars merely interrupt and disperse existing axonal connections and their evolving myelin deposition. These histopathological findings bridged an existing gap between birth asphyxia and status marmoratus. Similar disarray of myelination is typical of focal cortico-subcortical scarring in ulegyria (Borit and Herndon 1970). Grey nuclei affected by ischaemia may shrink, causing the putamen to lose its lateral convex border (Friede 1989).

Reviewing details of 43 neuropathological descriptions of status marmoratus recorded in the literature (Malamud 1950, Sylvester 1960, Schneider *et al.* 1975, Leech and Alvord 1977, Hayashi *et al.* 1991), one can recognize a pattern of regional involvement, subject to variability but nevertheless with some consistencies (Table 8.13). Thalamic injury can be safely used as an indicator of diencephalic damage. Putaminal necrosis and, to a slightly lesser extent, pallidal damage are other markers. Symmetry of the lesions is almost obligatory, obvious unilaterality being very rare (Malamud 1950). Damage has been recorded in various thalamic subregions, with occasional sparing of pulvinar and non-involvement of centromedian and intralaminar nuclei. The claustrum was reported to be necrotic in at least one infant (Sylvester 1960). Obvious predilection for the inferior colliculi within the quadrigeminal plate was mentioned by Schneider *et al.* (1975). Not surprisingly, unilateral status marmoratus can affect the caudate, putamen and lateral pallidum when 'total' arterial infarction occurs within the territory of the

TABLE 8.13

Target structures associated with status marmoratus

Diagnostic (i.e. most cases): thalamus, inferior collicle, inferior olive, basal pontine nuclei, hippocampus (Sommer's sector and subiculum), putamen, globus pallidus

Frequent (more than half of cases): brainstem reticular formation, cerebral cortex, caudate nucleus, dentate nucleus, cranial nerve nuclei, lateral geniculate, cerebral white matter, substantia nigra (pars compacta), cerebellar granular layer and Purkinje cells, subthalamus

Common (less than half of cases but not rare): amygdaloid complex

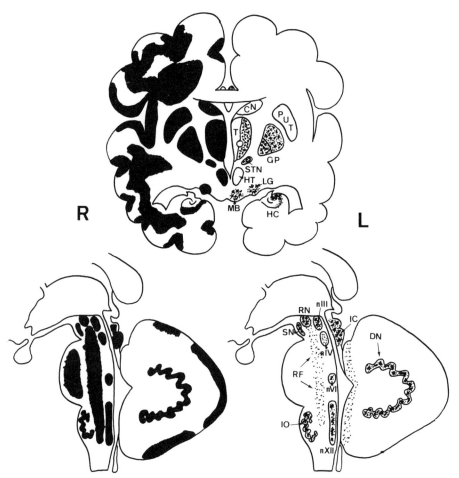

Fig. 8.28. Structural targets of neuronal loss in severe birth asphyxia of the 'cardiac arrest' type *(right)* and kernicterus *(left)*.

  (CN = caudate nucleus; T = thalamus; PUT = putamen; GP = globus pallidus; STN = subthalamic nucleus; HT = hypothalamus; LG = lateral geniculate; MB = mamillary body; HC = hippocampus; RN = red nucleus; SN = substantia nigra; RF = reticular formation; IC = inferior collicle; DN = dentate nucleus; IO = inferior olive.)

144

middle cerebral artery (Norman 1947). Trans-synaptic degeneration of thalamic neurons as a consequence of primary damage to cerebral white matter, cerebral cortex or cerebellum can be differentiated from initial thalamic injury by the absence of neuronal calcification.

In term neonates, differentiation from bilirubin-induced brain damage (Fig. 8.28) can usually be made on the basis of history and clinical findings (Rutherford *et al.* 1992). For detailed reviews of the neuropathological differences between postasphyxial and kernicteric nervous damage the reader is referred to Ahdab-Barmada and Moossy (1984), Wigglesworth (1984), Jellinger (1986*a*), Friede (1989), Turkel (1990) and Hayashi *et al.* (1991). Changes within cerebral or cerebellar white matter and cortical grey matter almost refute the diagnosis of pure kernicterus. Pivotal necrosis of the pallidum has suggested the eponym globo-luysian athetoid cerebral palsy, as opposed to the post-asphyxial thalamo-striate counterpart of status marmoratus (Hayashi *et al.* 1991).

Pathogenesis (Fig. 8.29)
The peculiar combination of necrotic changes within thalamus, striatum, pallidum and brainstem defies interpretation on a vascular basis (Azzarelli and Velasco 1987). For example, symmetrical infarction of the areas perfused by the anterior choroidal arteries, either because of its recurrent and long course or due to compression against the tentorium in the case of brain swelling, would not lead to damage of putamen, head of caudate, cerebral cortex or brainstem below midbrain level (Helgason *et al.* 1986, Jellinger 1986*a*). Deep venous thrombosis classically leads to haemorrhagic infarction (seen in a minority of cases of postasphyxial deep cerebral grey matter damage) and IVH. Sparing of the internal capsule, as regularly mentioned in reports of status marmoratus, militates against venous infarction involving both pallidum and thalamus in the same patient.

Whereas in the adult isolated or primordial pallidal necrosis (*e.g.* in carbon monoxide poisoning) is challenging the ancient 'pathoclisis' theory (Jellinger 1986*b*), in the context of birth or neonatal asphyxia at term a particular vulnerability of the aforementioned structures does seem to play a major pathogenetic role (Azzarelli and Velasco 1987). Several authors have detailed the basic pathophysiological alterations (Volpe 1987, Vannucci 1990*b*, Espinoza and Parer 1991, Pryds 1991, Garcia 1992, Siesjö 1992).

The fetal brainstem is a metabolically sophisticated structure, which is understandable in view of its phylogenetic cardiorespiratory function and also reflects early vestibular and acoustic stimulation (Gluckman *et al.* 1991). This obvervation is supported by a hierarchy of regional cerebral blood flow distribution: in the near-term fetal lamb for instance, flow to brainstem is double that to cerebral cortex or white matter (Szymonowicz *et al.* 1988). Following birth, cortical perfusion surmounts flow to the brainstem (Richardson 1991). The teleological assumption that a high perfusion rate is inherent to a high metabolic level has been substantiated by autoradiographic study of glucose and protein

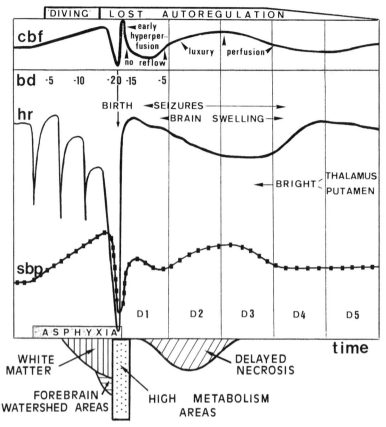

Fig. 8.29. Time course (in days) vs. clinical events in severe birth asphyxia (cbf = cerebral blood flow; bd = base deficit; hr = heart rate; sbp = systemic blood pressure). Brain areas vulnerable at certain stages in the sequence of events are shown underneath. High metabolism structures are basal ganglia, thalamus and brainstem reticular formation. Delayed necrosis preceding brain swelling presumably indicates excitotoxic and oxygen free radical injury. The latter event overlaps with clinical seizures and luxury perfusion.

metabolism and measurement of cerebral oxidative metabolism by comparison of venous and arterial metabolites (Abrams *et al.* 1984, Richardson *et al.* 1985, Abrams and Cooper 1987, Jones *et al.* 1988). This linkage of fetal cerebral blood flow to metabolism is not straightforward, as a low haemoglobin P_{50} (high oxygen affinity) could also account for an increase of perfusion (Jones *et al.* 1988). If present its underlying mechanism remains subject to speculation (Pryds 1991). Glucose-positron emission tomography in the healthy newborn human infant has established a relatively high level of metabolism in the thalamus as well as the sensorimotor cortex, cerebellar vermis and midbrain–brainstem region (Volpe *et al.* 1985, Chugani and Phelps 1986). The same areas have repeatedly proved to be targets of birth asphyxia, resulting in paracentral ulegyria, status marmoratus and gliosis within the brainstem (De Reuck 1977, Larroche 1977, Leech and Alvord 1977, Pape and Wigglesworth 1979, Volpe 1987, Levene 1988, Friede 1989).

In contrast to the experimental setting, it is not necessarily clear in human perinatal asphyxia to what extent there have been hypoxia, hypercarbia, lactic acidosis, hypotension and alterations of glucose metabolism. Iatrogenic influences (inotropic support with vaso-active drugs, different ventilation protocols with variable increase of central venous pressure) can also affect the brain. To understand the association of deep grey matter damage with leukomalacia and cerebral cortical injury in a substantial number of term neonates, one has to reflect on systemic and cerebro-vascular reactions to hypoxic hypoxia (low P_aO_2), hypotension and the presence of metabolic acidosis or myocardial failure.

During isolated hypoxic or anaemic hypoxia (low C_aO_2 = oxygen carrying capacity of arterial blood), brain vessels cope with marked reductions of oxygen delivery up to a critical level of P_aO_2 around 2.7kPa (20mmHg) (oxygen saturation around 50 per cent), when autoregulation starts to fail (Younkin *et al.* 1987) and metabolic acidosis gradually develops (Torrance and Wittnich 1992). Non-invasive exploration of the asphyxiated brain with phosphor-NMR spectroscopy supports this observation, documenting an actual threshold between 2.7 and 4.0kPa (20–30mmHg) (Delivoria-Papadopoulos and Chance 1988). Within 60 seconds of lowered C_aO_2, global brain flow will increase to keep a constant cerebral oxygen extraction rate (Jones *et al.* 1988). Cerebral blood flow is uneven, with preferential perfusion increase to brainstem > forebrain grey matter > forebrain white matter (Pryds 1991). Naloxone, an opioid antagonist, abolishes these selective perfusion changes (Lou *et al.* 1985). In newborn piglets phenobarbitone in anticonvulsant concentrations has been shown to blunt the global increase of cerebral blood flow during hypertension and hypoxia (Goddard-Finegold and Michael 1992). Inherent to this compensatory orchestration, cerebral white matter in the newborn infant may already be at risk of nutrient deprivation at this early stage of isolated hypoxia (Cavazutti and Duffy 1982) and during haemorrhagic hypotension with normal P_aO_2 and P_aCO_2 (Young *et al.* 1982).

In order to preserve cerebral blood flow during moderate asphyxia, term fetal animals increase systemic blood pressure in spite of a transient reduction in fetal heart rate (Hanson 1991). Mechanical compression of the head during delivery will contribute to this bradycardia. Meanwhile the 'diving reflex' assures perfusion to vital organs (brain, adrenal glands and heart) at the expense of gut, kidney and lungs. Umbilical venous blood is shifted away from the right liver lobe into the ductus venosus in order to deviate more oxygen across the foramen ovale into the systemic circulation. As long as autoregulatory mechanisms within the brain still function, the aforementioned regional distributory changes prevail, even with (?gradual) onset of moderate combined systemic acidosis (arterial pH >7.1) (Jones *et al.* 1988, Coplerud *et al.* 1989, Calvert *et al.* 1990, Gluckman *et al.* 1991). It is unclear what deleterious effects this overlap period with systemic acidosis and ongoing autoregulation of brain perfusion may incur.

Experiments in primates have established that the presence of brain acidosis and hypotension is essential for the development of brain necrosis in severe asphyxia (Ginsberg *et al*. 1974, Brann and Myers 1975, Myers 1975, Fenichel 1983, Myers *et al*. 1987, Volpe 1987). *In utero* the impending cardio-vascular collapse is heralded by late decelerations (Hanson 1991). Before the onset of severe bradycardia or cardiac arrest, cerebral autoregulation collapses leaving the whole brain dependent for perfusion on systemic blood pressure. As combined ventricular output falls, forebrain watershed areas will be subject to hypoperfusion: parasagittal (pericentral) parieto-occipital (sub)cortex, the depths of cerebral sulci, hippocampus and subiculum (Gilles 1969, Brann and Myers 1975, Takashima *et al*. 1978, Volpe 1987, Revesz and Geddes 1988, Gluckmann *et al*. 1991). There is evidence for a stepwise loss of cerebral autoregulation: pressure regulation before sensitivity to carbon dioxide before sensitivity to oxygen (Pryds 1991). Combined loss of regulatory response to pressure, carbon dioxide and oxygen carries a bad prognosis (Pryds *et al*. 1990).

The extent of brain necrosis will subsequently depend on several compounding factors: (i) the level and (ii) the duration of reduction of cerebral blood flow; (iii) regional differences in vulnerability to hypoperfusion; (iv) enhancement by factors increasing neuronal anaerobic glycolysis and lactic acidosis; (v) secondary intracranial effects of intracellular oedema and brain swelling, such as compression of the posterior cerebral artery; (vi) duration and severity of post-event hyperperfusion (vasogenic oedema and injury by oxygen free radicals); (vii) iatrogenic influences, both positive and negative; (viii) maturation phenomena (excitotoxic or oxygen-induced delayed neuronal death). For recent reviews the reader is referred to Volpe (1987), Lou (1988), Vannucci (1990*a*,*b*), Espinoza and Parer (1991), Garcia (1992), Siesjö (1992) and Kogure *et al*. (1993). Irreversibility of neuronal damage manifests with (i) a severe degree of cerebral lactic acidosis (Volpe 1987), (ii) a characteristic duration and pattern of electro-cortical changes (triphasic: suppression, epileptiform activity, resolution) (Watkins *et al*. 1988, Williams *et al*. 1990, Gluckman *et al*. 1991), and (iii) a prolonged second stage of intracellular oedema as measured by cerebral impedence (Rothman and Olney 1987, Gluckman *et al*. 1991). Loss of ionic homeostasis occurs from a cerebral blood flow level around 12mL/100g/min. in adult humans and animals. It is referred to as 'membrane failure', the end stage of neuronal dysfunction (Siesjö 1992). Evaluation of human brains after birth asphyxia by means of phosphorus MRI spectroscopy (Wyatt *et al*. 1989) has shown that the disruption in oxidative phosphorylation manifests hours after the insult, peaking at 2 to 3 days of age. This delay of neuronal death had already been suggested by experimental work (Pulsinelli *et al*. 1982).

What exactly happens at neuronal level during cardiac arrest is a matter of conjecture. Aforementioned animal work and observations in affected neonates and survivors with status marmoratus has confirmed selective vulnerability of the thalamus, brainstem and basal ganglia during the event. The current hypothesis is that peculiarities of neuronal function in the perinatal period can predispose to ischaemic damage. Whatever the exact mechanism, it is cardiac arrest or severe bradycardia (Apgar 0 or 1 at one minute) that damages these nuclei (Leech and Alvord 1977). The occasional observation of isolated deep grey matter and brainstem neuronal necrosis sparing cortex and white matter might be explained by abrupt cessation of perfusion and thus autoregulation without pre-existing (forebrain → deep structures) shift. In such situations, metabolic and not vascular factors could determine the end result.

Considering the complexity of cerebro-vascular changes preceding cardiac arrest, it is not surprising that the relevance of post-event alterations of perfusion has not been delineated. This contrasts with the better description of a reperfusion penumbra in focal arterial cerebral infarction (Macfarlane *et al.* 1991, Garcia 1992, Siesjö 1992). In the latter context, reperfusion of an infarcted area within four to eight hours can be expected to improve the final outcome, although it might also contribute to secondary oedema and free radical injury thus acting as a two-edged sword. Following global experimental brain ischaemia, an early (within minutes) and brief period of general reactive hyperaemia has been recorded (Pryds 1991). In paralysed ventilated piglets disconnected from the ventilator until bradycardic (<80 bpm) with a pH around 7.1, regional flow to thalamus and brainstem remained higher than baseline from onset of asphyxia well into the stage of recovery (Coplerud *et al.* 1989). If reactive hyperaemia exists in human birth asphyxia, one could expect haemorrhagic necrosis in thalamus, parasagittal cortex, striatum or brainstem within hours of the event.

Better defined is the 'no reflow' or vasospastic period probably affecting all brain areas for several hours (Levene 1988). During this period there is a gradual accumulation of intracellular oedema peaking on days 2 and 3, usually coinciding with intracranial hypertension.

After this stage a third one, referred to as 'luxury perfusion', occurs, detectable with Doppler ultrasound by finding a low resistance index (Lupton *et al.* 1988; Levene 1989; Gluckman *et al.* 1991; Williams *et al.* 1991, 1993). A late second period of hypoperfusion has been documented after this hyperaemic stage (Volpe *et al.* 1985, Mujsce *et al.* 1990). One major conclusion from extensive experimental work and clinical observation is that the delayed intracellular oedema reflects already established neuronal ischaemia and does not play an important role in its genesis (Vannucci *et al.* 1992). This has in part abolished steroid use in that context.

Recent animal experiments have focused on interruption of the cascade of neuronal events triggered by asphyxia through the use of drugs to control excitotoxic injury and free oxygen radical damage and to preserve normal ion flux across the cell's membrane (reviewed by Volpe 1987, Levene 1988, Hill and Volpe 1989, Vannucci 1990*b*, Peliowski and Finer 1992, Kogure *et al.* 1993, Palmer and Vannucci 1993). More might conceivably be gained by correct interpretation of the early signs of fetal distress and subsequent administration of drugs to the mother to manipulate fetal systemic and cerebral blood flow during parturition.

149

Clinical setting

The main obstetric antecedents of status marmoratus and asphyxial deep grey matter necrosis recognized in the living newborn infant are compared in Table 8.14. Similarities again warrant linkage of both nosological entities. Severe umbilical cord compression and abruptio placentae seem to be common causes, but mechanical problems during delivery are still contributing to severe intrapartum asphyxia of this type.

The severity of the initial insult is reflected in the very low Apgar score at one minute (usually 0 or 1). Actual cardiac arrest is common but not obligatory. Sylvester (1960) referred to the initial state of 'white asphyxia'. Delayed onset of initial breathing for at least 15 minutes in infants with echo-bright thalami was observed by Shen *et al.* (1986). The marked degree of early systemic metabolic acidosis in the course of these case histories was stressed by Voit *et al.* (1987).

Presenting features and temporary changes during the first days after severe birth asphyxia or postnatal cardiac arrest have been dealt with at length in several recent papers (Volpe 1987, Hill and Volpe 1989, Levene *et al.* 1989, Perlman 1989, Peliowski and Finer 1992). A misleading period of improvement has been described in the first hours after the event, with striking alertness and peculiar periodic breathing. After this a downhill course with apnoea progressing to respiratory arrest, intracranial hypertension and gradual loss of brainstem reflexes and cranial nerve function is typical. This dynamic process has been illustrated in case reports by Kotagal *et al.* (1983), Kreusser *et al.* (1984), Voit *et al.* (1987), and Roland *et al.* (1988). A severe grade of clinical encephalopathy—obligatory seizures and very often coma and signs of decerebration (Sarnat stage III)—has been described by all authors on day 2 or 3, when lesions of the basal ganglia have been apparent later in the neonatal period. Rutherford *et al.* (1992) commented on the tremulousness and abnormal feeding behaviour in the late neonatal period.

Radiological assessment

In theory there ought to be three types of haemorrhagic transformation of acutely ischaemic diencephalic and brainstem structures: (i) onset during reactive early hyperaemia → major bleeding within 24 hours; (ii) onset during 'luxury perfusion' → confluent petechial symmetrical haemorrhagic necrosis after 24 hours; (iii) new capillary formation from surrounding vital tissue → post-ischaemic high vascularity after a minimum of three to four days. There is some clinical support for the existence of each type.

At least four term newborn infants with autopsy-confirmed major early haemorrhage in the thalamus and/or basal ganglia had sonographic evidence of bleeding within 24 hours after birth (Kreusser *et al.* 1984, Hokazono *et al.* 1987, Voit *et al.* 1987, Hill and Volpe 1989). Haemorrhagic densities on ultrasound were as dense as bone in thalami and putamen. They spared the internal and external capsules. None of the infants had IVH. At post-mortem examination globi pallidi were haemorrhagic in three of the four, with bleeding in brainstem areas in two.

TABLE 8.14

Aetiology of status marmoratus and neonatal asphyxial damage to diencephalon and basal ganglia

	*Status marmoratus (N=33)**	*Deep grey matter necrosis in life (N=29)***
Birth asphyxia	27	27
Cord: nuchal	3	3
knotted	1	1
prolapsed	3	0
Abruptio placentae	2	7
Mechanical difficulties	15	5
Postnatal cardiac arrest	6	2

*Norman (1947), Malamud (1950), Sylvester (1960), Schneider *et al.* (1975), Dambska *et al.* (1976), Leech and Alvord (1977).
**Macpherson *et al.* (1969), Shewmon *et al.* (1981), Babcock and Ball (1983), Kotagal *et al.* (1983), Kreusser *et al.* (1984), Slovis *et al.* (1984), Kanarek and Gieron (1986), Okada *et al.* (1986), Shen *et al.* (1986), Voit *et al.* (1987), Colamaria *et al.* (1988), Roland *et al.* (1988), Cabanas *et al.* (1991), Rutherford *et al.* (1992).

The caudate nuclei were spared in all but one infant. CT confirmed diencephalic bleeding at 12 hours in one infant (Hokazono *et al.* 1987). Slit ventricles betrayed associated brain swelling in three: these were resuscitated stillborn infants with an arterial pH <7.0. In two the EEG at 9 and 16 hours was reported to be isoelectric. One other term infant was found collapsed shortly after delivery: at necropsy five days later, florid haemorrhagic necrosis symmetrically affected thalamus, putamen, globus pallidus, cerebral cortex and brainstem from midbrain to medulla (including inferior olives and pontine nuclei) (Leech and Brumback 1988).

Delayed haemorrhagic conversion of affected deep grey matter areas has been claimed repeatedly by the use of ultrasound and MRI without necropsy confirmation (Kotagal *et al.* 1983, Cabanas *et al.* 1991, Keeney *et al.* 1991, Pasternak *et al.* 1991, Rutherford *et al.* 1992). The absence of haemorrhagic density on concurrent uncontrasted CT scan virtually excludes genuine haemorrhage in some infants, although the ideal scanning time may have been missed. In others, opacification of affected areas on uncontrasted CT scan and before expected onset of dystrophic calcification would suggest haemorrhagic necrosis (Shewmon *et al.* 1981, Kotagal *et al.* 1983, Voit *et al.* 1987, Cabanas *et al.* 1991).

CASE 8.5

This firstborn infant presented with the occiput posterior at term and was subsequently delivered by emergency caesarean section after seven failed vacuum tractions (with three cup detachments) and three failed forceps tractions. Apgar scores were 1 and 6 at one and five minutes, and her birthweight was 3520g. Endotracheal ventilation was started at 15 minutes because of hypotonia and pallor. Before referral her arterial pH was 6.79 with a

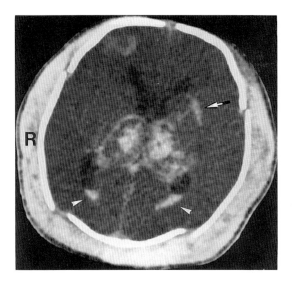

Fig. 8.30. Axial post-mortem scan in Case 8.5 on day 9: note almost symmetrical hyperdensity in thalamus and globus pallidus, left putaminal haemorrhage *(arrow)* and bilateral intraventricular haemorrhage *(arrowheads)*. There is extensive residual subgaleal haemorrhage.

P_aco_2 of 3kPa and a base deficit of 33mmol/L. On admission, hypovolaemic shock was suspected because of a huge subgaleal haemorrhage (occipitofrontal head circumference, 34cm at birth, increased to 41cm within hours). After infusion of 210mL of plasma expander the first systolic blood pressure >40mmHg was recorded 3.5 hours after birth. However, rapidly developing sclerema and persistent pulmonary hypertension were followed by disseminated intravascular (and intra-haematoma) coagulation, renal tubular necrosis, pneumothorax, hypoglycaemia and finally death on day 8 (body weight 7400g, brain weight 900g). Sonography on days 3 and 6 had shown absent diastolic flow in the intracranial arteries, with bilateral thalamic hyperdensity on day 6. The post-mortem CT scan is shown in Figure 8.30. Advanced cerebral softness precluded proper examination but confirmed clotted blood in ventricles and thalami.

These densities symmetrically engage the caudate nucleus, putamen and thalamus from the second week after the event to at least 10 months of age (Colamaria *et al.* 1988). They are fine and soft at first, with unusual linear and nodular appearance in the thalamic area (Fig. 8.30). Although they might in part reflect bleeding in the first two weeks of life, their subsequent persistence and contrast enhancement argue against it. According to Shewmon *et al.* (1981) they represent post-ischaemic hypervascularity and neuronal calcification. These authors also documented enhancement in brainstem areas. Certainly capillary invasion and neuronal encrustation can be endorsed by post-mortem descriptions of this type of injury (Norman 1947, Sylvester 1960, Schneider *et al.* 1975, Dambska *et al.* 1976, Voit *et al.* 1987, Roland *et al.* 1988). In the case of subtotal necrosis, glial reaction could contribute to this remnant density on brain images. Documentation of diencephalic calcium deposits has been achieved with plain X-rays at the end of the first month (Macpherson *et al.* 1969), with CT scan from 14 days on (Kanarek and Gieron 1986) (Fig. 8.31) and with ultrasound by recognition of acoustic shadowing from 13

152

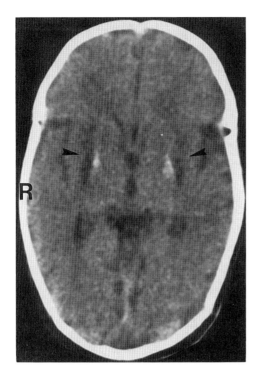

Fig. 8.31. Follow-up uncontrasted CT scan one month after resuscitated stillbirth with severe metabolic acidosis and seizures for several days: note symmetrical hypodensity of putamen, hyperdensity of globi pallidi and dilatation of third ventricle due to thalamic atrophy. There is disproportionate preservation of cerebral white matter and cortex.

days on (Voit *et al*. 1987). Together with disproportionate dilatation of the third ventricle, thalamic calcification can confidently be taken as suggestive of previous severe asphyxia (Roland *et al*. 1988). Residual putaminal lesions on CT were reported by Okada *et al*. (1986).

More descriptions are available of ultrasonographic correlates of diencephalic ischaemia. Both putaminal and thalamic hyperdensity were documented by Babcock and Ball (1983) in infants with abruptio placentae and neonatal seizures. These densities were symmetrical, but clearly less dense than those reported in the abovementioned cases with necropsy-confirmed haemorrhage. They are observed convincingly only from day 3 onwards (Slovis *et al*. 1984, Shen *et al*. 1986, Cabanas *et al*. 1991). Their presence in the thalamus has been confirmed up to seven months of age (Shen *et al*. 1986). The echodensities have a sharp margin, are homogeneous and become brighter as the structure involved shrinks. Sparing of pulvinar (postero-lateral thalamic) neurons may at first create the wrong impression of regional hypodensity (Cabanas *et al*. 1991). Concurrent uncontrasted CT scan might show hypodensity, contrasting with the 'bright thalami' on ultrasound, suggestive of non-haemorrhagic necrosis. Over the past three years I have documented bright thalami and putamina in several infants with severe birth asphyxia (Figs 8.32, 8.33). For a clear description of the anatomy of this region readers are referred to Naidich *et al*. (1986).

153

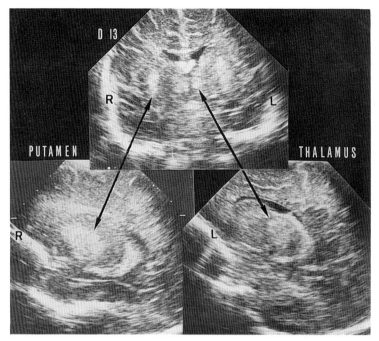

Fig. 8.32. Coronal *(top)* and parasagittal *(bottom)* ultrasound scans on day 13 in patient described in Fig. 8.31: note symmetrical hyperdensity of putamen *(right)* and medial thalamus *(left)*.

CASE 8.6

This firstborn child was delivered at 41 weeks of gestation by vacuum extraction with fundal pressure 45 minutes into the second stage of labour. There had been late fetal heart decelerations and a tight nuchal cord. Feto-placental bleeding was suspected but not proved. Apgar scores were 1 and 3 at one and five minutes; birthweight was 4000g. After bag and mask resuscitation both transcutaneous oxygen saturation and blood pressure were within normal limits. A capillary pH at 2 hours was 6.95, with P_cco_2 of 10kPa and base deficit 15mmol/L. At 3 hours twitching of both feet, lip-smacking and persistence of mixed respiratory and metabolic acidosis prompted endotracheal ventilatory support. Because X-ray indicated a small heart, plasma and additional bicarbonate were administered and he was referred to UZ Gent. The seizures persisted for two days, in spite of a sequential increase in anticonvulsant drug dosage. His encephalopathy was grade III (Sarnat 1976) for several days. There was no intracranial hypertension. In spite of the history he was able to feed normally by 14 days of age. By then his gaze was remarkably alert. Obvious tremor of both hands and the chin persisted until his discharge from hospital at age 3 weeks. On ultrasound (Fig. 8.33) slight brightness of both lateral thalami, sparing the pulvinar, was recorded on day 4, together with normal intracranial arterial flow velocities. Similar densities were not seen in the caudate nuclei. In spite of this the caudate heads underwent cystic change in the second week of life. CT scan on day 4 had shown only subarachnoid haemorrhage. EEG on days 4 and 12 did not show the burst–suppression pattern. Acute hypovolaemic shock and birth asphyxia possibly caused isolated deep grey matter damage in this infant, asymmetrically involving the caudate nuclei.

154

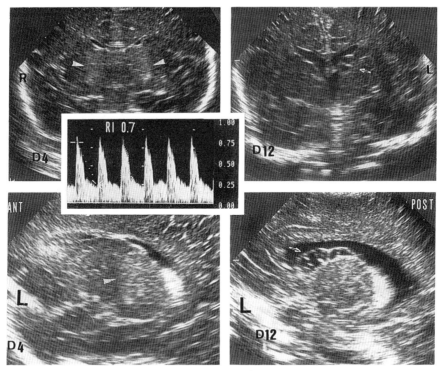

Fig. 8.33. Coronal *(top)* and left parasagittal *(bottom)* ultrasound scans in Case 8.6: *arrowheads* indicate mild thalamic hyperdensity; *arrows* point to cystic necrosis of head of left caudate nucleus in second week. *Inset:* normal Doppler resistance index in middle cerebral artery on day 4.

Though still not yet fully evaluated, there is little doubt that MRI will improve recognition and definition of deep grey matter damage in the neonatal period. Most data, however, do not relate to findings in the first post-event week. Direct comparison of early ultrasound and CT scans with late MRI scans against the pathological 'gold standard' has so far not been possible. Several studies on asphyxial damage from the second week on have referred to haemorrhagic necrosis in thalami, putamina and pallidi (Voit *et al.* 1987, Barkovich and Truwit 1990, De Vries *et al.* 1990, Keeney *et al.* 1991, Steinlin *et al.* 1991, Rutherford *et al.* 1992). This conclusion is based on sequential density changes typical of the temporal behaviour of blood clot (Gomori *et al.* 1985) and characteristic sites of damage. Thus, aberrant MRI densities have been shown to persist beyond infancy. Histological changes rendering interpretation of MRI scans difficult might be: (i) vascular congestion in the first hours; (ii) newly formed capillaries from about four days on after the acute episode; (iii) astroglial proliferation and microglial activation from three to four days on; (iv) neuronal microcalcification from 10 days on (Ellis *et al.* 1988). In the early stages of status marmoratus during infancy,

155

normal myelin formation disorganized by glial scarring may eventually contribute to changes in density on MRI (Friede and Schachenmayr 1977). Deposition of iron in basal ganglia neurons after interruption of their projection to the cerebral cortex has been suggested as an alternative to explain iron deposition in these nuclei in the absence of pre-existing haemorrhage (Dietrich *et al.* 1988).

Neurodevelopmental consequences
Despite apparent complexity, research in this field will add insight into the patterns of birth asphyxia. Recent investigation has confirmed the often gloomy prognosis for intact survival when cardio-pulmonary resuscitation in the delivery room has been needed (Perlman 1992).

Neuropathological confirmation of suggested abnormalities remains very important. Clearly the complexity of neuronal injury will never make birth asphyxia an ideal model for the clinical study of neurological sequelae. It is thought that associated extensive telencephalic damage with ensuing spasticity and severe mental retardation masks the athetotic picture associated with deep grey matter lesions (Volpe 1987). A clinical entity with neonatal hypotonia, infantile hypertonia with tremulousness, acceptable feeding behaviour and later athetoid cerebral palsy has been linked with bilateral cystic necrosis of the putamen (Burton *et al.* 1984, Rutherford *et al.* 1992). Evidence has also been produced that isolated pallidal necrosis will lead to dystonic cerebral palsy (Brun and Kyllerman 1979). MRI density changes in the pallidum throughout infancy might correlate with transient hypotonia, not leaving permanent sequelae (De Vries *et al.* 1990). On the other hand, delay in onset of dyskinetic cerebral palsy after 5 years of age has been traced back to birth asphyxia (Arvidsson and Hagberg 1990).

Cerebellar haemorrhage
Bleeding into cerebellar substance is quite common and well described in the preterm infant (Pape and Wigglesworth 1979, Reeder *et al.* 1982, Perlman *et al.* 1983, Volpe 1987).

Its recognition by ultrasound has been reported from the early 1980s on (Foy *et al.* 1982, Reeder *et al.* 1982), although only major lesions are detectable by this method. The sonograpic presentation and dimensions of structures in and around the posterior fossa have been adequately described by McLeary *et al.* (1984), Yousefzadeh and Naidich (1985), Helmke *et al.* (1987), and more recently Co *et al.* (1991) and Ichyama and Hayashi (1991). With CT scanning the lesions are easily detected, but coronal images are necessary to clarify the precise anatomical location (Scotti *et al.* 1981).

Both techniques together also made it possible to delineate some patterns of cerebellar haemorrhage in the term newborn infant (Table 8.15). Scotti *et al.* (1981) diagnosed four cerebellar haemorrhages in 91 infants with intracranial haemorrhage on CT scan and birthweight ≥2500g; Welch and Strand (1986) mentioned four instances in 24 term infants with traumatic intracranial haemorrhage; and

TABLE 8.15

Types of intracerebellar haemorrhage in the term newborn infant

1. Contusion due to occipital birth injury
2. Dissection of a major central tentorial haemorrhage into the superior cerebellar vermis
3. (Confluent) petechial haemorrhage in disturbances of coagulation
4. Associated with organic aciduria
5. During ECMO
6. Unspecified

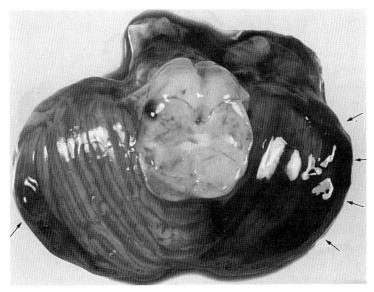

Fig. 8.34. Contusional damage *(arrows)* of surface of cerebellum in infant with occipital osteodiastasis and fatal liver trauma.

Sachs *et al.* (1987) recorded one cerebellar and 11 other intracranial haemorrhages in 23,000 term liveborn infants (the infant with cerebellar haemorrhage was delivered normally after a second stage lasting four hours).

The first type of cerebellar haemorrhage at term is associated with *occipital osteodiastasis* (Hemsath 1934, Wigglesworth and Husemeyer 1977). Both the anterior bony margin of the occipital squama as it is pushed into the posterior fossa and the retrocerebellar subdural haemorrhage associated with severe cases can cause contusional damage to the postero-inferior cerebellar surface (Fig. 8.34).

The second type, also associated with birth trauma, is described in its characteristic presentation and recognized on coronal CT scan by Scotti *et al.*

157

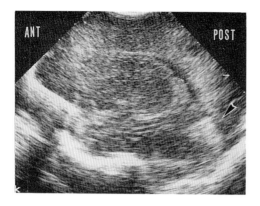

Fig. 8.35. Parasagittal ultrasound scan on day 6 in infant with temporal lobe haematoma and thrombocytopenia (Case 8.1): *arrowhead* points to CT-confirmed haemorrhage in left cerebellar hemisphere.

(1981), Menezes *et al.* (1983), Welch and Strand (1986) and De Campo (1989). Subdural haematoma collecting in the cisterna ambiens after *central tentorial trauma* or rupture of a cerebellar bridging vein can compress and displace the cerebellar vermis from above. The brainstem can be bowed forward when the haemorrhage is extensive (De Campo 1989). This kind of cerebellar injury can follow normal, breech or instrumental delivery.

A third variety is linked with some form of *haemorrhagic diathesis*, be it: (i) DIC, as seen in one infant with birth asphyxia, immune hydrops and frontal subarachnoid haematoma (Chessells and Wigglesworth 1970), and in a second with staphylococcal meningo-encephalitis (Larroche 1977); (ii) vitamin K deficiency (Chaou *et al.* 1984); or (iii) thrombocytopenia, as seen in Case 8.1 (Fig. 8.35). As in the preterm infant, the first lesions are perivascular and petechial in the subarachnoid, pial or cortical areas, but confluent large haemorrhages have been reported.

Three term newborn infants with *organic aciduria* (isovaleric, methylmalonic and propionic respectively), sudden neurological deterioration and apnoea due to either extensive symmetrical subarachnoid or unilateral parenchymal cerebellar haemorrhage have been described by Fischer *et al.* (1981) and Dave *et al.* (1984). The pathogenesis was possibly related to thrombocytopenia, but preceding exchange transfusion, bicarbonate infusion or hypoxia and metabolic acidosis might have been contributory in addition to a suggested specific metabolic vermal haemorrhagic necrosis. In the case described by Fischer *et al.* (1981) upward cerebellar herniation was the probable cause of death.

The fifth pattern was recently described in term infants under ECMO (Bulas *et al.* 1991). Interestingly, the haematomas in that setting are unilateral hemispheric, large, and remain hypodense on ultrasound during the phase of anticoagulation.

Finally, some parenchymal intracerebellar haemorrhages are *not classifiable* amongst the previous groups. Such a bleeding described by Toma *et al.* 1990, presented with pallor, tremor and hypotonia 24 hours after uneventful delivery of a

TABLE 8.16

Perinatal forms of brainstem haemorrhage*

1. Associated with mechanical birth trauma
2. Cardiac arrest type of ischaemic damage to diencephalic and brainstem structures, especially reticular formation
3. Focal infarcts
4. Petechial disseminated bleeding
5. Pial haemorrhage
6. Tumour
7. Vascular anomaly
8. Unspecified pathogenesis

term male. Subsequent development of a cerebellar cyst communicating with the fourth ventricle was documented by the use of ultrasound. These intracerebellar alterations must be differentiated from cavitary changes within peritentorial haemorrhages (Huang and Shen 1991).

Case history
CASE 8.7
This firstborn boy was born uneventfully at 37 weeks gestation. His mother was a tobacco smoker. The first stage lasted 13 hours, the second 20 minutes. Apgar scores were 7 and 10 at one and five minutes. His birthweight was 2700g and head circumference 34cm. He needed emergency ventilatory support after four hours because of unexplained apnoea. He was hypotonic, but showed repetitive unusual leg movements. The fontanelle felt normal. There was metabolic acidosis (base deficit 12mmol/L), hyponatraemia, anaemia (haemoglobin 12g/dL) and a serum fibrinogen of 0.6g/L with a normal platelet count. Primary haemostatic disorders were excluded and salicylates were undetectable in serum. Ultrasound showed a density in the upper cerebellar area. CT scan on day 3 confirmed the presence of a hetero-geneous parenchymal cerebellar density with moderate dilatation of the supratentorial ventricles. MRI on day 20 confirmed the cerebellar haematoma, and demonstrated dilatation and displacement of the fourth ventricle and remnant densities in the ambient cistern. In spite of transient stabilization with serial lumbar punctures and acetazolamide–furosemide treatment, ensuing post-haemorrhagic hydrocephalus required shunting on day 70. MRI and colour Doppler flow imaging both failed to reveal an underlying vascular anomaly. Direct angiography was debated but not undertaken.

Perinatal brainstem haemorrhage
Types of possible haemorrhages within midbrain, pons or medulla are listed in Table 8.16. Some items, like damage to diencephalon and brainstem in the 'cardiac arrest' type of acute asphyxia, occipital osteodiastasis, tumour and vascular anomaly are discussed separately. Ischaemic lesions are included because of their possible conversion to haemorrhage.

Traumatic brainstem damage
This type of injury to the hindbrain has been well described. Two classical patterns

TABLE 8.17

Brainstem haemorrhage due to birth trauma

Injury	Mode of delivery	
	Breech	Cephalic forceps
Occipital osteodiastasis	+++	++
Cerebellar herniation	++	++
Torsion	++[1]	++
Elongation/traction/stretch	+++	+[2]
Compression from flexion/extension	++	+
Lateroflexion	++	+++[3]
Arterial occlusion	++	++

+++ Typical; ++ common; + rare.
[1]Especially if forceps applied to aftercoming head.
[2]Isolated cases reported.
[3]On delivery of shoulders.

that lead to it are occipital osteodiastasis (see Chapter 6) and brain swelling with cerebellar herniation and haemorrhage of the pons around the foramen magnum (Pryse-Davies and Beard 1973, Larroche 1977). In addition the brainstem can be damaged by: (i) excessive traction or elongation of the nuchal region, forcing the brainstem and inferior cerebellum down into the foramen magnum and causing surface injury: (ii) compression of the brainstem at the foramen magnum due to abnormal antero-posterior flexion or extension of the neck; (iii) lateroflexion or torsion with either subsequent haemorrhage into the posterior columns of the medulla and the dorsal nerve roots, or stretch injury of the cerebellar peduncles (Table 8.17) (Towbin 1964, Yates 1973, Larroche 1977, Reid 1983). Finally, trauma to the vertebral artery or its branches, registered in about 15 per cent of perinatal autopsies when carefully checked, could lead to focal infarction of brainstem, posterior cerebrum or cerebellum (Yates 1959, 1973; Reid 1983). The well-known severe cord damage in breech or rotational forceps delivery is not covered in this study of intracranial lesions. Suffice it to say that even in spontaneous cephalic delivery damage to the cord and medulla has been reported on occasion, as a rule affecting the upper cord and brainstem rather than the cervico-thoracic spinal cord as in breech delivery (reviews in Shulman *et al.* 1971, Yates 1973). It is not unthinkable for axial ultrasound images to be capable of displaying haemorrhage into the upper brainstem, depending on the image quality (Helmke *et al.* 1987).

Disseminated petechial haemorrhage
As previously described (see p. 106), severe cerebro-venous congestion can lead to dispersed perivascular haemorrhages throughout the CNS. Larroche (1977) refers to asphyxia and immune fetal hydrops as main causes. Their presence in the

160

reticular formation of pons and medulla was acknowledged by pathologists before the Second World War (Holland 1937, Kehrer 1939). Though they were blamed for transient or permanent—often fatal—damage to the respiratory centres (Hirvensalo 1949), it is more likely that these punctiform lesions are agonal consequence rather than cause (Morison 1963). Their appearance is similar in asphyxial states and following difficult labour, as reviewed by Yates (1973).

Primary brainstem haemorrhage of unspecified cause
At least one term newborn infant recently reported seems to have suffered from major brainstem haemorrhage without a clear-cut pattern of injury (Blazer *et al.* 1989). This boy was delivered normally at 42 weeks gestation and immediately ventilated because of meconium aspiration. Apgar scores were 4 and 8 at one and five minutes. His birthweight was 3600g. Hypotonia of the legs was recorded in the delivery room. Bilateral diaphragmatic paralysis was documented on fluoroscopy within the first hours of life and necessitated continuing endotracheal support. The initially present sucking reflex disappeared at about 14 hours. On day 10 appearances compatible with a large brainstem haemorrhage were noted on CT scan, in the region of the upper medulla and lower pons. Clinical examination in the first weeks added evidence of damage to the hypoglossal nuclei, and fibrillation in the trapezius and sterno-cleido-mastoid muscles on EMG suggested accessory nucleus involvement as well. He was weaned from the ventilator at 3 months, but adequate diaphragmatic excursions were not established until the end of the first year. Gross motor development was retarded. According to Blazer *et al.* diaphragmatic palsy in this patient may have been caused by brainstem damage within the lower pons and upper medulla.

9
DIFFERENTIAL DIAGNOSIS: VASCULAR ANOMALIES

The various ways in which vascular intracranial anomalies manifest themselves in the newborn period are listed in Table 9.1.

Fetal brain damage recognized before or after birth can be secondary to hereditary proliferative vasculopathy leading to aqueductal stenosis and extreme hydrocephalus (Fowler *et al.* 1972, Harper and Hockey 1983), to posterior fossa leptomeningeal thickening with dilatation of all ventricles (Norman *et al.* 1981), or to cerebral hypoperfusion and postnecrotic calcification associated with a vein of Galen aneurysm (Norman and Becker 1974, Perez-Fontan *et al.* 1982).

Recently, non-immune fetal hydrops was added to the clinical spectrum of vein of Galen aneurysm (Ordorica *et al.* 1990, Strauss *et al.* 1991).

It can be anticipated that given a carefully documented family history one may diagnose silent anomalies in asymptomatic newborn infants by the use of colour Doppler ultrasound or MRI. Familial occurrence of arterio-venous malformations has been well documented in Ehlers–Danlos syndrome type IV, in Weber–Rendu–Osler syndrome, and as an isolated phenomenon. The orocutaneous telangiectatic dots typical of adults with Weber–Rendu–Osler disease can be a hint towards diagnosis in their newborn offspring. Anamnestic findings of relevance are subarachnoid cerebral haemorrhage in children or young adults, haemorrhage from pulmonary arterio-venous malformation, recurrent epistaxis and easy bruising.

In some newborn infants, cutaneous vascular lesions prompt a search for intracranial vascular anomalies: disseminated (miliary) haemangiomatosis (Holden and Alexander 1970, Heudes *et al.* 1990), extensive vascular hamartomatosis (Arienzo *et al.* 1987), cavernous haemangioma of the skin (Burns *et al.* 1991), Sturge–Weber disease, arteriectasis with subcutaneous arterial thrombosis (Ferry *et al.* 1974), engorged facial or periorbital veins in vein of Galen aneurysm, Wyburn–Mason syndrome (Patel and Gupta 1990), linear sebaceus naevus syndrome (Nuno *et al.* 1990) and von Hippel–Lindau angiomatosis (Larroche 1977).

The Kasabach–Merritt syndrome, even in the absence of dermatological signs, can point to hidden visceral and cerebral vascular anomalies (Holden and Alexander 1970, Ibarguen *et al.* 1988).

Congestive heart failure is characteristic of aneurysm of the vein of Galen or of large arterio-venous malformations without aneurysmal varix.

Some arterial aneurysms (Thompson and Pribram 1969, Pickering *et al.* 1970) and angiomas (Scott *et al.* 1992) will interfere with CSF circulation or cause focal neurological signs.

162

TABLE 9.1

**Clinical presentation of neonatal vascular
intracranial anomalies**

1. Prenatal brain damage, non-immune hydrops
2. Typical family history
3. Suggestive cutaneous anomalies
4. Kasabach–Merritt syndrome
5. Congestive heart failure
6. Mass effect within the brain
7. Intracranial haemorrhage

Finally, acute neurological dysfunction due to subarachnoid (either in one sylvian fissure or over the base of the brain), intraventricular or intraparenchymal haemorrhage can be due to rupture of an arterial aneurysm or to bleeding from an arterio-venous malformation, or be associated with microangiomatosis of the basal ganglia or with vein of Galen aneurysm (Fig. 9.1).

According to a recent review (Gordon and Isler 1989), the (alternating) hemiplegia typical of moyamoya disease has not been described in the perinatal period. Hemimegalencephaly can present with evidence of neonatal intracranial arterio-venous shunting without actual delineation of a vascular malformation (Walters *et al.* 1990). It is thought that diffuse cerebral dysplasia in this syndrome is associated with increased hemicerebral perfusion.

Arterial aneurysm
There have been several reports of rupture of a 'berry' aneurysm within the neonatal period and in early infancy. It has been documented in association with occipital encephalocele and cerebellar hypoplasia, agenesis of the corpus callosum (Garcia-Chavez and Moossy 1965), Weber–Rendu–Osler disease (Roy *et al.* 1990) and generalized arteriectasis (Ferry *et al.* 1974).

Two major patterns of haemorrhage characterize aneurysmal rupture, each occurring in about half the reported cases: near the midline, and on a peripheral branch.

If the sac is close to or on the circle of Willis, the subarachnoid blood collection will mainly affect the base of the brain and for some unspecified reason can be associated with intraventricular haemorrhage (Pickering *et al.* 1970, Lee *et al.* 1978). The initial signs are apnoea, focal or general seizures and intracranial hypertension. In addition, the site of the aneurysm, *e.g.* on the posterior inferior cerebellar artery (Pickering *et al.* 1970) may cause specific damage, *e.g.* due to compression and haemorrhagic necrosis of the medulla with ensuing respiratory arrest. Ventricular dilatation can lead to uncal herniation (Pickering *et al.* 1970).

When the sac is situated on a peripheral branch of the middle cerebral artery, a dome-shaped almost nodular haematoma will fill the arachnoid space in one sylvian fissure (Grode *et al.* 1978, Hungerford *et al.* 1981, McLellan *et al.* 1986, Roy *et al.*

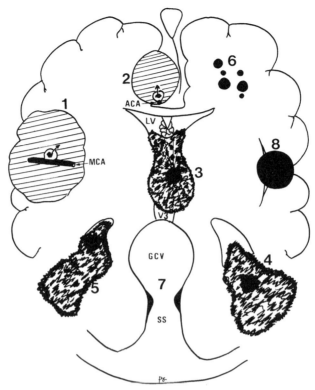

Fig. 9.1. Diagram indicating several vascular anomalies leading to neonatal intracranial haemorrhage: (1) rupture of a saccular aneurysm on a peripheral branch of the middle cerebral artery (MCA) with focal fronto-temporo-parietal subarachnoid haematoma; (2) rupture of a saccular aneurysm on a peripheral branch of the anterior cerebral artery (ACA) with focal interfrontal supracallosal subarachnoid haematoma; (3) thalamic and third ventricle (V3) haemorrhage from a midline arterio-venous malformation (AVM); (4) haemorrhage from a transcerebral AVM; (5) ruptured choroid plexus AVM; (6) multiple nodular lesions as in disseminated haemangiomatosis; (7) midline aneurysmal varix (GCV = great cerebral vein; SS = straight sinus); (8) lateral aneurysmal varix.

1990). Infants affected in this way can present with sudden pallor, inconsolable and loud crying, vomiting, sweatiness, focal clonic and/or general tonic fits, irritability and a tense fontanelle. Associated bleeding in the eye fundus, not necessarily unilateral, could raise suspicion of intracranial non-accidental shaking injury (McLellan *et al.* 1986) (Fig. 9.2). The cerebral ventricles can be normal but shifted by the haemorrhage or filled with blood after transcerebral dissection of the haematoma (Roy *et al.* 1990). In the latter infant a secondary arterial vasospastic episode was another suggested feature. The CT pictures of such unilateral subarachnoid haematomas are identical (Hungerford *et al.* 1981, McLellan *et al.* 1986): they are well-circumscribed, homogeneous and rounded opacities with a thin rim of attenuated brain substance where they border the skull. Differentiation has

164

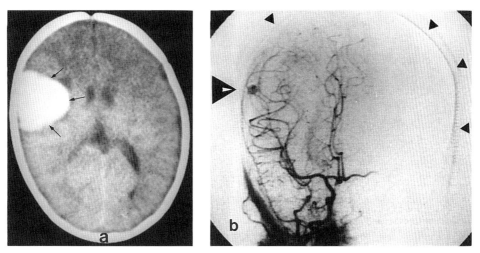

Fig. 9.2. CT scan *(left)* of 6-week-old girl with suspected non-accidental shaking injury: focal right fronto-parietal haematoma; corresponding angiogram *(right)* demonstrates aneurysm in distal ascending frontal branch of right middle cerebral artery. (McLellan *et al.* 1986, by permission.)

to be made from lobar temporal haemorrhage or a ruptured arterio-venous malformation. Treatment of a symptomatic lesion by complete resection has been successful (Grode *et al.* 1978).

Involvement of (a branch of) the anterior cerebral artery will lead to an interhemispheric haematoma above the corpus callosum (Frank and Zusman 1991).

Ferry *et al.* (1974) described a term male infant with varicosities on trunk and left arm, who presented with non-specific signs at age 6 weeks: fever, irritability, vomiting and restlessness. At 3 months the child was found semi-comatose with fever, right oculomotor nerve palsy, intracranial hypertension and right retinal haemorrhage. Lumbar CSF was blood-stained, and angiography revealed bilateral fusiform ectasia of the internal and external carotid arteries together with a large aneurysm of the basilar artery and additional ones on both posterior cerebral arteries. In spite of shunting for post-haemorrhagic hydrocephalus he died at 5 months of age. Post-mortem findings included aneurysmal dilatation of mesenteric, renal and iliac arteries with thrombosed subcutaneous arterial aneurysms. The actual site of the second haemorrhage was not mentioned. The inner part of the degenerated muscle media was replaced by myxoid tissue, and some fragmentation of the internal elastic membrane was also recorded. Menkes' disease was appropriately ruled out.

Arterio-venous malformation
In young infants the brain is the most common site of an arterio-venous

TABLE 9.2

TABLE 9.2
Characteristics of arterio-venous malformation vs. cavernous angioma*

	Arterio-venous malformation	*Cavernous angioma*
Vessels involved	Arteries, veins, arterialized transition vessels	Sinusoid capillary-like vessels with honeycomb appearance
Interstitial brain tissue	Rare glial cells	Absent
Hypertrophied feeding artery	Present	Absent
Dilated tortuous draining veins	Present	Possible
Angiography	Shows up unless thrombosed or recent bleeding	Occult, unless by prolonged contrast administration
Danger of haemorrhage (surgery or biopsy)	Present	Almost absent
Treatment	Excision if small and accessible; initial embolization if large	Excision if accessible

*Both can contain evidence of haemorrrhage, thrombosis and calcification on CT and MRI scan; angiography warranted for management of arterio-venous malformation, not cavernous angioma.

malformation (AVM), superceding hepatic and pulmonary localization (Knudson and Alden 1979). The anomaly is a mixture of hypertrophied arteries feeding into arterialized veins and drained by dilated tortuous veins without interposition of a capillary network. Small lesions arc fed by arteries with a proper function in the perfusion of brain substance distal to the AVM (vessels '*en passage*') (Stein and Wolfert 1980, Mohr *et al.* 1989). Up to 50 per cent of adult AVMs present with haemorrhage, most often intracerebral (around two-thirds of the cases) or subarachnoid (*ca.* one-third), with intraventricular bleeding in about 5 per cent only. The frequency of haemorrhage seems greater in small AVMs, and its risk is increased by location near the midline with central venous drainage and coverage by ependyma only, especially in the face of associated downstream venous obstruction (Miyasaka *et al.* 1992). Intranidus arterial aneurysm formation is also thought to increase the risk of haemorrhage (Arai *et al.* 1972). Most authors agree that, once bleeding has occurred, the chance of recurrence is high enough to warrant intervention (see review by Stein and Wolfert 1980).

Haemorrhagic stroke in childhood is often due to rupture within an arterio-venous anomaly, in contrast with the adult population where rupture of a saccular aneurysm is much more common (Hourihan *et al.* 1984, Mohr *et al.* 1989). Between one and two infants per 1000 livebirths probably carry an intracranial AVM, but clinical presentation in the neonatal period is rare.

Table 9.2 contrasts the characteristics of cavernous angioma with those of AVM. I could find only one report of a neonate with symptoms related to cavernous angioma in the literature (Prensky and Gado 1973). This concerned a boy with a swollen left eye and dilated pupil on day 10; he became irritable and

TABLE 9.3

Classification of perinatal arterio-venous brain anomalies

1. *Isolated arterio-venous fistulae* (vein of Galen varix, direct fistulae to another sinus or varix formation of a cerebral vein)

2. *Cerebral arterio-venous malformation (AVM)* (with deep venous drainage and possibly dilated great cerebral vein)
   —transcerebral
   —deep: small AVM
            large AVM (microangiomatosis)

3. *Choroid plexus AVM*
   —third ventricle (see p. 168)
   —lateral ventricle

4. *Cerebellar AVM*

5. *Brainstem AVM*

6. *Dural AVM*

started vomiting. Angiography documented a vascular malformation with sluggish circulation fed by the left internal and external carotid arteries. This cavernous angioma extended from the orbita into the middle cranial fossa. The anomaly regressed under steroid treatment and had disappeared on repeat angiograph at 8 months. The child was left with visual deficit of the left eye.

Table 9.3 presents an attempt at classification of relevant arterio-venous anomalies. Varix-forming midline fistulae will be discussed separately. The topographical distribution of AVMs seems to be proportional to the brain volume of that region, so that for instance the frontal lobes—roughly accounting for 30 per cent of brain mass—will carry 30 per cent of the malformations.

Transcerebral AVM is used to describe the wedge-shaped anomaly that extends from brain surface to ventricle margin (tip of the pyramid pointing to the ventricle). Its usual location is at the borderzone between major cerebral arteries. Feeding vessels belong to both their superficial and deep branches. This anatomical property can help in differentiating haemorrhage in AVM from lobar parenchymal bleeding. Drainage is via deep (*e.g.* internal cerebral) or cortical (*e.g.* middle cerebral) veins or a major sinus. Presentation in the newborn infant is usually dramatic, with intracranial hypertension, uncal herniation and coma (Beatty 1974, Hanigan 1990*a*, Uno *et al.* 1990). One should suspect bleeding from a giant AVM in infants with extensive cerebral haemorrhage and associated intraventricular or extracerebral haemorrhage. Complete removal of the lesion is possible in early infancy (Beatty 1974, Uno *et al.* 1990). Spontaneous obliteration of the arterio-venous shunt was accompanied by profound psychomotor retardation in the infant reported by Hanigan *et al.* (1990*a*).

Deep AVM may be the primary lesion in term newborn infants with intraventricular haemorrhage (Schum *et al.* 1979, Needell *et al.* 1983, Alonso *et al.* 1984, Heafner *et al.* 1985). In those reports, three of four children for whom birthweight was mentioned were macrosomic (birthweight >4000g), a finding also noted in infantile presentation of deep para-midline AVM (Ghram *et al.* 1988). These infants presented with uncontrollable crying and irritability (4/4), vomiting (2/4), intracranial hypertension (2/4) and hypertonia with hyperreflexia (3/4). Seizures were tonic, clonic or subtle, Acute ventricular distension may cause nystagmus and failure of upward gaze. Lumbar CSF will be blood-stained. If located within the roof of the third ventricle (possibly in choroid tissue), the brunt of haematoma formation will be in that ventricle, with relative sparing of the lateral ones (Schum *et al.* 1979, Heafner *et al.* 1985). Direct (Schum *et al.* 1979) or digital subtraction (Heafner *et al.* 1985) angiograms reveal the anomaly with its feeding posterior choroidal artery and its draining non-varicose internal or great cerebral vein. Non-involvement of the caudate nuclei, and absence of subependymal haemorrhage and of deep venous thrombosis will guide in differentiation from thalamo-ventricular haemorrhage.

A frontal transcallosal approach has been used with success for surgical resection (Heafner *et al.* 1985).

Congestive heart failure was the presenting sign in two infants reported by Needell *et al.* (1983), with AVM in the roof of the third ventricle and thalamus, drained by a dilated vein to a vein of Galen varix. On coronal ultrasound scan this angioma invaded the roof of the midline varix and third ventricle. The presence of direct arterio-venous fistulae into the varix was not commented on.

Two unrelated newborn infants with 'microangiomatosis of the basal ganglia' were reported by Alonso *et al.* (1984). Lenticulo-striate branches of the left middle cerebral artery fed these vascular malformations, predominantly drained by the basal vein. At surgery, a mass of gliotic tissue and newly formed vessels was removed from the left thalamic region in both infants. The angiographic appearance of microangioma, as suggested by Gerlach (1969), is of small, spotty, almost homogeneous areas of contrast uptake associated with small spherically coiled vessels and abnormal venous structures. Although the rarity of these lesions precludes formal conclusions, they may well be a distinct entity within the field of deep AVMs.

Choroid plexus AVM in the inferior horn of a lateral ventricle caused subarachnoid and cerebral haemorrhage in a male infant within the first hours of life (Wakai *et al.* 1990). The child presented with apnoeic spells and was noted to have signs of intracranial hypertension. On the second day of life he underwent surgery following documentation of a midline shift and intracerebral haemorrhage on CT. A vascular nodule ($2 \times 1 \times 0.5$cm) was removed from the centre of the cerebral haemorrhage. The neurological status at 7 months was described as normal. The neonatal choroid plexus angiomas described by Doe *et al.* (1972) are less convincing: they occurred symmetrically in two out of three newborn infants suffering from lethal cardiac anomalies or dying after major abdominal surgery, and the angiomas were not visible with the naked eye within the large glomi of the lateral ventricle choroid plexus.

Dural arteries feed about 10 to 15 per cent of supratentorial AVMs in adults, and almost half of posterior fossa AVMs (Newton and Cronqvist 1969). The feeders involved are branches of external (middle meningeal and occipital) and internal carotid (marginal tentorial) arteries, as well as meningeal tributaries from the posterior cerebral artery. The clinical features of dural AVM in infancy have been reviewed by Obrador *et al.* (1975) and Leland Albright *et al.* (1985). Presentation is with heart failure, ventriculomegaly due to venous hypertension, distended occipital scalp veins, cranial bruit, seizures and subarachnoid haemorrhage. In spite of attempted treatment by bilateral external carotid artery ligation, a supratentorial dural AVM with huge intracranial varix ended with early death due to heart failure in one infant (Gordon *et al.* 1977). Dural AVM may cause subarachnoid, subdural and intracerebral haemorrhage. A 500g fresh clot in a distended torcular varix mimicked posterior fossa haematoma in a term newborn boy, birthweight 4470g, with marked hydrocephalus (head circumference 47.5cm) and heart failure obvious from birth (Ross *et al.* 1986). The lesion made the brainstem bow forward underneath the frontal lobes, in spite of which the aqueduct was patent. An occipital dural malformation communicated with the straight sinus without involvement of the vein of Galen. Therapeutic possibilities and pitfalls on managing dural AVM were reviewed by the authors of the latter case history.

Diffuse neonatal haemangiomatosis
This disorder of unknown cause usually presents at birth with disseminated small bright red cutaneous angiomas, ranging in diameter from 0.1 to 2.5cm (Holden and Alexander 1970). The larger lesions are raised. In order to diagnose this condition at least three different internal organ tissues have to be affected by these capillary hamartomas with absence of pericytes (Burman *et al.* 1967). Heudes *et al.* (1990) reviewed 43 reported instances with the typical skin lesions. Presenting features included: (i) congestive heart failure usually in association with liver angiomas and cholestasis (Burman *et al.* 1967, Robinson and Hambleton 1977); (ii) mucosal haemorrhage presenting as faecal blood loss or haematuria; and (iii) Kasabach–Merritt syndrome (Holden and Alexander 1970). The condition has been diagnosed in association with a rare combination of midline anomalies: absent corpus callosum, ectopia cordis and abdominal midline raphe (Geller *et al.* 1991). Intracranial angiomas were reported in 13 of the infants, in association with focal neurological deficit, hydrocephalus or haemorrhage (Burman *et al.* 1967, Holden and Alexander 1970).

The erratic distribution of the lesions described defies topographical systematization, as they can be found in the cerebrum (8/43), cerebellum (5/43), choroid plexus, meninges, cranial nerves and spinal cord. The anomalies show up during angiography, can be traced within the intestines by technetium-99m pertechnetate isotope scanning and within the brain by contrasted CT or MRI scanning. In addition to symptomatic cardiac treatment, steroids have been advocated repeatedly where there is congestive heart failure, cholestasis, major mucosal

169

haemorrhage or widespread intralesional coagulation (Robinson and Hambleton 1977, Ibarguen *et al.* 1988, Özsoylu *et al.* 1989, Byard *et al.* 1991).

The cerebellar and cerebral angiomatous lesions described in a newborn infant with von Hippel–Lindau disease are akin to those of disseminated haemangiomatosis (Larroche 1977).

Hereditary haemorrhagic telangiectasia (Weber–Rendu–Osler disease)

Typical presentation of this autosomal dominant small venule disease is with recurrent epistaxis in the second or third decade of life. Punctate well-marginated flat red telangiectatic lesions, not always fading on compression, or raised pinhead angiomas cover the lips, palms, tongue, nasal mucosa and palate. These dermatological features can appear from early childhood on, but are very rare in the neonatal period. Snyder and Doan (1944) described a child with multiple large cutaneous telangiectasias obvious at birth, whose father and mother had the typical orocutaneous features. The child died at 2.5 months of age and telangiectasia in the floor of the fourth ventricle was documented at necropsy. A newborn infant presenting with ruptured berry aneurysm has been described above (Roy *et al.* 1990). Boynton and Morgan (1973) reported a well-documented family history in a newborn infant with congestive heart failure and early neonatal death from a vein of Galen varix fed by both posterior cerebral arteries and branches of anterior and middle cerebral arteries as well. An identical observation by Salazar *et al.* (1987) concerned an infant with a telangiectatic lesion on the lower lip, who presented with heart failure in the second week of life. His father had typical dermatological features. Survival was achieved following clipping of the feeding arteries at 4 weeks of age.

Cavernous angioma

Cavernous (haem)angiomas can be found almost everywhere in the brain and orbits (Yamasaki *et al.* 1986). They consist of sinusoid vessels with a single layer of endothelial cells, without a muscle media or elastica and not interposed by neural or glial tissue. These lesions tend to grow by recurrent bleeding and endothelialization of previous cystic haemorrhage remnants. Recognition with CT and especially MRI scanning is based on the absence of straightforward contrast enhancement, the presence of calcification (CT) and of old haemorrhage enclosing a rounded mass (haemosiderin on MRI) (Gomori *et al.* 1986, Rigamonti *et al.* 1987, Scott *et al.* 1992) (see Table 9.2). Some ring enhancement can be seen after prolonged contrast perfusion.

One of the youngest children reported with a purely intracranial cavernous angioma was 2 months old when he presented with macrocephaly and a calcified mass on top of the cerebellar tent (Yamasaki *et al.* 1986). The lesion was excised with good result.

An orbital mass extending into the left middle cranial fossa was described in a neonate presenting at 10 days of age with swelling of the left eye and a dilated pupil

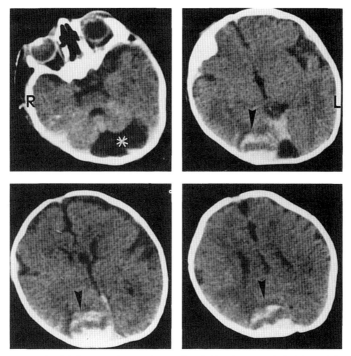

Fig. 9.3. Uncontrasted axial CT scans in case 9.1 on day 6, showing rounded right occipital hyperdensity attached to straight sinus *(arrowheads)*, right temporal lobe subpial haemorrhage *(arrow)*, retro-cerebellar cystic structure *(asterisk)* and absent corpus callosum.

(Prensky and Gado 1973). Angiography on day 21, performed because of irritability and vomiting, showed a lesion with sluggish circulation, perfused by normal arterial branches from the left internal and external carotid arteries and with large draining veins. Opacification did not occur until in the capillary and venous phase. After several months of systemic steroid treatment, the mass had disappeared on repeat angiography at 8 months, leaving the left eye amblyopic.

Venous angioma
Although I could trace no report of venous angioma diagnosed *in vivo* in the neonatal period, a personal case suggests that it may rarely be encountered.

Case history
CASE 9.1
This girl was referred following term delivery at home with birth asphyxia and poor details of the perinatal event. Birthweight was 2600g. She was ventilated for unspecified pulmonary disease. Dysmorphic features typical of trisomy 18 prompted karyotyping, and the diagnosis was confirmed. Ultrasound and CT scans suggested the existence of a peculiar haemorrhagic lesion in the right occipital area (Fig. 9.3). She died aged 7 days. At autopsy the falx was

TABLE 9.4

Anatomical variants of midline aneurysmal varix

1. *True aneurysmal varix of the median prosencephalic vein*
   —with direct arterio-venous fistula(e)
   —with arterio-venous fistula(e) to a common collector emanating from the varix

2. *Aneurysmal varix of the vein of Galen*
   (downstream of an arterio-venous malformation)

3. *Isolated varix of the vein of Galen*
   (with distal venous obstruction)

4. *Hybrid lesions* (mixtures of 1–3)

absent, a subpial haematoma was found in the right temporo-occipital area, and the density covering the right occipital lobe was histologically shown to be a venous angioma.

Midline cerebral aneurysmal varix (vein of Galen aneurysm)

The prominent vessel typical of what is currently referred to as pure vein of Galen aneurysm is an arterialized venous remnant of the median prosencephalic vein and therefore not really a dilated vein of Galen. It is thought that this vessel, temporarily draining the primitive choroid plexus, fails to regress normally between the seventh and 12th postconceptional week (30 to 100mm stage) (Raybaud *et al.* 1987, Velut 1987). There are unresolved questions about its origin, but it is clear that both primitive choroid and pineal tissue are implicated in the basic lesion (Velut 1987). Almost invariably the midline varix is the result of more distal arterio-venous shunting, different anatomical versions being possible (Table 9.4) (Litvak *et al.* 1960, Lasjaunias *et al.* 1987, Merland *et al.* 1987, Raybaud *et al.* 1987, Seidenwurm *et al.* 1991). The onset of symptoms is related to the degree of shunting in such a way that early presentation, as in the fetal or neonatal period, usually indicates considerable shunting. Males are predominantly affected but—apart from the association with hereditary haemorrhagic diathesis—a genetic basis has not yet been determined.

The varicose vessel is located in the midline behind the third ventricle and quadrigeminal plate, sitting on the cerebellar vermis. Some outward displacement of the lateral ventricles is most clearly seen on coronal ultrasound scans (Needell *et al.* 1983, Mansour *et al.* 1987, Saliba *et al.* 1987*b*). The mass is anechogenic and round with some irregular wall reflections in most cases (Fig. 9.4). It can prolong into a widely patent straight sinus and torcular, mimicking a tennis racket (Pellegrino *et al.* 1987, Picard *et al.* 1987, Strauss *et al.* 1991, Ginsberg *et al.* 1992). Echogenicity within the aneurysm is usually due to thrombus formation, either following treatment or as a spontaneous event (Picard *et al.* 1987, Saliba *et al.* 1987*b*, Beltramello *et al.* 1991). In half of those cases the thrombosis will be complete and prevent angiographic visualization, whereas a calcified rim could still

172

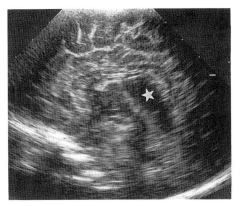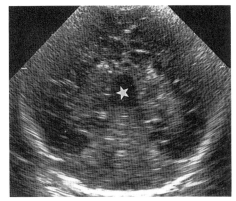

Fig. 9.4. Sagittal *(left)* and coronal *(right)* ultrasound scans of newborn girl with congestive heart failure: *asterisk* indicates midline varix of vein of Galen.

highlight its wall. Recognition of this event will obviate surgery. A post-thrombotic coagulopathy has been reported (Rosenberg and Nazar 1991). An unusual coincidence of midline aneurysmal varix and systemic air embolism may also induce echogenicity (Mehall *et al.* 1990). Differentiation from a dilated third ventricle pouch or midline arachnoidal cyst has been greatly facilitated by (colour) Doppler flow studies (Mansour *et al.* 1987, Saliba *et al.* 1987*a*, Schranz *et al.* 1988, Strauss *et al.* 1991, Dan *et al.* 1992). Within the sac continuous venous flow is captured, and turbulence is superimposed near the site(s) of arterial admixture. Striking elevation of intracranial venous pressure, obliteration of subarachnoid CSF pathways and residual changes due to previous subarachnoid bleeding will contribute to the ventricular dilatation often accompanying the anomaly. There is some doubt about aqueductal stenosis as an obligatory component of this hydrocephalus (Seiden-wurm *et al.* 1991). White matter atrophy might also contribute.

Though at any age a cranial bruit or subarachnoid haemorrhage can be the initial sign, the classical neonatal onset (over 95 per cent of cases) is with heart failure (Amacher and Shillito 1973, Knudson and Alden 1979, Hoffman *et al.* 1982, Maheut *et al.* 1987*a*, Nicholson *et al.* 1989, Ordorica *et al.* 1990, Strauss *et al.* 1991).

Fetal sonographic detection of nonimmune hydrops with cardiomegaly and hepatomegaly should invite the obstetrician to look for a major intracranial arterio-venous shunt (Vintzileos *et al.* 1986, Ordorica *et al.* 1990, Comstock and Kirk 1991, Strauss *et al.* 1991). The earliest reported gestational age at detection was 32 weeks. In other instances it will be hydrocephalus, microcephaly and/or brain necrosis with calcification that attract attention (Norman and Becker 1974, Perez-Fontan *et al.* 1982).

Neonatal high output heart failure implicates an obligatory search for occult arterio-venous shunts. Its presentation in midline cerebral aneurysmal varix has been repeatedly described (Stern *et al.* 1968, Holden *et al.* 1972, Stanbridge *et al.*

1983, Maheut *et al.* 1987*a*, Salazar *et al.* 1987, Saliba *et al.* 1987*a*, Pellegrino *et al.* 1987, O'Donnabhain and Duff 1989).

Intracranial haemorrhage as part of the neonatal clinical picture has occurred as petechial haemorrhages in the cerebral white matter (Stehbens *et al.* 1973), haemorrhagic white matter infarction (Stern *et al.* 1968), basal subdural haematoma (Lejeune *et al.* 1987), subarachnoid haemorrhage (Iannucci *et al.* 1979, Mickle and Quisling 1986) and intraventricular bleeding with disruption of the thalamus and basal ganglia (Norman and Becker 1974, Iannucci *et al.* 1979). The latter presentation may resemble thalamo-ventricular haemorrhage due to deep venous thrombosis. The origin of bleeding is notoriously difficult to trace in most cases.

For the time being, (digital subtraction) angiography is still warranted for detailed presurgical description of the anomaly. Treatment methods are hotly debated and will not be reviewed here. Almost invariably, infants surviving the neonatal ordeal are severely disabled, although recent developments in interventional radiological embolization do seem to promise a definite change in outcome (Lasjaunias *et al.* 1987, 1991; Merland *et al.* 1987; Picard *et al.* 1987; Friedman *et al.* 1991).

Lateral aneurysmal varix
Well documented cases of arterio-venous fistulization with prominent varix formation unrelated to deep cerebro-venous drainage have been documented in infants (Arai *et al.* 1972, Carrillo *et al.* 1984) and neonates (Stern *et al.* 1968, Tomlinson *et al.* 1992). The basic lesion is an arterio-venous fistula fed by one or more pial arteries causing varicose dilatation of a cerebral vein, drained by dilated venous structures to superior sagittal, straight, lateral or sigmoid sinus.

Heart failure, precipitated by cardio-pulmonary adaptive changes after birth, was the presenting fatal sign in a boy reported by Stern *et al.* (1968). At post-mortem examination a meningeal varix of the middle cerebral vein (1×1.5cm) in the upper part of the left central sulcus was fed by several hypertrophied branches of ipsilateral anterior and middle cerebral arteries; it drained to the superior sagittal sinus. Prenatal detection of hypodense unidentified masses within the cranium triggered neonatal investigations in the boy described by Tomlinson *et al.* (1992). Direct angiography disclosed a similar right middle cerebral vein varix (3.1cm diameter) fed by one anterior temporal branch of the right middle cerebral artery and drained via the enlarged vein of Trolard and inferior temporal veins to superior sagittal and transverse sinus respectively. Two branches of the right vertebral artery at the foramen magnum fed an additional right subtentorial varix (3.3cm diameter) with venous drainage to straight and sigmoid sinus. Following clipping of the right middle cerebral feeding artery and wire embolization of the varix at the end of the first month of life, the infant developed hyponatraemic seizures postoperatively. At 3 months of age the subtentorial anomaly was treated in a similar manner. In the meantime a juxtaductal aortic coarctation, detected early on, had become progressively narrower and was repaired by subclavian artery pedicle. At 1 year of age this boy did not have angiographic remnants of intracranial fistulae and showed only mild left hemiparesis. Multiple intracranial arterio-venous anomalies are uncommon outside Weber–Rendu–Osler and Wyburn–Mason syndromes.

Aortic coarctation could be secondary to haemodynamic changes induced by the shunt (Tomlinson *et al.* 1992).

10
DIFFERENTIAL DIAGNOSIS: INFECTION AND HAEMOSTATIC DEFECTS

Infection

A systematic review of brain infections at term is not the goal of this section. Descriptions of pathological (Berman and Banker 1966, Gilles *et al.* 1977, Larroche 1977, Rosenberg and Bernstein 1981, Wigglesworth 1984, Friede 1989, Singer 1991), clinical (Volpe 1987) and radiological findings (CT—New and Davis 1980; MRI—Zimmerman and Haimes 1988) will guide the interested reader. In some situations haemorrhagic brain lesions complicate systemic infection, whereas in others actual infection within the cranium causes brain damage sometimes mimicking or including bleeding as a secondary phenomenon.

Intracranial haemorrhage due to systemic effects of infection

The *haemorrhagic diathesis* accompanying disseminated intravascular coagulation can lead to pial and subarachnoid haematoma (Chessells and Wigglesworth 1970, Larroche 1977, Barson 1990, Govaert *et al.* 1992*b*). Similar circumstances have led to lobar cerebral haematoma (Fouché *et al.* 1982) or cerebellar haemorrhage.

Systemic disease associated with bacteraemia, such as hypotension, metabolic acidosis, asphyxia or persistent pulmonary hypertension, have been blamed for induction of *arterial cerebral infarction* (haemorrhagic in cases reported by Barmada *et al.* 1979, Hill *et al.* 1983, plus personal observations) and *white matter infarction* especially in group B streptococcal bacteraemia (Faix and Donn 1985, Colan 1986, Takashima *et al.* 1987).

General effects of infection have in the past been associated with *superficial cerebral venous thrombosis* (Byers and Hass 1933, Bailey and Hass 1958, Friede 1972). Asymmetrical haemorrhagic cerebral (sub)cortical necrosis could follow such an event.

Direct effects of intracranial infection

The sequence of events in neonatal *ventriculitis and leptomeningitis* has been reviewed by Berman and Banker (1966), Friede (1972), Gilles *et al.* (1977) and Daum *et al.* (1978). Some of the cortical infarctions may take the form of lobar haematomas. Thalamo-ventricular haemorrhage in association with listerial (De Vries *et al.* 1990) or group B streptococcal infections (Govaert *et al.* 1992*a*) is another possible consequence.

Haemorrhagic cerebral necrosis is a distinct separate entity, described in fulminating gram-negative (Cussen and Ryan 1967, Shortland-Webb 1968,

Larroche 1977) and viral (Pape and Wigglesworth 1979) CNS infection. The basic lesion is widespread vasculitis and haemorrhagic necrosis. Description of such lesions in life is yet to be produced.

Haemostatic defects
Term infants may develop intraventricular, cerebral parenchymal and subarachnoid haemorrhages due to anomalous haemostasis. However, the UZ Gent experience of primary haemostatic failure is very limited. One near-term infant developed bilateral intraventricular haemorrhages which were considered to be due to maternal salicylate ingestion; a second infant had an unexplained thrombocytopenia (see Table 1.3, p. 4). The contribution of clotting failure to some subgaleal haemorrhages is reviewed in Chapter 6. Of four infants with haemorrhage secondary to infection, three with disseminated intravascular coagulation (DIC) developed intracerebral haemorrhage.

Readers are thus referred elsewhere for discussion of the approach to identifying the different subtypes of haemorrhagic diathesis and their relevant clinical aspects (Oski and Naiman 1982, Buchanan 1986, Schlegel and Beaufils 1988, Stockman and Pochedly 1988, Caen 1989, Gibson 1989, Suzuki et al. 1991).

Major bleeding or thrombosis can lead to consumption of coagulant factors and platelets with secondary features of DIC. This has been reported in infants with subgaleal haemorrhage (Govaert et al. 1992c), superior sagittal sinus thrombosis (Leissring et al. 1968), thalamo-ventricular haemorrhage with deep venous thrombosis (Govaert et al. 1992a), and subdural haematoma (Welch and Strand 1986). Even two days after the event, infants compensating for a closed space haemorrhage may not have typical features of DIC: they may combine thrombocytopenia with elevated levels of fibrinogen and factor VIII with a short to normal activated partial thromboplastin time (Easa 1978). Useful tests to confirm ongoing DIC are detection of microangiopathic haemolytic anaemia, raised levels of fibrin degradation products, lowered plasma antithrombin III levels (bearing in mind the non-specificity of the latter finding as it is also found in shock of any cause), elevated fibrinopeptide A levels, elevated platelet derived ß-thromboglobulin or platelet factor 4 in plasma, prolongation of the thrombin clotting time and incoagulable state of the thrombelastogram (Vinazzer 1983, Fruchtman and Aledort 1986, Schmidt et al. 1986, Maki 1992). Erroneous interpretation of these changes could mislead the clinician into thinking that a bleeding disorder preceded, rather than followed, the haemorrhage.

11
MEDICO-LEGAL ASPECTS

Jonathan S. Wigglesworth

The low perinatal mortality and morbidity rates now seen in developed countries ensure that parents expect to give birth to healthy living infants. Unexpected death or impairment comes as a great shock and leads to feelings of guilt and anger, often directed toward medical or nursing staff of the hospital where the child was born.

In addition, the presence of a severely neurodevelopmentally disabled infant within a family may now result in major financial hardship. In a family where both parents would normally expect to be earning, the high dependency and recurring medical needs of a disabled child may mean the loss of a least one parental salary. At the same time it may be suggested that the developing child would benefit from sophisticated equipment, specific modes of treatment or alterations to the home which cannot be supplied through state medical care. Moreover, the constant disruption of family life due to the need for 24 hour care and interference with the simplest outside activities (*e.g.* the difficulty of shopping with a child who screams for hours on end) often result in family break-up. Given such a background, the increasing frequency of litigation in these cases is fully understandable. The majority of publications on the medico-legal aspects of such cases describe an outcome of cerebral palsy, the alleged causation most commonly being 'birth asphyxia'. Cases where cranial haemorrhage was a feature form a subset within the cerebral palsy group (Towbin 1986, Freeman and Nelson 1988, Shields and Schifrin 1988, Hall 1989, *Lancet* 1989).

The discovery of intracranial haemorrhage in the term infant may lead to consideration of a likely traumatic origin as discussed elsewhere in this volume. Any such suggestion will obviously encourage speculation as to possible negligent obstetric management.

However, haemorrhage within or externally to the cranium in a neonate of any gestation may be due to one of a variety of causes and always requires a careful analysis of possible causation irrespective of whether the child dies or survives and irrespective of whether or not there is evidence of negligent obstetric or paediatric management.

In this chapter I will outline the analysis of causation that is critical for the presentation of an expert opinion to solicitors acting either on behalf of the plaintiff or for a defending practitioner or health care agency, and will mention some aspects of alleged negligent management that a causation analysis may support or refute. From this it is possible to derive some of the principles of risk management that should be employed to minimize future claims.

Balance of probability

It is important to understand that the level of proof required for determining liability in cases of litigation for alleged medical negligence is very low. The test to be applied by the judge (or a jury in the USA) is that the injury resulted from a negligent act 'on the balance of probability': that is, with a probability greater than 50 per cent. The discovery of one minor piece of evidence on the nature or timing of a perinatal cranial lesion may completely change the balance of probability.

Traumatic haemorrhage

The diagnosis of haemorrhage as due to trauma carries an immediate implication of negligence. Obviously trauma is never the intended outcome or accompaniment of any delivery; it may also be possible in retrospect to propose alternative methods or timing of delivery that would have avoided the traumatic episode. It is thus difficult to defend claims of negligence in cases where trauma is proven to have occurred 'on balance of probability'.

Haemorrhage that may be of traumatic origin can occur at a number of sites (see Chapter 6). In most, other explanations are possible and the diagnosis of traumatic haemorrhage will usually depend on the exact pattern of bleeding or the circumstances of its occurrence.

Thus, subaponeurotic haemorrhage is claimed to develop with undue frequency in infants delivered by ventouse (Plauché 1979) but has also been claimed to be a manifestation of a bleeding tendency (Robinson and Rossiter 1968). Subperiosteal and subdural haemorrhages are almost invariably the result of trauma.

Subarachnoid haemorrhage is not normally thought to result from trauma, although the rupture of the unsupported bridging veins between the cerebral veins and the dural venous sinuses may occur within the subarachnoid as well as the subdural space (Pape and Wigglesworth 1979).

Intracerebral haemorrhage is also not often considered to be the consequence of trauma. Extensive haemorrhagic infarction of the cerebral hemispheres can develop in association with subdural haemorrhage by the mechanism described in Chapter 6.

Association between traumatic haemorrhage, asphyxia and ischaemia

As pointed out in a previous monograph in this series (Pape and Wigglesworth 1979), haemorrhage may only be part of a traumatic lesion. The distortion of the infant cranium that causes tentorial tears with subdural haemorrhage from ruptured bridging veins is also likely to cause widespread cerebral ischaemia. Further ischaemia and infarction can result from secondary interference with cerebral artery flow due to direct focal compression or generalized swelling of the contused cerebrum. In addition, the development of fetal asphyxia may render the infant more susceptible to later traumatic damage due to loss of tone in the musculature of the head and neck or venous engorgement.

For medico-legal purposes it may be very important to distinguish between the cerebral haemorrhage and ischaemia due to trauma and that due to prenatal asphyxia, even if this distinction has little significance for prognosis.

Diagnosis of traumatic lesions

Diagnosis in life

Most traumatic lesions affecting the infant CNS occur at the time of birth. The cranial distortion that can cause a tentorial tear during a forceps delivery must occur in most instances during traction or rotation of the head very shortly before delivery. In the case of the aftercoming head of an infant presenting by the breech, any cranial trauma would be virtually at the moment of delivery. Most infants who have suffered a purely traumatic lesion appear completely healthy at birth immediately after the event. Apgar scores are often normal, and it may be several hours before suspicion of any damage is aroused. At some time within the first 24 hours the infant may be noted to have become pale or lethargic. Local swelling or obvious bruising round the head may become apparent, the fontanelle may become tense, and convulsions may develop. There is likely to be evidence of continued bleeding in the form of a falling haematocrit, and imaging studies may reveal some characteristic pattern of traumatic intracranial haemorrhage.

The differential diagnosis in most instances is intrapartum asphyxia. The infant who has suffered pure asphyxia shortly before birth characteristically has a depressed Apgar score. S/he is usually hypotonic at birth, with delayed onset of respiration. The hypotonic phase is succeeded by hypertonia, and there may be development of convulsions usually between 12 and 24 hours of age.

In the developed stage, by 24 hours it may be impossible, on clinical grounds, to distinguish between hypoxic–ischaemic encephalopathy due to birth asphyxia and similarly extensive haemorrhagic and ischaemic brain damage due to trauma.

Although the early clear period can be helpful as an aid to recognizing traumatic injury, considerable difficulty may arise in those cases where trauma was superimposed on preceding asphyxia. There are also instances where severe trauma was induced sufficiently early in labour for the infant's state to have deteriorated by the time of birth. Such instances include those where a series of procedures were attempted in order to effect delivery (*e.g.* ventouse followed by forceps and final recourse to caesarean section). Other traumatic events associated with poor state at birth have been prolonged intrapartum scalp haemorrhage associated with multiple fetal blood sampling and cervico-medullary spinal cord transection or infarction associated with Kielland forceps rotation.

Accurate diagnosis of most lesions should now be possible in life with modern ultrasound, CT and MRI scanning equipment.

Post-mortem diagnosis

Post-mortem examination by a specialist perinatal pathologist is strongly recommended in all cases of unexpected perinatal death. This is particularly important if death of an apparently normally formed term infant occurs at or soon after delivery.

If the parents are blaming the hospital for the death it may be necessary to involve the coroner: ideally the examination is then performed by a regional perinatal pathologist on behalf of the coroner. The technique of performing post-mortem examinations in such cases will not be described here.

Photographs and X-rays are an important part of such a post-mortem examination. It is also critical that the pathologist should be sufficiently skilled and confident of her/his technique as to distinguish fresh haemorrhage and fractures or fracture dislocations (*e.g.* separation of squamous and lateral parts of the occipital bone) from the effects of disruption caused during the dissection procedure. Examination of the upper cervical spinal cord from the posterior aspect is important in any case of death following rotational forceps delivery.

Careful gross and microscopic examination of the brain is important, but is often inadequately performed. The brain should be fixed intact, but may be sampled fairly rapidly for histology if time is critical. My own practice is to fix the brain in 4 per cent buffered formaldehyde solution for 2 to 7 days before cutting coronal sections. If the shorter time is employed I cut thick coronal sections and fix for a further 24 hours before taking blocks for histology. Gross lesions are photographed, and sections from at least six areas including frontal lobe, temporal lobe with hippocampus, thalamus, midbrain, pons, cerebellum and medulla are taken, in addition to several levels of the spinal cord and any gross lesions. The importance of such sampling is to assess whether there is underlying anoxic–ischaemic damage apart from any traumatic lesion.

Assessment of causation and timing when negligence is alleged
A paediatrician, paediatric neurologist or pathologist may be asked to provide a report on probable causation and timing of a cerebral lesion resulting in death or permanent disability.

One problem is the considerable time delay between the inception of brain damage, however caused, and the requirement to search for causative factors on medico-legal grounds. In the UK currently there is no time limit within which proceedings must be commenced in cases of alleged birth injury. Surviving disabled infants can sue in their own right, and thus legal aid is granted irrespective of parental income. A child born ten or more years ago who developed hypoxic–ischaemic encephalopathy will not have been investigated by modern imaging studies. It may be found on an initial search of the records that a diagnosis of birth asphyxia or (less frequently) cranial trauma was made on purely clinical grounds and little attempt was made to exclude other possible diagnoses.

Assessments should be approached with no pre-existing bias, irrespective of whether they have been requested by solicitors acting for the plaintiff or for the defendants. In making an assessment of causation there is no possible short cut. It is essential to work through the obstetric background including ultrasound assessments of fetal growth, prepartum and intrapartum cardio-tocographic records, intrapartum acid–base studies and the normality of progress of labour as shown on the partogram. Descriptions of operative delivery by ventouse, forceps or caesarean section are obviously important but frequently are brief and uninformative. The paediatrician or pathologist may be aided in some of the specific details of obstetric management by the opinion of an obstetric expert, but should be able to make a separate analysis of the normality or otherwise of pregnancy and labour as a whole.

The state of the infant at birth and the changes observed in the first 24 hours of life are of major importance, particularly in making the distinction between asphyxial damage induced during labour, trauma during delivery or pre-existing brain abnormality due to malformation or prenatal brain injury (*e.g.* haemorrhage or infarction during the latter part of pregnancy).

Initial measurements of weight, length and head circumference form an important baseline against which any later changes may be set. Certain serial measurements can be critical in cases where no hard copies of sequential imaging studies are available. Thus, a series of normal haemoglobin measurements combined with a single record of a clear CSF make it difficult to claim 'on balance of probability' that the infant suffered a traumatic delivery. Swelling around the head noted in such a case would almost certainly be a caput succedaneum comprising mainly oedema with very little blood.

If there was evidence of haemorrhage in the form of a falling haemoglobin level, this may well have been assumed due to cranial trauma during the process of delivery. However, a careful analysis of the records may indicate a different pattern of injury. Some fetal scalp sampling analysers give a reading of haemoglobin as well as acid–base data. A progressive fall in the haemoglobin reading, overlooked at the time, has on occasion indicated that neonatal scalp swelling and anaemia were due to vascular trauma by a scalp electrode or sampling needle.

Alternatively, sudden neonatal collapse associated with a slowly increasing head swelling and falling haemoglobin level has indicated a subaponeurotic bleed in a case previously ascribed to asphyxial brain damage (personal case).

A series of full blood counts can provide a pattern of fluctuations in nucleated red cells, white cells or platelets that can suggest or refute a range of possibilities from feto-maternal haemorrhage (or feto-fetal haemorrhage in monochorial twins—Fusi *et al.* 1991) to infection, congenital thrombocytopenia or secondary haemostatic failure.

Sequential acid–base studies give an initial measure of the severity of any asphyxial component, since a large base deficit takes some time to clear even with rapid and effective neonatal resuscitation.

The timing of a fall in urinary output and rise in blood urea gives an indication of the timing of renal tubular damage due to shock.

Changes in glucose, electrolytes and 'liver function' tests may all provide critical information in individual cases. The results of tests carried out in the neonatal period will usually have been correctly interpreted at the time. However, the significance of some neonatal findings may be overlooked at a later stage when attempts are being made to account for the established pattern of disability revealed at 2 to 3 years of age. In addition, the precise timing of a lesion may not have seemed so important in the early neonatal period as it becomes years later when litigation proceedings are commenced.

A paediatric neurological assessment of a surviving child at several years of age, when the pattern of physical and mental disablement is becoming well established, can also be of major assistance in delineating the likely sites of major damage. This is perhaps of less help in cases of severe birth trauma than in those of an alleged asphyxial causation, as the cerebral contusion or shock associated with trauma may lead to a wide range of patterns of focal or generalized ischaemic brain injury.

Imaging studies using realtime ultrasound, CT or MRI are the nearest to an anatomical examination of the brain, spinal cord and meninges that can be performed in the living infant. It is most helpful in later assessment if sequential imaging studies have been carried out in the early days, weeks and months of life. If CT and MRI scans have been performed there is seldom a problem in obtaining hard copies to examine at a later date. Neonatal ultrasound studies in contrast are often performed with mobile machines and reported on the basis of the appearance on the monitor at the time without retaining photographic copies. This is especially the case if the initial findings were negative. The reports of such examinations written in the notes are seldom of help for later assessment. In instances where copies have been kept they can be of major importance. For instance, in one case re-examination of a scan originally regarded as negative revealed evidence of massive established cerebral necrosis very shortly after birth, indicating that damage had developed before admission of the mother to hospital in labour (personal case). In another infant admitted to hospital following acute collapse at several weeks of age, the presence of a completely normal ultrasound scan taken soon after admission effectively refuted a claim by forensic pathologists at a later inquest that the haemorrhagic brain atrophy found at post-mortem examination could have occurred during birth (personal case).

All is not lost if no imaging studies were performed in the neonatal period in an infant who is several years of age at the time of assessment. The final anatomical pattern of brain damage often clearly indicates the nature of the original lesion. MRI studies have shown developmental anomalies of neuronal migration as a cause of persistent epilepsy in children of more than 6 years old. A CT scan revealed a pattern characteristic of periventricular leukomalacia in a child aged 9 years in whom brain damage was alleged to be due to pertussis immunization (personal case). Such studies will of course be of no help in those cases where the question is one of establishing the time of damage to within hours or days rather than its nature.

In the event of death of an infant at or at any time after birth the post-mortem findings become of critical importance. Unfortunately there are still relatively few pathologists with skills, time and facilities to perform a post-mortem examination to the standards desirable to answer later medico-legal questions. If death occurs at or soon after birth the possibility of later medico-legal involvement is often not considered. Even if the examination has been performed on behalf of the coroner it is seldom that the brain will have received the level of attention I outlined above as my own standard approach. If the child survived some months or years and died after litigation had commenced it is more likely that the brain will have been preserved for study.

Study of the post-mortem report may give useful information on organ weights (indicating patterns of fetal growth), details of recent traumatic lesions (but see my comments on cranial dissection above) and asphyxial lesions such as meconium inhalation and haemorrhages. The value of the information provided by the report varies considerably according to the skills of the pathologist. The report should, however, indicate what material was processed for histological study and whether the brain was retained. As part of a causation analysis all this material should be carefully re-examined by an experienced perinatal or paediatric pathologist. The type of finding that proves useful is the demonstration of established anoxic–ischaemic cerebral lesions in an infant thought to have died as a result of acute traumatic or asphyxial damage, or the recognition of acute renal tubular necrosis as confirmation of a recent episode of shock. I have experienced a case where an infant thought to have severe mental retardation as a result of cerebral atrophy, diagnosed on CT and allegedly due to events at birth, died at several years of age with a brain that could not be recognized as structurally abnormal on gross and microscopic study. In such a case the possibility of causation by a major asphyxial or traumatic event at birth can be confidently excluded. Perinatal brain damage resulting in long-term disability is associated with extensive neuronal necrosis that leaves clearly recognizable macroscopic and histological scars if not areas of gross atrophy.

In cases of alleged trauma, photographic evidence obtained at the time of post-mortem examination can be of considerable help. In one case a moderately preterm infant, who collapsed shortly after birth and died at 1 week of age, was found to have a large depressed cranial fracture. Later argument centred round possible causation of the fracture at forceps delivery or, as alleged by the parents, by the infant's head accidentally striking a weighing scale when being carried toward it to record the birthweight. A photograph taken at the post-mortem examination revealed a clean semicircular edge to the fracture that precisely mirrored the end of one of the flat metal bars supporting the plastic scale pan. A photograph of the scales showed loss of the rubber cups that normally cover the ends of the metal supports (personal case).

Relation of causation to negligence and liability
As mentioned above, establishment of liability depends on convincing the court

that, on balance of probability, the damage suffered by the plaintiff was caused by a negligent act. Without the causal link, the separate demonstration of negligence and presence of damage are insufficient to support a claim.

In some instances the demonstration of a convincing cause may itself be indicative of negligence and leave little room for defence, as in the case of the infant banged on the scales. In others the demonstration of a cause leaves open the question of timing in relation to a recognized act of negligence. In the case of trauma it may be relevant to question as to whether it can ever be defended. There are instances where an abnormality of the infant almost inevitably implicates trauma. In a study on cases of fatal congenital arthrogryposis, Quinn *et al.* (1991) found a high frequency of severe and multiple birth trauma. In one infant, for instance, there was massive subdural haemorrhage associated with tentorial tears as well as bilateral fractures of the humeri. These infants were characterized by fixed deformities of the limbs, poor muscle development, thin cranium and long bones, a combination of features that undoubtedly rendered them at greatly increased risk of severe birth trauma. This group of infants included all the most severe cases of traumatic intracranial haemorrhage seen at perinatal post-mortem examination at Hammersmith Hospital over a 10 year period (Wigglesworth 1988). Undoubtedly the occurrence of birth trauma in this group could be stoutly defended if litigation was threatened. In the more frequent situation of an apparently normally developed infant, severe traumatic damage is difficult to defend. If cranial fracture or intracranial haemorrhage follow a forceps delivery there is a tendency to accept that *res ipse loquitor* (the fact speaks for itself) however much the obstetrician protests of the care with which s/he managed the delivery.

The importance of timing as a link between causation and liability arises when it becomes apparent that an intracranial haemorrhage is likely to be of asphyxial rather than traumatic origin. Secondary bleeding into areas of brain infarction is now well recognized; the lesions may resemble those of bleeding into areas of traumatic contusion. In a case where on analysis the lesions are considered to be of asphyxial cause the obstetric experts may recognize a time at which good obstetric practice would demand immediate delivery. They may concede that management was negligent if delivery was not in fact achieved until some hours later.

If neonatal imaging studies or post-mortem examination of the brain indicate that the cerebral lesions were already fully developed by the time it became appropriate to expedite delivery, then the link between causation and negligence will not have been established and liability cannot be proved. It is often quite impossible retrospectively to time the occurrence of a non-traumatic brain lesion to the level of precision demanded. In some instances the stage of development of the cerebral lesions puts their time of onset many hours before the critical period. The possibility of making such an assessment is a good reason for taking the series of brain block samples that I have listed above, as these encompass most of the areas where asphyxial injury is liable to be detected. In the surviving infant with brain examination limited to imaging studies, the separation of time of onset of the lesion and the critical time when delivery should have been achieved would have to be many hours, if not days, for it to be possible to mount a defence on this basis. Without the benefit of histology it will usually have to be conceded that maintenance of the infant *in utero* after development of the primary episode of asphyxial damage may well have allowed further extension of the initial lesion.

Implications for risk management strategies

Development of risk management strategies is an essential response to the recent enormous increase in medical litigation. It does not involve defensive medicine in the sense of carrying out unnecessary tests but does involve specific targeting for improvements in investigation and record keeping of those areas where litigation is most likely to arise.

In terms of the area discussed in this chapter the following recommendations would seem worthwhile.

Any infant who develops signs of encephalopathy that could be due to either trauma or asphyxia should have imaging studies by real-time ultrasound or CT scan performed as soon as possible to provide an initial baseline and show whether prenatal damage is present. Copies of all ultrasound scans should be kept with the notes or X-rays.

The reason for any specific procedures, obstetric or neonatal, particularly if non-standard, should always be stated in the notes. Neonatal records are usually far better than obstetric records in this and other respects. A period of missing observations in the case notes, such as lack of fetal heart rate records over a significant period, are extremely difficult to defend at a later stage.

Paediatricians should be extremely careful to avoid labelling the neurologically disabled infants in their care as having suffered severe birth asphyxia or trauma if they have not personally studied the obstetric records. Letters from paediatricians to colleagues detailing 'severe fetal anoxia' when no evidence for such an event can be deduced from obstetric records have on more than one occasion been instrumental in starting or prolonging unjustified claims. There is an obvious tendency when faced with a severely disabled child to feel outrage at the lurid tale of obstetric mismanagement that may be detailed by the parents. Full examination of the facts reveals that such outrage is not always justifiable, and it is better to employ descriptive terms of known events such as 'delayed onset of respiration' or 'neonatal encephalopathy' rather than those that imply a particular unproven causation.

If an infant or child dies in circumstances that suggest the possibility of litigation, it is important to get a skilled post-mortem examination with photographic and radiological records as well as full examination of the brain.

REFERENCES

Freeman, J.M., Nelson, K.B. (1988) 'Intrapartum asphyxia and cerebral palsy.' *Pediatrics*, **82**, 240–249.

Fusi, L., McFarland, P., Fisk, N., Wigglesworth, J.S. (1991) 'Acute twin–twin transfusion: a possible mechanism for brain-damaged survivors after intrauterine death of a monochorionic twin.' *Obstetrics and Gynecology*, **78**, 517–520.

Hall, D.M.B. (1989) 'Birth asphyxia and cerebral palsy.' *British Medical Journal*, **299**, 279–282.

Lancet (1989) 'Cerebral palsy, intrapartum care, and a shot in the foot.' *Lancet*, **2**, 1251–1252. *(Editorial.)*

Pape, K.E., Wigglesworth, J.S. (1979) *Haemorrhage, Ischaemia and the Perinatal Brain. Clinics in Developmental Medicine No. 69/70.* London: Spastics International Medical Publications.

Plauché, W.C. (1979) 'Fetal cranial injuries related to delivery with the Malmström vacuum extractor.' *Obstetrics and Gynecology*, **53**, 750–757.

Quinn, C.M., Wigglesworth, J.S., Heckmatt, J. (1991) 'Lethal arthrogryposis multiplex congenita: a pathological study of 21 cases.' *Histopathology*, **18**, 155–162.

Robinson, R.J., Rossiter, M.A. (1968) 'Massive subaponeurotic haemorrhage in babies of African origin.' *Archives of Disease in Childhood*, **43**, 684–687.

Shields, J.R., Schifrin, B.S. (1988) 'Perinatal antecedents of cerebral palsy.' *Obstetrics and Gynecology*, **71**, 899–905.

Towbin, A. (1986) 'Obstetric malpractice litigation: the pathologist's view.' *American Journal of Obstetrics and Gynecology*, **155**, 927–935.

Wigglesworth, J.S. (1988) 'Trauma and the developing brain.' *In:* Kubli, E., Patel, N., Schmidt, W. (Eds) *Perinatal Events and Brain Damage in Surviving Children.* Berlin: Springer-Verlag, pp. 64–69.

12
CONCLUSIONS

(1) There are major problems in *defining birth trauma* as it is currently documented in surviving newborn infants. The proposal outlined in Chapters 2 and 4 is open to criticism. In the meantime, publication should be encouraged of clinico-pathological studies, especially those focusing on radiological findings in the living term infant.

(2) If one includes subarachnoid haemorrhage, the estimated *incidence* of intracranial haemorrhage among living term neonates is more than 2 per cent. Serious haemorrhages (*i.e.* more than just primary subarachnoid) affect between two and four per 1000 term liveborn infants per year. From the data presented in this monograph it appears that in Flanders at least half of these serious haemorrhages are probably due to mechanical birth trauma, be it isolated or in combination with variable birth asphyxia. Some estimated incidence figures are given in Table 12.1.

(3) A subdivision into two categories of haemorrhage at term, superficial and deep, seems to be appropriate. The underlying cause in *superficial haemorrhage* is trauma during delivery; in addition birth asphyxia is contributory in a proportion of primary subarachnoid haemorrhages, whereas haemorrhagic diathesis precedes most instances of subarachnoid haematoma. *Deep bleeding* (intraventricular, parenchymal, in haemorrhagic stroke or haemorrhagic leukomalacia, in basal ganglia/thalamus/brainstem) can be associated with mechanical difficulties during parturition, but should prompt an active search for asphyxial causes, haemorrhagic diathesis, infection, vascular anomalies or tumour.

(4) Given the limitations of retrospective study and often partial description of the reviewed case histories, the relationship between *mode of delivery* and some types of haemorrhage does offer some idea about the obstetric background of those lesions (Table 12.2).

(5) As explained in detail in the introductory chapters, *vacuum delivery* is the preferred method of instrumental assistance in Flanders. Subgaleal bleeding is strongly related with this mode of delivery. Cephalhaematoma and primary subarachnoid haemorrhage are also frequently diagnosed following vacuum delivery, and epidural, intradural, central tentorial and basal subdural haemorrhages are not uncommonly associated. Vacuum delivery can lead to growing synchondrosal rupture and thrombosis of the superior sagittal sinus.

TABLE 12.1

Estimated yearly incidence of cranial haemorrhage in term liveborn infants

Type of lesion	Incidence (per 1000 deliveries)
Cephalhaematoma	20
Subgaleal haemorrhage	0.5–1.0 (5–10/1000 vacuum deliveries)
Epidural haemorrhage	0.1–0.5
Subarachnoid haemorrhage	20 (50–60/1000 instrumental deliveries)
Supratentorial subdural haemorrhage	<0.5
Central tentorial damage	~1
Fatal cranial birth trauma	0.1–0.5

TABLE 12.2

Mode of delivery vs. selected types of intracranial haemorrhage

Type of haemorrhage	Normal	Breech	Caesarean	Instrumental
Convexity subdural	+++	+	+	++++
Basal subdural	+++	++	+	++++
Central tentorial	+++	+++	+	++++
Epidural	+	+++	+	++++
Subarachnoid	+	+	++	++++

++++ Frequently associated; +++ commonly associated; ++ occasionally associated; + rarely associated.

There is circumstantial evidence for the potentiality of bone injury due to ventouse traction. (i) The incidence of cephalhaematoma, a direct lesion of outer periosteum, is higher following vacuum than forceps delivery. (ii) A depressed skull fracture can be reduced with vacuum application without traction. (iii) Dural membrane injury of falx and/or tentorium has been well documented following both types of instrumental traction, and can be explained as the consequence of skull compression. For the ventouse, a direct elevating effect on the falx has been suggested in addition.

(6) To understand direct *cause and effect relations* it is necessary to study peak and total tractional force, level of the engaged vertex at the onset of traction, number of pulls, fetal arterial Doppler velocity changes during labour (cerebral and peripheral), quantifiable abnormalities in cardiotocography and fetal electro-encephalography, umbilical artery blood gases, Apgar scores and arterial blood gases within the first hour of life. These data will have to be matched with serial cerebral ultrasound examination (both real time and with Doppler) and both early (first days) and late (late neonatal period) brain imaging results (CT, MRI, spectroscopy).

TABLE 12.3

Neurological sequelae of mechanical cranial birth trauma

1. Associated birth asphyxia
2. Associated haemorrhagic shock due to subgaleal bleeding, possibly leading to persistent pulmonary hypertension and disseminated intravascular coagulation
3. Direct brain contusion or compression, as underneath a skull fracture with depressed margin
4. Arterial cerebral infarction due to oedema and vessel compression, spasm or thrombosis
5. Impression of the occipital squama with ensuing superficial venous thrombosis and (sub)cortical cerebral infarction
6. Growing skull or syndesmosal injury with cerebral erosion
7. Venous stasis and intraventricular or thalamo-ventricular haemorrhage
8. Iatrogenic and nosocomial consequence of intensive care
9. Late consequences: syringomyelia, cerebellar dysfunction, infantile convexity subdural haematoma

(7) It is notoriously difficult to differentiate the impact of birth trauma and asphyxia on *ultimate neurological damage*. In addition to generalized hypoxic–ischaemic damage, some distinct patterns of brain necrosis can follow mechanical trauma to the fetal head during delivery (Table 12.3).

(8) The most frequent cause of fatal cranial birth trauma, in both the UZ Gent and Hammersmith Hospital populations, was instrumental and not breech delivery. Mechanical assistance of delivery is a potential cause of fetal and neonatal death.

(9) Although there is indirect evidence for the existence of a sequence from trauma through haemorrhage to arterial infarction, documentation in life of the pathogenetic intermediate is still lacking.

(10) Hypoxic–ischaemic damage to deep grey matter and brainstem can be recognized by ultrasound and MRI. Better anatomical definition of the lesions in life is a task for the future. Early recognition, within minutes to hours of the event, will be necessary for the implementation of treatment that might prevent further brain damage. Cerebrovascular changes during asphyxia *in utero* should be investigated with the aim of eventual attempts at controlling vascular changes.

The almost obligatory involvement of thalamic substructures during acute total asphyxia may suggest other mechanisms than glutamate-induced neuronal injury, since there is no current evidence for a high glutamate turnover in those areas.

Acquired prenatal brain damage and rare fetal neurodegenerative processes should always be kept in mind when discussing the morphological brain findings of infants asphyxiated at birth.

(11) A detailed search for *clotting anomalies* is essentially part of the approach to almost any cranial haemorrhage in a term newborn infant. Prenatal salicylate use

by the mother may contribute to serious intracranial haemorrhage around the time of birth.

(12) In selected instances an unexpected and morphologically peculiar intracranial haemorrhage is indicative of a *vascular anomaly*. Colour Doppler flow imaging, MRI and thereafter direct angiography are the tools for clarifying such a problem.

ACKNOWLEDGEMENTS

In the past few years I have enjoyed the privilege of working with grand persons who made this effort possible. Jules Leroy, Professor of Paediatrics at Gent University Hospital, has generated renewed scientific thrust in the department, thus permitting growth of several subspecialities like our Neonatal Intensive Care Unit, run by Piet Vanhaesebrouck. Jonathan Wigglesworth, Professor of Perinatal Pathology at Hammersmith Hospital, gave encouragement in my concept. He has been a patient teacher during many post-mortem examinations with me as an inquisitive bystander. Discussions of aspects of medico-legal situations he was involved in have encouraged me to carry on, as they made me realize how crucially important simple clinical observations are in that context. If in anyone's, I am in his debt most of all.

A wealth of colleagues have stimulated by discussing relevant topics as part of our clinical duties in Gent: Piet Vanhaesebrouck, Claudine de Praeter, Koen Smets, Dietbrant Carton, Paul Defoort, Eric Achten, Jacques Caemaert, Dirk Voet, Professor Marcel Afschrift, Professor Luc Calliauw and Professor Erik van de Velde. The lively atmosphere created by the junior and visiting perinatal pathologists at Hammersmith Hospital was most helpful: John Bridger, Peter Ozua, Afaf El-Hag and Chris Wright. At the Heartlink ECMO unit in Leicester, Gale Pearson, Alan Fenton and Richard Reece have been most helpful in the conception of the section on brain lesions related to extracorporeal membrane oxygenation.

Some logistical help has been provided by Rosanne Weytens, Christelle Maes and Erik Vandevelde in Gent and by Christine White, Jay Bhundia, William Thompson-Ambrose and Lee Knight in London. Lieven Verbeke has been as constructive as before.

Dr Pamela Davies, editing this book for Mac Keith Press, must have suffered from my language weaknesses and relatively youthful age. To her and all those mentioned above I express sincere gratitude. The same goes to all paediatricians and obstetricians referring sick newborn infants to our neonatal unit in Gent and to the neonatal nurses and other staff who shared responsibility in caring for these children. The figures used by courtesy are very helpful for documentation of relevant events and I feel grateful to all these authors.

For me this work is important enough to halt and thank my parents, Emilienne and Remi, and parents-in-law, Angele and Jean-Louis, for their support. My gratitude to Myriam is beyond expression.

REFERENCES*

Abrams, R.M., Cooper, R.J. (1987) 'Effect of ketamine on local cerebral glucose utilization in fetal sheep.' *American Journal of Obstetrics and Gynecology*, **156**, 1018–1023.
—— Ito, M., Frisinger, J.E., Patlak, C.S., Pettigrew, K.D., Kennedy, C. (1984) 'Local cerebral glucose utilization in fetal and neonatal sheep.' *American Journal of Physiology*, **246**, R608–R618.
Abroms, I.F., McLennan, J.E., Mandell, F. (1977) 'Acute neonatal subdural hematoma following breech delivery.' *American Journal of Diseases of Children*, **131**, 192–194.
Adam, R., Greenberg, J.O. (1978) 'The mega cisterna magna.' *Journal of Neurosurgery*, **48**, 190–192.
Aguero, O., Alvarez, H. (1962) 'Fetal injury due to the vacuum extractor.' *Obstetrics and Gynecology*, **19**, 212–217.
Ahdab-Barmada, M., Moossy, J. (1984) 'The neuropathology of kernicterus in the premature neonate: diagnostic problems.' *Journal of Neuropathology and Experimental Neurology*, **43**, 45–55.
Ahuja, G.L., Willoughby, M.L.N., Kerr, M.M., Hutchison, J.H. (1969) 'Massive subaponeurotic haemorrhage in infants born by vacuum extraction.' *British Medical Journal*, **2**, 743–745.
Allan, W.C., Riviello, J.J. (1992) 'Perinatal cerebrovascular disease in the neonate.' *Pediatric Clinics of North America*, **39**, 621–650.
Alonso, A., Taboada, D., Alvarez, J.A., Vidal-Sampedro, J., Vieito, X. (1984) 'Spontaneous hematomas caused by microangiomatosis of the basal ganglia.' *Child's Brain*, **11**, 202–211.
Alvarez, L.A., Maytal, J., Shinnar, S. (1986) 'Idiopathic external hydrocephalus: natural history and relationship to benign familial macrocephaly.' *Pediatrics*, **77**, 901–907.
Amacher, A.L., Shillito, J. (1973) 'The syndromes and surgical treatment of the great vein of Galen.' *Journal of Neurosurgery*, **39**, 89–98.
Amiel-Tison, C., Sureau, C., Shnider, S.M. (1988) 'Cerebral handicap in full-term neonates related to the mechanical forces of labour.' *Baillière's Clinical Obstetrics and Gynaecology*, **2**, 145–165.
Amit, M., Camfield, P.R. (1980) 'Neonatal polycythemia causing multiple cerebral infarcts.' *Archives of Neurology*, **37**, 109–110.
Ando, M., Takashima, S., Mito, T. (1988) 'Endotoxin, cerebral blood flow, amino acids and brain damage in young rabbits.' *Brain and Development*, **10**, 365–370.
Aoki, N. (1983) 'Epidural haematoma communicating with cephalhaematoma in a neonate.' *Neurosurgery*, **13**, 55–57.
—— (1990) 'Epidural haematoma in the newborn infant: therapeutic consequences from the correlation between haematoma content and computed tomography features.' *Acta Neurochirurgica*, **106**, 65–67.
—— Mizutani, H., Masuzawa, H. (1985) 'Unilateral subdural–peritoneal shunting for bilateral chronic subdural hematomas in infancy.' *Journal of Neurosurgery*, **63**, 134–137.
—— Toyofuku, T., Komiya, K. (1986) 'Cerebellar infarction.' *Neuropediatrics*, **17**, 124–128.
Appleton, R.E., Lee, R.E.J., Hey, E.N. (1990) 'Neurodevelopmental outcome of transient neonatal intracerebral echodensities.' *Archives of Disease in Childhood*, **65**, 27–29.
Apuzzio, J.J., Pelosi, M.A., Ganesh, V.V. (1984) 'Fetal heart bradycardia associated with the vacuum extractor.' *Obstetrics and Gynecology*, **29**, 496–497.
Arai, H., Sugiyama, Y., Kawakami, S., Miyazawa, N. (1972) 'Multiple intracranial aneurysms and vascular malformations in an infant.' *Journal of Neurosurgery*, **37**, 357–360.
Arienzo, R., Ricco, C.S., Romeo, F. (1987) 'A very rare fetal malformation: the cutaneous widespread vascular hamartomatosis.' *American Journal of Obstetrics and Gynecology*, **157**, 1162–1163.
Armstrong, D., Norman, M.G. (1974) 'Periventricular leukomalacia.' *Archives of Disease in Childhood*, **49**, 367–375.
Armstrong, D.L., Goddard, J., Schwartz, M., Stenbach, W. (1980) 'Another look at the pathology of intraventricular hemorrhage.' *In: Perinatal Intracranial Hemorrhage Conference*. Washington, DC: Ross Laboratories, Professional Services Dept., pp. 1–21.

*Contains bibliography for Chapters 1–6, 8–10 and 12. References for Chapters 7 and 11 can be found at the end of those chapters.

Arvidsson, J., Hagberg, B. (1990) 'Delayed-onset dyskinetic "cerebral palsy" – a late effect of perinatal asphyxia?' *Acta Paediatrica Scandinavica*, **79**, 1121–1123.

Asindi, A.A., Stephenson, J.B., Young, D.G. (1988) 'Spastic hemiparesis and presumed prenatal embolisation.' *Archives of Disease in Childhood*, **63**, 68–69.

Aso, K., Scher, M.S., Barmada, M.A. (1990) 'Cerebral infarcts and seizures in the neonate.' *Journal of Child Neurology*, **5**, 224–228.

Awon, M.P. (1964) 'The vacuum extractor—experimental demonstration of distortion of the fetal skull.' *Journal of Obstetrics and Gynaecology of the British Commonwealth*, **74**, 634–636.

Azzarelli, B., Velasco, M. (1987) 'Rostral and caudal patterns in perinatal "anoxic" central nervous system damage.' *Journal of Neuropathology and Experimental Neurology*, **46**, 385. *(Abstract no. 160.)*

Babcock, D.S., Ball, W. (1983) 'Postasphyxial encephalopathy in full-term infants: ultrasound diagnosis.' *Radiology*, **148**, 417–423.

Bachmann, K.D., Friedmann, G., Weiden, H., Springmann, L., Schmidt, E., Bolte, A. (1968) 'Pathologische befunde bei Neugeborenen nach Entbindung durch Vakuumextraktion.' *Geburtshilfe und Frauenheilkunde*, **28**, 1090–1103.

Bailey, O.T. (1959) 'Results of long survival after thrombosis of the superior sagittal sinus.' *Neurology*, **9**, 741–746.

—— Hass, G.M. (1958) 'Dural sinus thrombosis in early life.' *Journal of Pediatrics*, **11**, 755–772.

Balériaux, D., Ticket, L., Dony, D., Jeanmart, L. (1980) 'The contribution of CT to perinatal intracranial hemorrhage including that accompanying apparently uncomplicated delivery at full-term.' *Neuroradiology*, **19**, 273–277.

Baram, T.Z., Butler, I.J., Nelson, M.D., McArdle, C.B. (1988) 'Transverse sinus thrombosis in newborns: clinical and magnetic resonance imaging findings.' *Annals of Neurology*, **24**, 792–794.

Barkovich, A., Truwit, C.H. (1990) 'Brain damage from perinatal asphyxia: correlation of MR findings with gestational age.' *American Journal of Neuroradiology*, **11**, 1087–1096.

Barmada, M.A., Moossy, J., Schuman, R.M. (1979) 'Cerebral infarcts with arterial occlusion in neonates.' *Annals of Neurology*, **6**, 495–502.

Barson, A.J. (1983) 'The changing pattern of perinatal pathology.' *In:* Chiswick, M.L. (Ed.) *Recent Advances in Perinatal Medicine*. London: Churchill Livingstone, pp. 1–20.

—— (1990) 'A postmortem study of infection in the newborn from 1976 to 1988.' *In:* De Louvois, J., Harvey, D. (Eds) *Perinatal Practice, Vol. 6. Infection in the Newborn*. Chichester: John Wiley, pp. 13–34.

Baumann, R.J., Carr, W.A., Shuman, R.M. (1987) 'Patterns of cerebral arterial injury in children with neurological disabilities.' *Journal of Child Neurology*, **2**, 298–306.

Beatty, R.A. (1974) 'Surgical treatment of a ruptured intracerebral arteriovenous malformation in a newborn.' *Pediatrics*, **53**, 571–572.

Bejar, R., Coen, R.W., Ekpoudia, I., James, H.E., Gluck, L. (1985) 'Real time ultrasound diagnosis of hemorrhagic pathological conditions in the posterior fossa of preterm infants.' *Neurosurgery*, **16**, 281–289.

Beltramello, A., Perini, S., Mazza, C. (1991) 'Spontaneously healed vein of Galen aneurysm: clinical radiological features.' *Child's Nervous System*, **7**, 129–134.

Ben-Ami, T., Yousefzadeh, D., Backus, M., Reichman, B., Kessler, A., Hammerman-Rozenberg, C. (1990) 'Lenticulostriate vasculopathy in infants with infections of the central nervous system: sonographic and Doppler findings.' *Pediatric Radiology*, **20**, 575–579.

Beneke, R. (1910) 'Ueber Tentoriumzerreißungen bei der Geburt, sowie die Bedeutung der Duraspannung für chronische Gehirnerkrankungen.' *Muenchener Medizinische Wochenschrift*, **4**, 2125–2127.

Bergman, I., Bauer, R.E., Barmada, M.A., Latchaw, R.E., Taylor, H.G., David, R. Painter, M.J. (1985) 'Intracerebral hemorrhage in the full-term neonatal infant.' *Pediatrics*, **75**, 488–496.

Berman, P.H., Banker, B.Q. (1966) 'Neonatal meningitis. A clinical and pathological study of 29 cases.' *Pediatrics*, **38**, 6–24.

Bignami, A., Ralston, H.J. (1968) 'Myelination of fibrillary astroglial processes in long term Wallerian degeneration. The possible relationship to status marmoratus.' *Brain Research*, **11**, 710–713.

Billard, C., Dulac, O., Diebler, C. (1982) 'Ramollissement cérébral ischémique du nouveau-né.' *Archives Françaises de Pédiatrie*, **39**, 677–683.

194

Bird, G.C. (1982) 'The use of the vacuum extractor.' *Clinics in Obstetrics and Gynecology*, **9**, 641–661.

Bjarke, B., Herin, P., Blombäek, M. (1974) 'Neonatal aortic thrombosis. A possible clinical manifestation of congenital antithrombin III deficiency.' *Acta Paediatrica Scandinavica*, **63**, 297–301.

Bladin, P.F., Berkovic, S.F. (1984) 'Striatocapsular infarction: large infarcts in the lenticulostriate arterial territory.' *Neurology*, **34**, 1423–1430.

Blanc, J.F., Langue, J., Bochu, M., DutrugeSalle, B. (1982) 'Les hémorragies intra-cérébrales chez le nouveau-né à terme.' *Archives Françaises de Pédiatrie*, **39**, 251–253.

Blank, N.K., Strand, R., Gilles, F.H., Palakshappa, A. (1978) 'Posterior fossa subdural hematomas in neonates.' *Archives of Neurology*, **35**, 108–111.

Blazer, S., Hemli, J.A., Sujov, P.O., Braun, J. (1989) 'Neonatal bilateral diaphragmatic paralysis caused by brain stem haemorrhage.' *Archives of Disease in Childhood*, **64**, 50–52.

Blennow, G., Svenningsen, N.W., Gustafsson, B., Sunden, B., Cronquist, S. (1977) 'Neonatal and prospective follow-up study of infants delivered by vacuum extraction.' *Acta Obstetricia et Gynaecologica Scandinavica*, **56**, 189–192.

Bogousslavsky, J. (1992) 'The plurality of subcortical infarction.' *Stroke*, **23**, 629–631.

Boon, W.H. (1961) 'Vacuum extraction in obstetrics.' *Lancet*, **2**, 662.

Borit, A., Herndon, R.M. (1970) 'The fine structure of plaques fibromyéliniques in ulegyria and in status marmoratus.' *Acta Neuropathologica*, **14**, 304–311.

Boynton, R.C., Morgan, B.C. (1973) 'Cerebral arteriovenous fistula with possible hereditary telangiectasia.' *American Journal of Diseases of Children*, **125**, 99–101.

Brand, M., Saling, E. (1988) 'Obstetrical factors and intracranial hemorrhage.' *In:* Kubli, F., Patel, N., Schmidt, W., Linderkamp, O. (Eds) *Perinatal Events and Brain Damage in Surviving Children*. Berlin: Springer-Verlag, pp. 216–227.

Brann, A.W., Myers, R.E. (1975) 'Central nervous system findings in the newborn monkey following severe *in utero* partial asphyxia.' *Neurology*, **25**, 327–338.

Brenner, B., Fishman, A., Goldsher, D., Schreibman, D., Tavory, S. (1988) 'Cerebral thrombosis in a newborn with a congenital deficiency of antithrombin III.' *American Journal of Hematology*, **27**, 209–211.

Bret, A.J., Coiffard, P. (1961) 'Les ancêtres des ventouses obstétricales.' *Revue Française de Gynécologie et d'Obstétrique*, **56**, 535–553.

Brill, C.B., Jarath, V., Black, P. (1985) 'Occipital interhemispheric acute subdural hematoma treated by lambdoid suture tap.' *Neurosurgery*, **16**, 247–251.

Brockerhoff, P., Brand, M., Ludwig, B. (1981) 'Untersuchungen zur Häufigkeit perinataler Hirnblutungen und deren Abhängigkeit von Geburtsverlauf mit Hilfe der cranialen Computer-tomographie.' *Geburtshilfe und Frauenheilkunde*, **41**, 597–600.

Brückmann, H., Kotlarek, F., Biniek, R., Roßberg, C. (1989) 'Stammganglieninfarkte im Kindesalter, klinisch-neuroradiologische Befunde und Differentialdiagnose.' *Klinische Pädiatrie*, **201**, 78–85.

Brun, A., Kyllerman, M. (1979) 'Clinical, pathogenic and neuropathological correlates in dystonic cerebral palsy.' *European Journal of Pediatrics*, **131**, 93–104.

Buchan, G.C., Alvord, E.C. (1969) 'Diffuse necrosis of subcortical white matter associated with bacterial meningitis.' *Neurology*, **19**, 1–9.

Buchanan, G.R. (1986) 'Coagulation disorders in the neonate.' *Pediatric Clinics of North America*, **33**, 203–220.

Burger, P.C., Graham, D.G., Burch, J.G., Hackel, D.B. (1978) 'Hemorrhagic cerebral white matter infarction with cerebral deep venous thrombosis and hypoxia.' *Archives of Pathology and Laboratory Medicine*, **102**, 40–42.

Burman, D., Mansell, P.W.A., Warin, R.P. (1967) 'Miliary haemangiomata in the newborn.' *Archives of Disease in Childhood*, **42**, 193–197.

Burns, A.J., Kaplan, L.C., Mulliken, J.B. (1991) 'Is there an association between hemangioma and syndromes with dysmorphic features?' *Pediatrics*, **88**, 1257–1267.

Burry, V.F., Hellerstein, S. (1966) 'Septicemia and subperiosteal cephalhematomas.' *Journal of Pediatrics*, **69**, 1133–1135.

Burton, K., Farrell, K., Calne, D.B. (1984) 'Dystonia and basal ganglia lesions: is there a correlation with putaminal dysfunction?' *Neurology*, **34** (Suppl. 1), 130.

Butler, N.R., Alberman, E.D. (1969) *Perinatal Problems. The Second Report of the 1958 British*

Perinatal Mortality Survey. Edinburgh: E. & S. Livingstone.
—— Bonham, D.G. (1963) *Perinatal Mortality: The First Report of the 1958 British Perinatal Mortality Survey.* Edinburgh: E. & S. Livingstone.
Byard, R.W., Burrows, P.E., Izakawa, T., Silver, M.M. (1991) 'Diffuse infantile haemangiomatosis: clinicopathological features and management problems in five fatal cases.' *European Journal of Pediatrics*, **150**, 224–227.
Byers, R.K., Hass, G.M. (1933) 'Thrombosis of the dural venous sinuses in infancy and childhood.' *American Journal of Diseases of Children*, **45**, 1161–1183.
Cabanas, F., Pellicer, A., Perez-Higueras, A., Garcia-Alix, A., Roche, C., Quero, J. (1991) 'Ultrasonographic findings in thalamus and basal ganglia in term asphyxiated infants.' *Pediatric Neurology*, **7**, 211–215.
Caen, J.P. (1989) 'Platelet disorders.' *Baillière's Clinical Haematology*, **2**, 503–747.
Calvert, S.A., Widness, J.A., Oh, W., Stonestreet, B.S. (1990) 'The effects of acute uterine ischemia on fetal circulation.' *Pediatric Research*, **27**, 552–556.
Camfield, P.R., Camfield, C.S. (1987) 'Neonatal seizures: a commentary on selected aspects.' *Journal of Child Neurology*, **2**, 244–251.
Cammermeyer, J. (1953) 'Agonal nature of the cerebral ring hemorrhages.' *Archives of Neurology and Psychiatry*, **70**, 54–63.
Carpenter, M.B. (1950) 'Athetosis and the basal ganglia: review of literature and study of 42 cases.' *Archives of Neurology and Psychiatry*, **63**, 875–901.
Carrillo, R., Carreira, L.M., Prada, J., Rosas, C., Egas, G. (1984) 'Giant aneurysm arising from a single arteriovenous fistula in a child.' *Journal of Neurosurgery*, **60**, 1085–1088.
Carson, S.C., Hertzberg, B.S., Bowie, J.D., Burger, P.C. (1990) 'Value of sonography in the diagnosis of intracranial hemorrhage and periventricular leukomalacia.' *American Journal of Roentgenology*, **155**, 595–601.
Carter, L.P., Pittman, H.W. (1971) 'Posterior fossa subdural hematoma of the newborn.' *Journal of Neurosurgery*, **34**, 423–426.
Cartwright, G.W., Culbertson, K., Schreiner, R.L., Garg, B.P. (1979) 'Changes in clinical presentation of term infants with intracranial hemorrhage.' *Developmental Medicine and Child Neurology*, **21**, 730–737.
Cavazutti, M., Duffy, T.E. (1982) 'Regulation of local cerebral blood flow in normal and hypoxic newborn dogs.' *Annals of Neurology*, **11**, 247–257.
Chalmers, J.A. (1971) *The Obstetric Vacuum Extractor.* London: Lloyd-Luke.
Chandra, S.A., Gilbert, E.F., Viseskul, C., Strother, C.M., Haning, R.V., Javid, M.J. (1990) 'Neonatal intracranial choriocarcinoma.' *Archives of Pathology and Laboratory Medicine*, **114**, 1079–1082.
Chaou, W-T., Chou, M-L., Eitzmann, D.V. (1984) 'Intracranial hemorrhage and vitamin K deficiency in early infancy.' *Journal of Pediatrics*, **105**, 880–884.
Chaplin, E.R., Goldstein, G.W., Norman, D. (1979) 'Neonatal seizures, intracerebral hematoma, and subarachnoid hemorrhage in full-term infants.' *Pediatrics*, **63**, 812–815.
Chasnoff, I.J., Bussey, M.E., Savich, R. (1986) 'Perinatal cerebral infarction and maternal cocaine use.' *Journal of Pediatrics*, **108**, 456–459.
Chessells, J.M., Wigglesworth, J.S. (1970) 'Secondary haemorrhagic disease of the newborn.' *Archives of Disease in Childhood*, **45**, 539–543.
Chiswick, M.L., James, D.K. (1979) 'Kielland's forceps: association with neonatal morbidity and mortality.' *British Medical Journal*, **1**, 7–9.
Choux, M., Grisoli, F., Peragut, J.C. (1975) 'Extradural hematomas in children: 104 cases.' *Child's Brain*, **1**, 337–347.
—— Lena, G., Genitori, L. (1986) 'Intracranial hematomas.' *In:* Raimondi, A.J., Choux, M., DiRocco, C. (Eds) *Head Injuries in the Newborn and Infant.* New-York: Springer-Verlag, pp. 203–216.
Chugani, H.T., Phelps, M.E. (1986) 'Maturational changes in cerebral function in infants determined by [18]FDG positron emission tomography.' *Science*, **231**, 840–843.
Churchill, J.A., Stevenson, L., Habhab, G. (1966) 'Cephalhematoma and natal brain injury.' *Obstetrics and Gynecology*, **27**, 580–584.
Clancy, R., Malin, S., Larague, D., Baumgart, S., Younkin, D. (1985) 'Focal motor seizures heralding

196

stroke in full-term neonates.' *American Journal of Diseases of Children*, **139**, 601–606.

Close, P.J., Carty, H.M. (1991) 'Transient gyriform brightness on non-contrast enhanced computed tomography (CT) brain scan of seven infants.' *Pediatric Radiology*, **21**, 189–192.

Co, E., Raju, T.N., Aldana, O. (1991) 'Cerebellar dimensions in assessment of gestational age in neonates.' *Radiology*, **181**, 581–585.

Cocker, J., George, S.W., Yates, P.O. (1965) 'Perinatal occlusion of the middle cerebral artery.' *Developmental Medicine and Child Neurology*, **7**, 235–243.

Cohen, D.L. (1978) 'Neonatal subgaleal hemorrhage in hemophilia.' *Journal of Pediatrics*, **93**, 1022–1023.

Coker, S., Beltran, R., Fine, M. (1987) 'Neonatal posterior fossa subdural hematoma.' *Clinical Pediatrics*, **26**, 375–376.

Colamaria, V., Curatolo, P., Cusmai, R., Della Bernardina, B. (1988) 'Symmetrical bithalamic hyperdensities in asphyxiated full-term newborns: an early indicator of status marmoratus.' *Brain and Development*, **10**, 57–59.

Colan, R.V. (1986) 'Gelatin sign: ultrasonographic evidence of cerebral necrosis in infants.' *Pediatrics*, **77**, 774–777.

Comstock, C.H., Kirk, J.S. (1991) 'Arteriovenous malformations. Locations and evolution in the fetal brain.' *Journal of Ultrasound Medicine*, **10**, 361–365.

Cooper, N.A., Lynch, M.A. (1979) 'Delayed haemorrhagic disease of the newborn with extradural haematoma.' *British Medical Journal*, **1**, 164–165.

Coplerud, J.M., Wagerle, C.L., Delivoria, M. (1989) 'Regional cerebral blood flow response during and after acute asphyxia in newborn piglets.' *Journal of Applied Physiology*, **66**, 2827–2832.

Cottrill, C.M., Kaplan, S. (1973) 'Cerebral vascular accidents in cyanotic congenital heart disease.' *American Journal of Diseases of Children*, **125**, 484–487.

Craig, W.S. (1938) 'Intracranial haemorrhage in the newborn.' *Archives of Disease in Childhood*, **13**, 89–124.

Critchley, E.R. (1968) 'Observations on retinal haemorrhages in the newborn.' *Journal of Neurology, Neurosurgery and Psychiatry*, **31**, 259–262.

Cushing, H. (1905) 'Concerning surgical intervention for the intracranial hemorrhages of the newborn.' *American Journal of Medical Science*, **130**, 563–581.

Cussen, L.J., Ryan, G.B. (1967) 'Hemorrhagic cerebral necrosis in neonatal infants with enterobacterial meningitis.' *Journal of Pediatrics*, **71**, 771–776.

Cyr, R.M., Usher, R.H., McLean, F.H. (1984) 'Changing patterns of birth asphyxia and trauma over 20 years.' *American Journal of Obstetrics and Gynecology*, **148**, 490–498.

Dambska, M., Laure-Kamionowska, M., Schmidt-Sidor, B. (1989) 'Early and late neuropathological changes in perinatal white matter damage.' *Journal of Child Neurology*, **4**, 291–298.

Dan, U., Shalev, E., Greif, M., Weiner, E. (1992) 'Prenatal diagnosis of fetal brain arteriovenous malformation: the use of color Doppler imaging.' *Journal of Clinical Ultrasound*, **20**, 149–151.

Daum, R.S., Scheifele, D.W., Syriopoulou, V.P., Averill, D., Smith, A.L. (1978) 'Ventricular involvement in experimental *Hemophilus influenzae* meningitis.' *Journal of Pediatrics*, **93**, 927–930.

Dave, P., Curless, R.G., Steinman, L. (1984) 'Cerebellar hemorrhage complicating methylmalonic and propionic acidemia.' *Archives of Neurology*, **41**, 1293–1296.

De Campo, M. (1989) 'Neonatal posterior fossa haemorrhage: a difficult ultrasound diagnosis.' *Australasian Radiology*, **33**, 150–153.

De Courten, G.M., Rabinowicz, T. (1981) 'Intraventricular hemorrhage in premature infants: reappraisal and new hypothesis.' *Developmental Medicine and Child Neurology*, **23**, 389–403.

De Gersem, R., De Laet, P., Vanhaesebrouck, P., Van Werveke, S., Leroy, J. (1984) 'Intracraniële bloeding bij pasgeborene na pre-partum inname van salicylaat door de moeder.' *Tijdschrift voor Geneeskunde*, **40**, 1197–1200.

De Girolami, U., Crowell, R.M., Marcoux, F.W. (1984) 'Selective necrosis and total necrosis in focal cerebral ischemia. Neuropathologic observations on experimental middle cerebral artery occlusion in the Macaque monkey.' *Journal of Neuropathology and Experimental Neurology*, **43**, 57–71.

De la Fuente, A. (1991) 'Locking and reverse molding of the fetal skull.' *Pediatric Pathology*, **11**, 271–280.

Delivoria-Papadopoulos, M., Chance, B. (1988) '^{31}P NMR spectroscopy in the newborn.' *In:* Guthrie, R.D. (Ed.) *Clinics in Critical Care Medicine, No. 14. Neonatal Intensive Care.* New York:

Churchill-Livingstone, pp. 153–179.

Del Toro, J., Louis, P.T., Goddard-Finegold, J. (1991) 'Cerebrovascular regulation and neonatal brain injury.' *Pediatric Neurology*, **7**, 3–12.

Deonna, T., Oberson, R. (1974) 'Acute subdural hematoma in the newborn.' *Neuropädiatrie*, **5**, 181–190.

—— Prod'hom, L-S. (1980) 'Temporal lobe epilepsy and hemianopsia in childhood of perinatal origin.' *Neuropädiatrie*, **11**, 85–90.

De Reuck, J.C. (1977) 'The significance of the arterial angioarchitecture in perinatal cerebral damage.' *Acta Neurologica Belgica*, **77**, 65–94.

—— Chattha, A.S., Richardson, E.P. (1972) 'Pathogenesis and evolution of periventricular leukomalacia in infancy.' *Archives of Neurology*, **27**, 229–236.

De Vries, L.S. (1987) *Ischaemic Lesions in the Premature Infant: Correlation of Imaging and Outcome.* (Thesis, University of Utrecht.)

—— Larroche, J.C., Levene, M.I. (1988a) 'Intracranial haemorrhage.' *In:* Levene, M.I., Bennett, M.J., Punt, J. (Eds) *Fetal and Neonatal Neurology and Neurosurgery.* London: Churchill-Livingstone.

—— Wigglesworth, J.S., Regev, R., Dubowitz, L.M.S. (1988b) 'Evolution of periventricular leukomalacia during the neonatal period and infancy: correlation of imaging and postmortem findings.' *Early Human Development*, **17**, 205–219.

—— Dubowitz, L.M.S., Dubowitz, V., Pennock, J.M. (1990) *Brain Disorders in the Newborn.* London: Wolfe Medical.

—— Smet, M., Goemans, W., Wilms, G., Devlieger, H., Casaer, P. (1992) 'Unilateral thalamic haemorrhage in the preterm and full-term newborn.' *Neuropediatrics*, **23**, 153–156.

Dietrich, R.B., Bradley, W.G. (1988) 'Iron accumulation in the basal ganglia following severe ischemic–anoxic insults in children.' *Radiology*, **168**, 203–206.

Dische, M.R., Gooch, W.M. (1981) 'Congenital toxoplasmosis.' *In:* Rosenberg, H.S., Bernstein, J. (Eds) *Perspectives in Pediatric Pathology, Vol. 6: Infectious Diseases.* New York: Masson, pp. 83–113.

Doe, F.D., Shuangshoti, S., Netsky, M.G. (1972) 'Cryptic hemangioma of the choroid plexus. A cause of intraventricular hemorrhage.' *Neurology*, **22**, 1232–1239.

Dolfin, T., Skidmore, M.B., Fong, K.W., Hoskins, E.M., Shennan, A.T., Hill, A. (1984) 'Diagnosis and evolution of periventricular leukomalacia: a study with real time ultrasound.' *Early Human Development*, **9**, 105–109.

Donat, J.F., Okazaki, H., Kleinberg, F., Reagan, T.J. (1978) 'Intraventricular hemorrhages in full-term and premature infants.' *Mayo Clinic Proceedings*, **53**, 437–441.

Dorsic, D., Altenburg, H., Herter, T. (1983) 'Diagnosis and treatment of cystic non-tumorous lesions of the posterior fossa in children.' *Advances in Neurosurgery*, **11**, 299–301.

Draaisma, J.M., Rotteveel, J.J., Meekma, R., Geven, W.B. (1991) 'Neonatal dural sinus thrombosis.' *Tijdschrift voor Kindergeneeskunde*, **59**, 64–67.

Dubose Ravenel, S. (1979) 'Posterior fossa hemorrhage in the term newborn: report of two cases.' *Pediatrics*, **64**, 39–42.

Dubowitz, L.M.S., Levene, M.I., Morante, A., Palmer, P., Dubowitz, V. (1981) 'Neurologic signs in neonatal intraventricular hemorrhage: a correlation with real-time ultrasound.' *Journal of Pediatrics*, **99**, 127–133.

—— Bydder, G.M., Mushin, J. (1985) 'Developmental sequence of periventricular leukomalacia: correlation of ultrasound, clinical and nuclear magnetic resonance functions.' *Archives of Disease in Childhood*, **60**, 349–355.

Duchon, M.A., De Mund, M.A., Brown, R.H. (1988) 'Laboratory comparison of modern vacuum extractors'. *Obstetrics and Gynecology*, **71**, 155–158.

Dunn, D.W. (1982) 'Acute subdural hematoma after subdural punctures.' *American Journal of Diseases of Children*, **136**, 371–372.

Easa, D. (1978) 'Coagulation abnormalities associated with localized hemorrhage in the neonate.' *Journal of Pediatrics*, **92**, 989–994.

Edvinsson, L., Lou, H.C., Tvede, K. (1986) 'On the pathogenesis of regional cerebral ischemia in intracranial hemorrhage: a causal influence of potassium?' *Pediatric Research*, **20**, 478–480.

Ehlers, H., Courville, C.B. (1936) 'Thrombosis of internal cerebral veins in infancy and childhood.'

Journal of Pediatrics, **8**, 600–623.

Eick, J.J., Miller, K.D., Bell, K.A., Tutton, R.H. (1981) 'Computed tomography of deep cerebral venous thrombosis in children.' *Radiology*, **140**, 399–402.

Ellis, S.S., Montgomery, J.R., Wagner, M., Hill, R.M. (1974) 'Osteomyelitis complicating neonatal cephalhematoma.' *American Journal of Diseases of Children*, **127**, 100–102.

Ellis, W.G., Goetzman, B.W., Lindenberg, J.A. (1988) 'Neuropathologic documentation of prenatal brain damage.' *American Journal of Diseases of Children*, **142**, 858–866.

Emery, J.L. (1972) 'Locking and reverse moulding of the fetal skull related to cerebral birth trauma.' *Nederlands Tijdschrift voor Verloskunde en Gynecologie*, **2**, 13–23.

Emmanouilides, G.C., Hoy, R.C. (1967) 'Transumbilical aortography and selective arteriography in newborn infants.' *Pediatrics*, **39**, 337–343.

Ennis, M., Vincent, C.A. (1990) 'Obstetric accidents: a review of 64 cases.' *British Medical Journal*, **300**, 1365–1367.

Eskes, J.K.A.B., Martinez, A., De Haan, J., Briet, J.W., Jongsma, H.W. (1975) 'Pressure on the hydrocephalic fetal head during the first stage of labour.' *European Journal of Obstetrics, Gynecology and Reproductive Biology*, **4/5**, 171–176.

Esparza, J., Portillo, J.M., Mateos, F., Lamas, E. (1982) 'Extradural hemorrhage in the posterior fossa in neonates.' *Surgical Neurology*, **17**, 341–343.

Espinoza, M.I., Parer, J.T. (1991) 'Mechanisms of asphyxial brain damage, and possible pharmacologic interventions, in the fetus.' *American Journal of Obstetrics and Gynecology*, **164**, 1582–1591.

Evrard, P., Gressens, P., Volpe, J.J. (1992) 'New concepts to understand the neurological consequences of subcortical lesions in the premature brain.' *Biology of the Neonate*, **61**, 1–3.

Fahmy, K. (1971) 'Cephalhematoma following vacuum extraction.' *Journal of Obstetrics and Gynaecology of the British Commonwealth*, **78**, 369–372.

Faix, R.G., Donn, S.M. (1983) 'Immediate management of the traumatized infant.' *Clinics in Perinatology*, **10**, 487–505.

—— —— (1985) 'Association of septic shock caused by early-onset group B streptococcal sepsis and periventricular leukomalacia in the infant.' *Pediatrics*, **76**, 415–419.

Fenichel, G.M. (1983) 'Hypoxic–ischemic encephalopathy in the newborn.' *Archives of Neurology*, **40**, 261–266.

—— Webster, D.L., Wong, W.K.T. (1984) 'Intracranial hemorrhage in the term newborn.' *Archives of Neurology*, **41**, 30–34.

Ferry, P.C., Kerber, C., Peterson, D., Gallo, A.A. (1974) 'Arteriectasis, subarachnoid hemorrhage in a three-month-old infant.' *Neurology*, **24**, 494–500.

Fischer, A.Q., Chall, V.R., Burton, B.K., McLean, W.T. (1981) 'Cerebellar hemorrhage complicating isovaleric acidemia: a case report.' *Neurology*, **31**, 746–748.

—— Anderson, J.C., Shuman, R.M. (1988) 'The evolution of ischemic cerebral infarction in infancy: a sonographic evaluation.' *Journal of Child Neurology*, **3**, 105–109.

Fischer, E.G., Strand, R.D., Gilles, F.H. (1972) 'Cerebellar necrosis simulating tumor in infancy.' *Journal of Pediatrics*, **81**, 98–100.

Fishman, M.A., Percy, A.K., Cheek, W.R., Speer, M.E. (1981) 'Successful conservative management of cerebellar hematomas in term neonates.' *Journal of Pediatrics*, **98**, 466–468.

Fitzhardinge, P.M., Flodmark, O., Fitz, C.R., Ashby, S. (1981) 'The prognostic value of computed tomography as an adjunct to assessment of the term infant with postasphyxial encephalopathy.' *Journal of Pediatrics*, **99**, 777–781.

Flodmark, O., Becker, L.E., Harwood-Nash, D.C., Fitzhardinge, P.M., Fitz, C.R., Chuang, S.H. (1980*a*) 'Correlation between computed tomography and autopsy in premature and full-term neonates that have suffered perinatal asphyxia.' *Radiology*, **137**, 93–103.

—— Fitz, C., Harwood-Nash, D.C. (1980*b*) 'CT diagnosis and short-term prognosis of intracranial hemorrhage and hypoxic–ischemic brain damage in neonates.' *Journal of Computer Assisted Tomography*, **4**, 775–787.

Fouché, S., Sevely, A., Rolland, M., Manelfe, C., Regnier, C. (1982) 'Hémorragies intracérébrales non-traumatiques du nouveau-né à terme.' *Pédiatrie*, **37**, 185–193.

Fowler, M., Dow, R., White, T.A., Greer, C.H. (1972) 'Congenital hydrocephalus–hydrencephaly in five siblings, with autopsy studies: a new disease.' *Developmental Medicine and Child Neurology*, **14**, 173–188.

Foy, P., Dubbins, P.A., Waldroup, L., Graziani, L., Goldberg, B.B., Berry, R. (1982) 'Ultrasound demonstration of cerebellar hemorrhage in a neonate.' *Journal of Clinical Ultrasound*, **10**, 196–198.

Frank, E., Zusman, E. (1991) 'Aneurysms of the distal anterior cerebral artery in infants.' *Pediatric Neurosurgery*, **16**, 179–182.

Frantzen, E., Jacobsen, H.H., Therkelsen, J. (1962) 'Cerebral artery occlusions in children due to trauma to the head and neck.' *Neurology*, **11**, 695–700.

French, B.N. Dublin, A.B. (1977) 'Infantile chronic subdural hematoma of the posterior fossa diagnosed by computerized tomography.' *Journal of Neurosurgery*, **47**, 949–952.

Friede, R.L. (1972) 'Subpial hemorrhage in infants.' *Journal of Neuropathology and Experimental Neurology*, **31**, 548–556.

—— (1973) 'Cerebral infarcts complicating neonatal leptomeningitis.' *Acta Neuropathologica*, **23**, 245–253.

—— (1989) *Developmental Neuropathology*. Berlin: Springer-Verlag.

—— Schachenmayr, W. (1977) 'Early stages of status marmoratus.' *Acta Neuropathologica*, **38**, 123–127.

Friedman, D.M., Madrid, M., Berenstein, A., Choi, I.S., Wisoff, J.H. (1991) 'Neonatal vein of Galen malformations: experience in developing a multidisciplinary approach using an embolization treatment protocol.' *Clinical Pediatrics*, **30**, 621–629.

Fruchtman, S., Aledort, L.M. (1986) 'Disseminated intravascular coagulation.' *Journal of the American College of Cardiology*, **8**, 159B–167B.

Fujii, K., Lenkey, C., Rhoton, A.L. (1980) 'Microsurgical anatomy of the choroidal arteries: lateral and third ventricles.' *Journal of Neurosurgery*, **52**, 165–188.

Fujimoto, S., Yokochi, K., Togari, H., Nishimura, Y., Imukai, K., Futamura, M., Sobagima, H., Suzuki, S., Wada, Y. (1992) 'Neonatal cerebral infarction: symptoms, CT findings and prognosis.' *Brain and Development*, **14**, 48–52.

Fujita, K., Matsuo, N., Mori, O., Koda, N., Mukai, E., Okabe, Y., Shirakawa, N., Tamai, S., Itagane, Y., Hibi, I. (1992) 'The association of hypopituitarism with small pituitary, invisible pituitary stalk, type 1 Arnold–Chiari malformation, and syringomyelia in seven patients born in breech position: a further proof of birth injury theory on the pathogenesis of "idiopathic hypopituitarism".' *European Journal of Pediatrics*, **151**, 266–270.

Gaissie, G., Roberts, M.S., Bouldin, T.W., Scatliff, J.H. (1990) 'The echogenic ependymal wall in intraventricular hemorrhage: sonographic–pathologic correlation.' *Pediatric Radiology*, **20**, 297–300.

Gama, C.H., Fenichel, G.M. (1985) 'Epidural hematoma of the newborn due to birth trauma.' *Pediatric Neurology*, **1**, 52–53.

Garcia, J.H. (1992) 'The evolution of brain infarcts. A review.' *Journal of Neuropathology and Experimental Neurology*, **51**, 387–393.

Garcia-Chavez, C., Moossy, J. (1965) 'Cerebral artery aneurysm in infancy: association with agenesis of the corpus callosum.' *Journal of Neuropathology*, **24**, 492–501.

Geirsson, R.T. (1988) 'Birth trauma and brain damage.' *Baillière's Clinical Obstetrics and Gynaecology*, **2**, 195–212.

Geller, J.D., Topper, S.F., Hashimoto, K. (1991) 'Diffuse neonatal haemangiomatosis: a new constellation of findings.' *Journal of the American Academy of Dermatology*, **24**, 816–818.

Gerlach, J. (1969) 'Intracerebral hemorrhage caused by microangiomas.' *Progress in Neurological Surgery*, **3**, 363–369.

Ghram, M., Trabelsi, M., Hammou-Jeddi, A., Bardi, I., Laouati, M., Touibi, S., Bennaceur, B., Gharbi, H.A. (1988) 'Insuffisance cardiaque secondaire à une malformation artério-veineuse de la région de l'ampoule de Galien. Traitement par embolisation endovasculaire.' *Pédiatrie*, **43**, 677–682.

Gibson, B. (1989) 'Neonatal haemostasis. Regular review.' *Archives of Disease in Childhood*, **64**, 503–506.

Gilles, F.H., Murphy, S.F. (1969) 'Perinatal telencephalic leucoencephalopathy.' *Journal of Neurology, Neurosurgery and Psychiatry*, **32**, 404–413.

—— Shillito, J. (1970) 'Infantile hydrocephalus: retrocerebellar subdural hematoma.' *Journal of Pediatrics*, **76**, 529–537.

—— Jammes, J.L., Berenberg, W. (1977) 'Neonatal meningitis. The ventricle as a bacterial reservoir.'

Archives of Neurology, **34**, 560–562.

Ginsberg, H.G., Coulon, R.A., Culpepper, W.S., Wood, B.P. (1992) 'Vein of Galen "aneurysm" draining an arteriovenous malformation.' *American Journal of Diseases of Children*, **146**, 349–350.

Ginsberg, M.D., Myers, R.E., McDonagh, B.F. (1974) 'Experimental carbon monoxide encephalopathy in the primate.' *Archives of Neurology*, **30**, 209–216.

Glauser, T.A., Rorke, L.B., Weinberg, D.M., Clancy, R.R. (1990) 'Acquired neuropathological lesions associated with the hypoplastic left heart syndrome.' *Pediatrics*, **85**, 991–1000.

Gluckman, P.D., Williams, C.E., Gunn, A.J. (1991) 'Brain stem and cerebral function in the fetus: its assessment and the impact of asphyxia.' *In:* Hanson, M.A. (Ed.) *The Fetal and Neonatal Brain Stem.* Cambridge: Cambridge University Press, pp. 185–210.

Goddard-Finegold, J., Michael, L.H. (1992) 'Brain vasoactive effects of phenobarbital during hypertension and hypoxia in newborn pigs.' *Pediatric Research*, **32**, 103–106.

Goetting, M.G., Sowa, B. (1990) 'Retinal hemorrhage after cardiopulmonary resuscitation in children: an etiologic re-evaluation.' *Pediatrics*, **85**, 585–588.

Gomori, J.M., Grossman, R.I., Goldberg, H.I., Zimmerman, R.A., Bilaniuk, L.T. (1985) 'Intracranial hematomas: imaging by high-field MR.' *Radiology*, **157**, 87–93.

—— —— Hackney, D.B., Zimmerman, R.A., Bilaniuk, L.T. (1986) 'Occult cerebral vascular malformations: high-field MR imaging.' *Radiology*, **158**, 707–713.

Gordon, I.J., Shah, B.L., Hardman, D.R., Chameides, L. (1977) 'Giant dural supratentorial arteriovenous malformation.' *American Journal of Roentgenology*, **129**, 734–736.

Gordon, N., Isler, W. (1989) 'Childhood moyamoya disease.' *Developmental Medicine and Child Neurology*, **31**, 98–107.

Gould, S.J., Howard, S., Hope, P.L., Reynolds, E.O.R. (1987) 'Periventricular intraparenchymal cerebral haemorrhage in preterm infants: the role of venous infarction.' *Journal of Pathology*, **151**, 197–202.

Gouyon, J.B., Alison, M., Nivelon, J-L. (1981) 'Conservative management of cerebellar hematomas in neonates.' *Journal of Pediatrics*, **90**, 827–828.

—— Cinquin, A.M., Sautreaux, J.L., Thierry, A., Giroud, M., Alison, M. (1985) 'L'hématome extradural du nouveau-né. Complication rare d'un accouchement par forceps.' *Archives Françaises de Pédiatrie*, **42**, 333–334.

Govaert, P., Van de Velde, E., Vanhaesebrouck, P., De Praeter, C., Leroy, J. (1990a) 'CT diagnosis of neonatal subarachnoid haemorrhage.' *Pediatric Radiology*, **20**, 139–142.

—— Vanhaesebrouck, P., Calliauw, L. (1990b) 'On the management of neonatal tentorial damage. Eight case reports and a literature review.' *Acta Neurochirurgica*, **106**, 52–64.

—— Oostra, A., Matthijs, D., Vanhaesebrouck, P., Leroy, J. (1991) 'How idiopathic is idiopathic external hydrocephalus?' *Developmental Medicine and Child Neurology*, **33**, 273–276.

—— Achten, E., Vanhaesebrouck, P., De Praeter, C., Van Damme, J. (1992a) 'Deep cerebral venous thrombosis in thalamo-ventricular haemorrhage of the term newborn.' *Pediatric Radiology*, **22**, 123–127.

—— Leroy, J., Caemaert, J., Wood, B. (1992b) 'Extensive neonatal subarachnoid hematoma.' *American Journal of Diseases of Children*, **146**, 635–636.

—— Vanhaesebrouck, P., De Praeter, C. (1992c) 'Traumatic neonatal intracranial bleeding and stroke.' *Archives of Disease in Childhood*, **67**, 840–845.

—— —— —— Moens, K., Leroy, J. (1992d) 'Vacuum extraction, bone injury and neonatal subgaleal bleeding.' *European Journal of Pediatrics*, **151**, 532–535.

—— Voet, D., Achten, E., Vanhaesebrouck, P., Van Rostenberghe, H., Van Gijsel, D., Afschrift, M. (1992e) 'Non-invasive diagnosis of superior sagittal sinus thrombosis in a neonate.' *American Journal of Perinatology*, **9**, 201–204.

Graeb, D.A., Dolman, C.L. (1986) 'Radiological and pathological aspects of dural arteriovenous fistulas.' *Journal of Neurosurgery*, **64**, 962–967.

Gresham, E.L. (1975) 'Birth trauma.' *Pediatric Clinics of North America*, **22**, 317–328.

Grode, M.L., Saunders, M., Carton, C.A. (1978) 'Subarachnoid hemorrhage secondary to ruptured aneurysms in infants.' *Journal of Neurosurgery*, **64**, 962–967.

Gröntoft, O. (1953) 'Intracerebral and meningeal haemorrhages in perinatally deceased infants. II: Meningeal haemorrhages.' *Acta Obstetricia et Gynaecologica Scandinavica*, **3**, 458–498.

Gross, R.E. (1945) 'Arterial embolism and thrombosis in infancy.' *American Journal of Diseases of*

Children, **70**, 61–73.

Gudinchet, F., Dreyer, J-L., Payot, M., Duvoisin, B., Laurini, R. (1991) 'Imaging of neonatal arterial thrombosis.' *Archives of Disease in Childhood*, **66**, 1158–1159.

Guekos-Thöni, U., Boltshauser, E., Mieth, D., Isler, W. (1980) 'Intracranial haemorrhage in the term infant confirmed by computer tomography.' *Helvetica Paediatrica Acta*, **35**, 531–544.

Gugliantini, P., Caione, P., Fariella, G., Rivosechi, M. (1980) 'Post traumatic leptomeningeal cysts in infancy.' *Pediatric Radiology*, **9**, 11–14.

Guzzetta, F., Shackelford, G.D., Volpe, S., Perlman, J.M., Volpe, J.J. (1986) 'Periventricular intraparenchymal echodensities in the premature newborn: critical determinant of neurologic outcome.' *Pediatrics*, **78**, 995–1006.

Haddad, J., Messer, J., Aranda, J. (1992) 'Periventricular haemorrhagic infarction associated with subependymal germinal matrix haemorrhage in the premature newborn.' *European Journal of Pediatrics*, **151**, 63–65.

Halsey, A.B., Stoddard, R.A. (1984) 'Neonatal cerebral infarction.' *Journal of Pediatrics*, **104**, 957–958.

Hambleton, G., Wigglesworth, J.S. (1976) 'Origin of intraventricular haemorrhage in the preterm infant.' *Archives of Disease in Childhood*, **51**, 651–659.

Hanigan, W.C., Brady, T., Medlock, M., Smith, E.B. (1990a) 'Spontaneous regression of giant arteriovenous fistulae during the perinatal period.' *Journal of Neurosurgery*, **73**, 954–957.

—— Morgan, A.M., Stahlberg, L.K., Hiller, J.L. (1990b) 'Tentorial hemorrhage associated with vacuum extraction.' *Pediatrics*, **85**, 534–539.

Hansen, K.N., Pedersen, H., Petersen, M.B. (1987) 'Growing skull fracture—rupture of coronal suture caused by vacuum extraction.' *Neuroradiology*, **29**, 502.

Hanson, M. (1991) 'The control of the fetal circulation.' *In:* Hanson, M.A. (Ed.) *The Fetal and Neonatal Brain Stem.* Cambridge: Cambridge University Press, pp. 59–86.

Harper, C., Hockey, A. (1983) 'Proliferative vasculopathy and an hydranencephalic–hydrocephalic syndrome: a neuropathological study of two siblings.' *Developmental Medicine and Child Neurology*, **25**, 232–244.

Hauck, A.J., Bambara, J.F., Edwards, W.D. (1990) 'Embolism of brain tissue to the lung in a neonate.' *Archives of Pathology and Laboratory Medicine*, **114**, 217–218.

Hausbrandt, F., Meier, A. (1936) 'Zur Kenntnis der geburtstraumatischen und extrauterin erworbenen Schäden des Zentralnervensystems bei Neugeborenen.' *Frankfurter Zeitschrift für Pathologie*, **49**, 21–62.

Hayashi, T., Harada, K., Honda, E., Utsunomyia, H., Hashimoto, T. (1987) 'Rare neonatal intracerebral hemorrhage.' *Child's Nervous System*, **3**, 161–164.

—— Satoh, J., Sakamoto, K., Morimatsu, Y. (1991) 'Clinical and neuropathological findings in severe athetoid cerebral palsy: a comparative study of globo-Luysian and thalamo-putaminal groups.' *Brain and Development*, **13**, 47–51.

Hayden, C.K., Shattuck, K.E., Richardson, C.J., Ahrendt, D.K., House, R., Swischuk, L.E. (1985) 'Subependymal germinal matrix hemorrhage in full-term neonates.' *Pediatrics*, **75**, 714–718.

Headings, D.L., Glasgow, L.A. (1977) 'Occlusion of the internal carotid artery complicating *Haemophilus influenzae* meningitis.' *American Journal of Roentgenology*, **150**, 897–902.

Heafner, M.D., Duncan, C.C., Kier, E.L., Ment, L.R., Scott, D.T., Kolaski, R., Sorgen, C. (1985) 'Intraventricular hemorrhage in a term neonate secondary to a third ventricular AVM.' *Journal of Neurosurgery*, **63**, 640–643.

Helgason, C., Caplan, L.R., Goodwin, J., Hedges, T. (1986) 'Anterior choroidal artery-territory infarction.' *Archives of Neurology*, **43**, 681–686.

Helmke, K., Winkler, P., Kock, C. (1987) 'Sonographic examination of the brain stem area in infants.' *Pediatric Radiology*, **17**, 1–6.

Hemsath, F.A. (1934) 'Birth injury of the occipital bone with a report of thirty-two cases.' *American Journal of Obstetrics and Gynecology*, **27**, 194–203.

Hernansanz, J., Munoz, F., Rodriguez, D., Soler, C., Principe, C. (1984) 'Subdural hematomas of the posterior fossa in normal-weight newborns.' *Journal of Neurosurgery*, **61**, 972–974.

Hernanz-Schulman, M., Cohen, W., Geniesen, N.B. (1988) 'Sonography of cerebral infarction in infancy.' *American Journal of Roentgenology*, **150**, 897–902.

Heudes, A.M., Boullie, M.C., Lauret, P., Mallet, E. (1990) 'Hemangiomatose néonatale miliaire.' *Archives Françaises de Pédiatrie*, **47**, 135–138.

Hickl, E-J., Grässel, G., Kugler, J., Fröschl, J., Fendel, H. (1969) 'Neurologische, ophtalmologische und radiologische Untersuchungen bei Neugeborenen nach Vakuumextraktion.' *Archiv für Gynäkologie*, **207**, 41–42.

Hill, A., Volpe, J.J. (1989) 'Perinatal asphyxia: clinical aspects.' *Clinics in Perinatology*, **16**, 435–457.

—— Martin, D.J., Daneman, A., Fitz, C.R. (1983) 'Focal ischemic cerebral injury in the newborn: diagnosis by ultrasound and correlation with computed tomographic scan.' *Pediatrics*, **71**, 790–793.

Hirvensalo, M. (1949) 'On hemorrhages of the medulla oblongata and the pons and on respiratory disorders in premature infants.' *Acta Paediatrica Scandinavica*. Suppl. 73.

Hoffman, H.J., Chuang, S., Hendrick, E.B., Humphreys, R.P. (1982) 'Aneurysm of the vein of Galen. Experience at the Hospital for Sick Children, Toronto.' *Journal of Neurosurgery*, **57**, 316–322.

Hokazono, Y., Yokochi, K., Ohtani, Y., Inukai, K., Takashima, S. (1987) 'A premature infant with a bilateral thalamostriatal hemorrhage: brain imaging and pathology.' *Acta Paediatrica Japonica*, **29**, 867–871.

Holden, A.M., Fyler, D.C., Shillito, J., Nadas, A.S. (1972) 'Congestive heart failure from intracranial arteriovenous fistula in infancy.' *Pediatrics*, **49**, 30–39.

Holden, K.R., Alexander, F. (1970) 'Diffuse neonatal hemangiomatosis.' *Pediatrics*, **46**, 411–421.

Holland, E. (1937) 'Birth injury in relation to labor.' *American Journal of Obstetrics and Gynecology*, **33**, 1–18.

Hooper, R. (1969) *Patterns of Acute Head Injury*. London: Edward Arnold.

Hope, P.L., Gould, S.J., Howard, S., Hamilton, P.A., Costello, A.M.deL., Reynolds, E.O.R. (1988) 'Precision of ultrasound diagnosis of pathologically verified lesions in the brain of very preterm infants.' *Developmental Medicine and Child Neurology*, **30**, 457–471.

Horie, M., Yokuchi, K., Inukai, K., Kito, H., Ogawa, J. (1988) 'Computed tomographic findings in full-term infants with good prognosis.' *Brain and Development*, **10**, 100–105.

Hourihan, M.D., Gates, P.C., McAllister, V.L. (1984) 'Subarachnoid hemorrhage in childhood and adolescence.' *Journal of Neurosurgery*, **60**, 1163–1166.

Huang, C-C., Shen, E-Y. (1991) 'Tentorial subdural hemorrhage in term newborns: ultrasonographic diagnosis and clinical correlates.' *Pediatric Neurology*, **7**, 171–177.

—— Ho, M-Y., Shen, E-Y. (1987) 'Sonographic changes in a parasagittal cerebral lesion in an asphyxiated newborn.' *Journal of Clinical Ultrasound*, **15**, 68–70.

Hungerford, G.D., Marzluff, J.M., Kempe, L.G., Powers, J.M. (1981) 'Cerebral arterial aneurysm in a neonate.' *Neuroradiology*, **21**, 107–110.

Hurst, R.W., Kerns, S.R., McIlhenny, J., Park, T.S., Cail, W.S. (1989) 'Neonatal dural venous sinus thrombosis associated with central venous catheterization: CT and MR studies.' *Journal of Computer Assisted Tomography*, **13**, 504–507.

Iannucci, A.M., Buonanna, F., Rizzuto, N., Mazza, C., Virenza, C., Maschio, A. (1979) 'Arteriovenous aneurysm of the vein of Galen.' *Journal of the Neurological Sciences*, **40**, 29–37.

Ibarguen, E.S., Sharp, H.L., Snyder, C.L., Ferrell, R.N., Leonard, A.S. (1988) 'Hemangiomatosis of the colon and peritoneum.' *Clinical Pediatrics*, **27**, 425–430.

Ichiyama, T., Hayashi, T. (1991) 'Ultrasonic measurements of the posterior cranial fossa structures in neonates and infants.' *European Journal of Pediatrics*, **150**, 719–721.

Ingraham, F.D., Matson, D.D. (1954) *Neurosurgery of Infancy and Childhood*. Springfield: Charles C. Thomas.

Inoue, Y., Takemoto, K., Miyamoto, T., Yoshikawa, N., Taniguchi, S., Saiwai, S., Nashimura, Y., Komatsu, T. (1980) 'Sequential computed tomographic scans in acute cerebral infarction.' *Radiology*, **135**, 655–661.

Jellinger, K. (1986a) '(Exogenous) striatal necrosis.' *Handbook of Clinical Neurology*, **49**, 465–491.

—— (1986b) 'Exogenous lesions of the pallidum.' *Handbook of Clinical Neurology*, **49**, 499–518.

Jocelyn, L.J., Casiro, O.G. (1992) 'Neurodevelopmental outcome of term infants with intraventricular hemorrhage.' *American Journal of Diseases of Children*, **146**, 194–197.

Johnsen, S., Greenwood, R., Fishman, M.A. (1973) 'Internal cerebral vein thrombosis.' *Archives of Neurology*, **28**, 205–207.

Jones, M.D., Traystman, R.J. (1984) 'Cerebral oxygenation of the fetus, newborn and adult.' *Seminars in Perinatology*, **8**, 205–216.

—— Koehler, R.C., Traystman, R.J. (1988) 'Regulation of cerebral blood flow in the fetus, newborn and adult.' *In:* Guthrie, R.D. (Ed.) *Clinics in Critical Care Medicine: Neonatal Intensive Care*. New

York: Churchill Livingstone, pp. 123–152.

Kagwa-Nyanzi, J.A., Alpidousky, V.K. (1972) 'Subaponeurotic haemorrhage in newborn infants.' *Clinical Pediatrics*, **11**, 224–227.

Kanarek, K.S., Gieron, M.A. (1986) 'Computed tomography demonstration of cerebral calcification in postasphyxial encephalopathy.' *Journal of Child Neurology*, **1**, 56–60.

Kanfer, A. (1990) 'Coagulation factors in nephrotic syndrome.' *American Journal of Nephrology*, **10** (Suppl. 1), 63–68.

Kappelle, L.J., Willemse, J., Ramos, L.M.P., Van Gijn, J. (1989) 'Ischaemic stroke in the basal ganglia and internal capsule in childhood.' *Brain and Development*, **11**, 283–292.

Keeney, S.E., Adcock, E.W., McArdle, C.B. (1991) 'Prospective observations of 100 high-risk neonates by high-field (1.5 Tesla) magnetic resonance imaging of the central nervous system. I. Intraventricular and extracerebral lesions. II. Lesions associated with hypoxic–ischemic encephalopathy.' *Pediatrics*, **87**, 421–430; 431–438.

Kehrer, E. (1939) *Die intrakraniellen Blutungen bei Neugeborenen.* Stuttgart: Ferdinand Enke Verlag.

Kelly, J.V., Sines, G. (1966) 'An assessment of the compression and traction forces of obstetrical forceps.' *American Journal of Obstetrics and Gynecology*, **96**, 521–537.

Kendall, N., Woloshin, H. (1952) 'Cephalhematoma associated with fracture of the skull.' *Journal of Pediatrics*, **41**, 125–132.

Klesh, K.W., Murphy, T.F., Scher, M.S., Buchanan, D.E., Maxwell, E.P., Guthrie, R.D. (1987) 'Cerebral infarction in persistent pulmonary hypertension of the newborn.' *American Journal of Diseases of Children*, **141**, 852–857.

Knowlson, G.T., Marsden, H.B. (1978) 'Aortic thrombosis in the newborn period.' *Archives of Disease in Childhood*, **53**, 164–166.

Knudson, M.R.P., Alden, E.R. (1979) 'Symptomatic arteriovenous malformation in infants less than 6 months of age.' *Pediatrics*, **64**, 238–241.

Koch, T.K., Jahnke, S.E., Edwards, M.S.B., Davis, S.L. (1985) 'Posterior fossa hemorrhage in term newborns.' *Pediatric Neurology*, **1**, 96–99.

Koeppen, A.H., Dentinger, M.P. (1988) 'Brain hemosiderin and superficial siderosis of the central nervous system.' *Journal of Neuropathology and Experimental Neurology*, **47**, 249–270.

Kogure, K., Hossmann, K-A., Siesjö, B.K. (1993) *Neurobiology of Ischemic Brain Damage. Progress in Brain Research Vol. 96.* Amsterdam: Elsevier.

Kopelman, A.E. (1990) 'Blood pressure and cerebral ischemia in very low birth weight infants.' *Journal of Pediatrics*, **116**, 1000–1002.

Kotagal, S., Toce, S.S., Kotagel, P., Archer, C.R. (1983) 'Symmetric bithalamic and striatal hemorrhage following perinatal hypoxia in a term infant.' *Journal of Computer Assisted Tomography*, **7**, 353–355.

Kotlarek, F., Rodewig, R., Brüll, D. (1981) 'Computed tomographic findings in congenital hemiparesis in childhood and their relation to etiology and prognosis.' *Neuropediatrics*, **12**, 101–109.

Kozinn, P.J., Rits, N.D., Horowitz, A.W. (1965) 'Scalp hemorrhage as an emergency in the newborn.' *Journal of the American Medical Association*, **194**, 567–568.

Kreusser, K.L., Schmidt, R.E., Shackelford, G.D., Volpe, J.J. (1984) 'Value of ultrasound for identification of acute hemorrhagic necrosis of thalamus and basal ganglia in an asphyxiated term infant.' *Annals of Neurology*, **16**, 361–363.

Kriewall, T.J., McPherson, G.K. (1981) 'Effects of uterine contractility on the fetal cranium.' *In:* Milunsky, A., Friedman, E.A., Gluck, L. (Eds.) *Advances in Perinatal Medicine.* New York: Plenum, pp. 295–356.

Krishnamoorthy, K.S., Shannon, D.C., De Long, G.R., Todres, I.D., Davis, K.R. (1979) 'Neurologic sequelae in the survivors of neonatal intraventricular hemorrhage.' *Pediatrics*, **64**, 233–237.

Kuban, K.C.K., Gilles, F.H. (1985) 'Human telencephalic angiogenesis.' *Annals of Neurology*, **17**, 539–548.

Kuhn, M.J., Couch, S.M., Binstadt, D.H., Rightmire, D.A., Morales, A., Khanna, N.N., Long, S.D. (1992) 'Prenatal recognition of central nervous system complications of alloimmune thrombocytopenia.' *Computerized Medical Imaging and Graphics*, **16**, 137–142.

Kundrat, H. (1890) 'Ueber die intermeningealen Blutungen Neugeborener.' *Wiener Klinische Wochenschrift*, **3**, 887–889.

Lacey, D.J., Terplan, K. (1982) 'Intraventricular hemorrhage in full-term neonates.' *Developmental*

Medicine and Child Neurology, **24**, 332–337.

Lam, A., Cruz, G.B., Johnson, I. (1991) 'Extradural hematoma in neonates.' *Journal of Ultrasound Medicine*, **10**, 205–209.

Larroche, J-C. (1977) *Developmental Pathology of the Neonate*. Amsterdam: Elsevier.

—— (1984) 'Perinatal brain damage.' *In:* Adams, J.H., Corsellis, J.A.N., Duchen, L.W. (Eds) *Greenfield's Neuropathology. 4th Edn.* London: Edward Arnold, pp. 451–489.

—— (1991) 'The central nervous system.' *In:* Wigglesworth, J.S., Singer, D.B. (Eds) *Textbook of Fetal and Perinatal Pathology*. Oxford: Blackwell Scientific, pp. 775–838.

Lasjaunias, P., Terbrugge, K., Piske, R., Lopez Ibor, L., Manelfe, C. (1987) 'Dilatation de la veine de Galien.' *Neurochirurgie*, **33**, 315–333.

—— Garcia-Monaco, R., Rodesch, G., Terbrugge, K., Zerah, M., Tardieu, M., De Victor, D. (1991) 'Vein of Galen malformation. Endovascular management of 43 cases.' *Child's Nervous System*, **7**, 360–367.

Laub, M.C., Ingrisch, H. (1986) 'Increased periventricular echogenicity (periventricular halos) in neonatal brain: a sonographic study.' *Neuropediatrics*, **17**, 39–43.

Laufe, L.E. (1971) 'Divergent and crossed obstetric forceps. Comparative study of compression and traction forces.' *Obstetrics and Gynecology*, **38**, 885–887.

Laurent, J.P., Molinali, G.F., Oakley, J.C. (1976) 'Primate model of cerebral hematoma.' *Journal of Neuropathology and Experimental Neurology*, **35**, 560–568.

Lauridsen, L., Pless, J., Uhrenholdt, A. (1962) 'Vacuum extraction. A follow-up study.' *Journal of Obstetrics and Gynaecology of the British Commonwealth*, **69**, 1019–1021.

Leblanc, R., O'Gorman, A.M. (1980) 'Neonatal intracranial hemorrhage.' *Journal of Neurosurgery*, **53**, 642–651.

Lee, Y.J., Kandall, S.R., Ghali, V.S. (1978) 'Intracerebral arterial aneurysm in a newborn.' *Archives of Neurology*, **35**, 171–172.

Leech, R.W., Alvord, E.C. (1974) 'Morphologic variations in periventricular leukomalacia.' *American Journal of Pathology*, **74**, 591–602.

—— —— (1977) 'Anoxic–ischemic encephalopathy in the human neonatal period.' *Archives of Neurology*, **34**, 109–113.

—— Brumback, R.A. (1988) 'Massive brain stem necrosis in the human neonate: presentation of three cases with review of the literature.' *Journal of Child Neurology*, **3**, 258–262.

Lefkowitz, L.L. (1936) 'Extradural hemorrhage as a result of birth trauma.' *Archives of Pediatrics*, **53**, 404–407.

Lehman, O., Andersson, H., Hannsson, G., Malmström, T., Ryba, W. (1963) 'Postnatal subgaleal haematomas.' *Acta Obstetricia et Gynaecologica Scandinavica*, **42**, 358–366.

Leijon, I. (1980) 'Neurology and behaviour of newborn infants delivered by vacuum extraction.' *Acta Paediatrica Scandinavica*, **69**, 625–631.

Leissring, J.C., Vorlicky, L.N., Alto, P. (1968) 'Disseminated intravascular coagulation in a neonate.' *American Journal of Diseases of Children*, **115**, 100–106.

Lejeune, J.P., Brévière, G.M., Krivosic, Y., Saboori, K., Dhellemmes, P. (1987) 'Aspects macroscopiques de deux anévrysmes de l'ampoule de Galien révélés par une asystolie aigue.' *Neurochirurgie*, **33**, 341–344.

Leland Albright, A., Latchaw, R.E., Price, R.A. (1985) 'Posterior dural arteriovenous malformations in infancy.' *Neurosurgery*, **13**, 129–135.

Levene, M.I. (1988) 'The asphyxiated newborn infant.' *In:* Levene, M.I., Bennett, M.J., Punt, J. (Eds) *Fetal and Neonatal Neurology and Neurosurgery*. London: Churchill Livingstone, pp. 370–382.

—— Fenton, A.C., Evans, D.H., Archer, L.N.J., Shortland, D.B., Gibson, N.A. (1989) 'Severe birth asphyxia and abnormal cerebral blood flow velocity.' *Developmental Medicine and Child Neurology*, **31**, 427–434.

Levkoff, A.H., Macpherson, R.I., Wood, B.P. (1992) 'Unrecognized subaponeurotic hemorrhage.' *American Journal of Diseases of Children*, **146**, 833–834.

Levy, S.R., Abroms, I-F., Marshall, P.C., Rosquete, E.E. (1985) 'Seizures and cerebral infarction in the full-term newborn.' *Annals of Neurology*, **17**, 366–370.

Lindgren, L. (1960) 'The causes of fetal head moulding in labour.' *Acta Obstetricia et Gynaecologica Scandinavica*, **39**, 46–62.

Lindvall, M., Edvinsson, L., Owman, C. (1977) 'Histochemical study on regional differences in the cholinergic nerve supply of the choroid plexus from various laboratory animals.' *Experimental Neurology*, **55**, 152–159.

Litvak, J., Yahr, M., Ransohoff, J. (1960) 'Aneurysms of the great vein of Galen and midline cerebral arteriovenous anomalies.' *Journal of Neurosurgery*, **17**, 945–954.

Loeser, J.D., Kilburn, H.L., Jolley, T. (1976) 'Management of depressed skull fracture in the newborn.' *Journal of Neurosurgery*, **44**, 62–64.

Lou, H.C. (1988) 'The "lost autoregulation hypothesis" and brain lesions in the newborn: an update.' *Brain and Development*, **10**, 143–146.

—— Tweed, W.A., Davies, J.M. (1985) 'Preferential blood flow increase to the brain stem in moderate neonatal hypoxia: reversal by naloxone.' *European Journal of Pediatrics*, **144**, 225–227.

Ludwig, B., Brand, M., Brockerhoff, P. (1980) 'Post-partum CT examination of the heads of full-term infants.' *Neuroradiology*, **20**, 145–154.

Lupton, B.A., Hill, A., Roland, E.H., Whitfield, M.F., Flodmark, O. (1988) 'Brain swelling in the asphyxiated term newborn: pathogenesis and outcome.' *Pediatrics*, **82**, 139–146.

Lye, W.C., Tan, C.C. (1991) 'Multiple arterial thromboses in nephrotic syndrome.' *Nephrology, Dialysis and Transplantation*, **6**, 55–56.

MacDonald, R.L., Weir, B.K.A., Runzer, T.D., Grace, M.G.A., Findlay, J.M., Saito, K., Cook, D.A., Mielke, B.W., Kanamaru, K. (1991) 'Etiology of cerebral vasospasm in primates.' *Journal of Neurosurgery*, **75**, 415–424.

Macfarlane, R., Moskowitz, M.A., Sakas, D.E., Tasdemiroglu, E., Wei, E.P., Kontos, H.A. (1991) 'The role of neuroeffector mechanisms in cerebral hyperperfusion syndromes.' *Journal of Neurosurgery*, **75**, 845–855.

Machin, G.A. (1975) 'A perinatal mortality survey in south-east London, 1970–1973: the pathological findings in 726 necropsies.' *Journal of Clinical Pathology*, **28**, 428–434.

Macpherson, R.I., Hoogstraten, J., Tjaden, R. (1969) 'Calcification of the basal ganglia in infancy.' *Journal of the Canadian Association of Radiologists*, **20**, 159–164.

Magilner, A.D., Wertheimer, I.S. (1980) 'Preliminary results of a computed tomography study of neonatal hypoxia–ischemia.' *Journal of Computer Assisted Tomography*, **4**, 457–463.

Maheut, J., Santini, J.J., Barthez, M.A., Billard, C. (1987*a*) 'Symptomatologie clinique de l'anévrysme de l'ampoule de Galien. Résultats d'une enquête nationale.' *Neurochirurgie*, **33**, 285–290.

—— —— —— —— (1987*b*) 'Anévrysme de l'ampoule de Galien. Résultats thérapeutiques de l'étude multicentrique nationale.' *Neurochirurgie*, **33**, 337–340.

Maki, M. (1992) 'Bedside diagnosis of acute obstetrical DIC.' *In:* Suzuki, S., Hathaway, W.E., Bonnar, J., Sutor, A.H. (Eds) *Perinatal Thrombosis and Hemostasis*. Tokyo: Springer-Verlag, pp. 11–20.

Maki, Y., Shirai, S. (1975) 'Angiographic findings in intraventricular hemorrhage in newborn infants.' *Acta Radiologica*, Suppl. 347, 167–174.

Malamud, N. (1950) 'Status marmoratus: a form of cerebral palsy following either birth injury or inflammation of the central nervous system.' *Journal of Pediatrics*, **37**, 610–619.

Malmström, T., Jansson, I. (1965) 'Use of the vacuum extractor.' *Acta Obstetricia et Gynaecologica Scandinavica*, **8**, 893–913.

Mannino, F.L., Trauner, D.A. (1983) 'Stroke in neonates.' *Journal of Pediatrics*, **102**, 605–610.

—— —— (1984) 'Neonatal cerebral infarction: reply.' *Journal of Pediatrics*, **104**, 957–958. *(Letter.)*

Mansour, H., Veyrac, C., Couture, A. (1987) 'Place de l'échographie cérébrale dans le diagnostic de l'anévrysme de la veine de Galien.' *Neurochirurgie*, **33**, 345–348.

Mantovani, J-F., Gerber, J.F. (1984) 'Idiopathic neonatal cerebral infarction.' *American Journal of Diseases of Children*, **138**, 359–362.

Marciniak, E., Wilson, H.D., Marlar, R.A. (1985) 'Neonatal purpura fulminans: a genetic disorder related to the absence of protein C in blood.' *Blood*, **65**, 15–20.

Marsh, E.E., Biller, J., Adams, H.P., Kaplan, J.M. (1991) 'Cerebral infarction in patients with nephrotic syndrome.' *Stroke*, **22**, 90–93.

Martin, D.J., Hill, A., Fitz, C.R. (1983) 'Hypoxic ischemic cerebral injury in the neonatal brain: a case report of sonographic features with computed tomographic correlations.' *Pediatric Radiology*, **13**, 307–312.

Martinez-Lage, J.F., Esteban, J.A., Perez, M.M., Pozanski, M. (1984) 'Craniostenosis secondary to calcified subperiosteal hematoma: case report.' *Neurosurgery*, **15**, 703–704.

McIlwaine, G. (1980) 'Perinatal mortality enquiries at regional level.' *In:* Chalmers, I., McIlwaine, G.

206

(Eds) *Perinatal Audit and Surveillance. Proceedings of the Eighth Study Group of the Royal College of Obstetricians and Gynaecologists, London*, pp. 124–132.

McLaurin, R.L., Isaacs, E., Lewis, H.P. (1971) 'Results of nonoperative treatment in 15 cases of infantile subdural hematoma.' *Journal of Neurosurgery*, **34**, 753–759.

McLeary, R.D., Kuhns, L.R., Barn, M. (1984) 'Ultrasonography of the fetal cerebellum.' *Radiology*, **151**, 439–442.

McLellan, N.J., Prasad, R., Punt, J. (1986) 'Spontaneous subhyaloid and retinal haemorrhages in an infant.' *Archives of Disease in Childhood*, **61**, 1130–1132.

McMurdo, S.K., Brant-Zawadzki, M., Bradley, W.G., Chang, G.Y., Berg, B.O. (1986) 'Dural sinus thrombosis: study using intermediate field strength MR imaging.' *Radiology*, **161**, 83–86.

Mealey, J. (1968) *Pediatric Head Injuries*. Springfield: C.C. Thomas.

Mehall, C.J., Amundson, G.M., Wood, B.P. (1990) 'Systemic air embolism within a vein of Galen malformation.' *American Journal of Diseases of Children*, **144**, 95–96.

Meidell, R., Marinelli, P.V., Randall, V., Pettett, G. (1983) 'Intracranial parenchymal hemorrhage in a full-term infant.' *Clinical Pediatrics*, **22**, 780–783.

Meier, A. (1938) 'Sinusthrombose als geburtstraumatische Folge.' *Zeitschrift für Kinderheilkunde*, **59**, 556–558.

Menezes, A.H., Smith, D.E., Bell, W.E. (1983) 'Posterior fossa hemorrhage in the term neonate.' *Neurosurgery*, **13**, 452–456.

Ment, L.R., Duncan, C.C., Ehrenkranz, R.A. (1984) 'Perinatal cerebral infarction.' *Annals of Neurology*, **16**, 559–568.

—— Stewart, W.B., Duncan, C.C., Cole, J., Pitt, B.R. (1985) 'Beagle puppy model of perinatal cerebral infarction: acute changes in cerebral blood flow and metabolism during haemorrhagic hypotension.' *Journal of Neurosurgery*, **63**, 441–447.

—— Duncan, C.C., Ehrenkranz, R.A. (1987) 'Perinatal cerebral infarction.' *Seminars in Perinatology*, **11**, 142–154.

Merland, J.J., Laurent, A., Rufenacht, D., Reizine, D. (1987) 'Malformation artério-veineuse de la région de l'ampoule de Galien.' *Neurochirurgie*, **33**, 349–352.

Merry, G.S., Stuart, G. (1979) 'Extradural hematoma in the neonate.' *Journal of Neurosurgery*, **51**, 713–714.

Mickle, J.P., Quisling, R.G. (1986) 'The transtorcular embolization of vein of Galen aneurysms.' *Journal of Neurosurgery*, **64**, 731–735.

Miller, G.M., Black, V.D., Lubchenco, L.O. (1981) 'Intracerebral hemorrhage in a term newborn with hyperviscosity.' *American Journal of Diseases of Children*, **135**, 377–378.

Mitchell, W., O'Tuama, L. (1980) 'Cerebral intraventricular hemorrhages in infants: a widening age spectrum.' *Pediatrics*, **65**, 35–39.

Miyasaka, Y., Yada, K., Ohwada, T., Kitahara, T., Kurata, A., Irikura, K. (1992) 'An analysis of the venous drainage system as a factor in hemorrhage from arteriovenous malformations.' *Journal of Neurosurgery*, **76**, 239–243.

Mohr, J.P., Stein, B.M., Hilal, S.K. (1989) 'Arteriovenous malformations.' *In:* Vinken, P.J., Bruyn, G.W., Klawans, H.L. (Eds) *Handbook of Clinical Neurology. Revised Series 10, Vol. 54. Vascular Diseases, Part II*. Amsterdam: Elsevier, pp. 361–393.

Moloy, H.C. (1942) 'Studies on head molding during labor.' *American Journal of Obstetrics and Gynecology*, **44**, 762–768.

Molteni, B., Oleari, G., Fedrizzi, E., Bracchi, M. (1987) 'Relation between CT patterns, clinical findings and etiological factors in children born at term, affected by congenital hemiparesis.' *Neuropediatrics*, **18**, 75–80.

Monset-Couchard, M., De Bethmann, O., Radvanyi-Bouvet, M-F., Papin, C., Bordarier, C., Relier, J-P. (1988) 'Neurodevelopmental outcome in cystic periventricular leukomalacia (CPVL) (30 cases).' *Neuropediatrics*, **19**, 124–131.

Montoya, F., Couture, A., Frerebeau, P., Bonnet, H. (1987) 'Hémorragie intraventriculaire chez le nouveau-né à terme: origine thalamique.' *Pédiatrie*, **42**, 205–209.

Moolgaoker, A.S., Ahamed, S.O.S., Payne, P.R. (1979) 'A comparison of different methods of instrumental delivery based on electronic measurements of compression and traction.' *Obstetrics and Gynecology*, **54**, 299–308.

Morison, J.E. (1963) *Foetal and Neonatal Pathology. 2nd Edn*. London: Butterworths.

Mujsce, D.J., Christensen, M.A., Vannucci, R.C. (1990) 'Cerebral blood flow and edema in perinatal hypoxic–ischemic brain damage.' *Pediatric Research*, **27**, 450–453.

Myers, R.E. (1975) 'Fetal asphyxia due to umbilical cord compression.' *Biology of the Neonate*, **26**, 21–43.

—— De Courten-Myers, G.M., Wagner, K.R. (1987) 'Physiopathology and biochemistry of perinatal asphyctic brain injury.' *In:* Yabuuchi, H., Watanabe, K., Okada, S. (Eds) *Neonatal Brain and Behaviour.* Nagoya: University of Nagoya Press, pp. 1–26.

Naidich, T.P. (1986) 'Sonography of the internal capsule and basal ganglia in infants. Part II: Localization of pathologic processes in the sagittal section through the caudothalamic groove.' *Radiology*, **161**, 615–621.

Nanba, E., Eda, I., Takashima, S., Ohta, S., Ohtani, K., Takeshita, K. (1984) 'Intracranial hemorrhage in the full-term neonate and young infant: correlation of the location and outcome.' *Brain and Development*, **6**, 435–443.

Natelson, S.E., Sayers, M.P. (1973) 'The fate of children sustaining severe head trauma during birth.' *Pediatrics*, **51**, 169–174.

Naujoks, H. (1934) *Die Geburtsverletzungen des Kindes.* Stuttgart: Ferdinand Enke.

Needell, G.S., Brewer, W.H., Kodroff, M.B., Fernandez, R.E. (1983) 'Midline cerebral arterio-venous anomalies: ultrasound diagnosis.' *Pediatric Radiology*, **13**, 72–76.

Nesbitt, R.E.L. (1957) *Perinatal Loss in Modern Obstetrics.* Philadelphia: E.A. Davis.

Neuweiler, W., Onwudiwe, E.U. (1967) 'Retinahaemorrhagien beim Neugeborenen.' *Gynecologia*, **163**, 308–310.

New, P.F.J., Davis, K.R. (1980) 'The role of CT scanning in diagnosis of infections of the central nervous system.' *In:* Remington, J.S., Swartz, M.N. (Eds) *Current Clinical Topics in Infectious Diseases.* New York: McGraw-Hill.

Newton, T.H., Cronquist, S. (1969) 'Involvement of dural arteries in intracranial arteriovenous malformations.' *Radiology*, **93**, 1071–1078.

—— Gooding, C.A. (1975) 'Compression of superior sagittal sinus by neonatal calvarial molding.' *Radiology*, **115**, 635–639.

Nicholson, A.A., Hourihan, M.D., Hayward, C. (1983) 'Arteriovenous malformations involving the vein of Galen.' *Archives of Disease in Childhood*, **64**, 1653–1655.

Norman, M.G. (1972) 'Antenatal neuronal loss and gliosis of the reticular formation, thalamus and hypothalamus.' *Neurology*, **22**, 910–916.

—— Becker, L.E. (1974) 'Cerebral damage in neonates resulting from arteriovenous malformation of the vein of Galen.' *Journal of Neurology, Neurosurgery and Psychiatry*, **37**, 252–258.

—— Thurber, L.A., Woolley, H.E. (1981) 'Abnormal leptomeninges and vessels causing fetal hydrocephalus: diagnosis of hydrocephalus at 19 weeks gestation by ultrasound.' *Acta Neuropathologica*, **54**, 283–285.

Norman, R.M. (1947) 'Etat marbré of the corpus striatum following birth injury.' *Journal of Neurology, Neurosurgery and Psychiatry*, **10**, 12–25.

Nuno, K., Mihara, M., Shimao, S. (1990) 'Linear sebaceus nevus syndrome.' *Dermatologica*, **181**, 221–223.

Nwaesi, C.G., Allen, A.C., Vincer, M.J., Brown, S.J., Stinson, D.A., Evans, J.R., Byrne, J.M. (1984) 'Periventricular infarction diagnosed by ultrasound. A postmortem correlation.' *Journal of Pediatrics*, **105**, 106–110.

Obrador, S., Soto, M., Silvela, J. (1975) 'Clinical syndromes of arteriovenous malformations of the transverse sigmoid sinus.' *Journal of Neurology, Neurosurgery and Psychiatry*, **38**, 436–451.

O'Brien, M.J., Ash, J.M., Gilday, D.L. (1979) 'Radionuclide brain-scanning in perinatal hypoxia/ischemia.' *Developmental Medicine and Child Neurology*, **21**, 161–173.

O'Donnabhain, D., Duff, D.F. (1989) 'Aneurysms of the vein of Galen.' *Archives of Disease in Childhood*, **64**, 1612–1617.

O'Driscoll, K., Meagher, D., MacDonald, D., Geoghegan, F. (1981) 'Traumatic intracranial haemorrhage in firstborn infants and delivery with obstetric forceps.' *British Journal of Obstetrics and Gynaecology*, **88**, 577–578.

Oelberg, D.G., Temple, D.M., Haskins, S., Bigelow, R.H., Adcock, E.W. (1988) 'Intracranial hemorrhage in term or near term newborns with persistent pulmonary hypertension.' *Clinical Pediatrics*, **27**, 14–17.

208

Okada, M., Yokochi, K., Suzuki, K. (1986) 'Sequential computed tomography in severely asphyxiated infants.' *Acta Paediatrica Japonica*, **28**, 202–208.

Okada, Y., Yamaguchi, T., Minematsu, K., Miyashita, T., Sawada, T., Sadoshima, S., Fujishima, M., Omae, T. (1989) 'Hemorrhagic transformation in cerebral embolism.' *Stroke*, **20**, 598–603.

Okuno, T., Takao, T., Ito, M., Konishi, Y., Mikawa, H., Nakano, Y. (1980) 'Infarction of the internal capsule in children.' *Journal of Computer Assisted Tomography*, **4**, 770–774.

Olsen, T.S., Lassen, N.A. (1984) 'A dynamic concept of middle cerebral artery occlusion and cerebral infarction in the acute stage based on interpreting severe hyperemia as a sign of embolic migration.' *Stroke*, **15**, 458–468.

Ordorica, S.A., Marks, F., Frieden, F.J., Hoskins, I.A., Young, B.K. (1990) 'Aneurysm of the vein of Galen: a new cause for Ballantyne syndrome.' *American Journal of Obstetrics and Gynecology*, **162**, 1166–1167.

Oski, F.A., Naiman, J.L. (1982) *Hematological Problems in the Newborn*. Philadelphia: W.B. Saunders.

Özsoylu, S., Irken, G., Gürgey, A. (1989) 'High dose intravenous methylprednisolone for Kasabach–Merritt syndrome.' *European Journal of Pediatrics*, **148**, 403–405.

Palma, P.A., Miner, M.E., Moriss, F.H., Adcock, E.W., Denson, S.E. (1979) 'Intraventricular hemorrhage in the neonate born at term.' *American Journal of Diseases of Children*, **133**, 941–944.

Palmer, C., Vannucci, R.C. (1993) 'Potential new therapies for perinatal cerebral hypoxia–ischemia.' *Clinics in Perinatology*, **20**, 411–432.

Pape, K.E., Wigglesworth, J.S. (1979) *Haemorrhage, Ischaemia and the Perinatal Brain*. Clinics in Developmental Medicine No. 69/70. London: Spastics International Medical Publications.

Papile, L-A., Burstein, J., Burstein, R., Koffler, H. (1978) 'Incidence and evolution of subependymal and intraventricular hemorrhage: a study of infants with birth weights less than 1,500 gm.' *Journal of Pediatrics*, **92**, 529–534.

Parag, K.B., Somers, S.R., Seedat, Y.K., Byrne, S., Da-Cruz, C.M., Kenajer, G. (1990) 'Arterial thrombosis in nephrotic syndrome.' *American Journal of Kidney Disease*, **15**, 176–177.

Pasternak, J.F., Predey, T.A., Mikhael, M.A. (1991) 'Neonatal asphyxia: vulnerability of basal ganglia, thalamus and brainstem.' *Pediatric Neurology*, **7**, 147–149.

Patel, U., Gupta, S.C. (1990) 'Wyburn–Mason syndrome: a case report and review of the literature.' *Neuroradiology*, **31**, 544–546.

Patronas, N.J., Duda, E.E., Mirfakhrace, M., Wollman, R.L. (1981) 'Superior sagittal sinus thrombosis diagnosed by computed tomography.' *Surgical Neurology*, **15**, 11–14.

Pavlakis, S.G., Gould, R.J., Zito, J.L. (1991) 'Stroke in children.' *Advances in Pediatrics*, **38**, 151–179.

Peeters, S., Vandenplas, Y., Jochmans, K., Bougatef, K., De Waele, M., De Wolf, D. (1993) 'Myocardial infarction in a neonate with hereditary antithrombin III deficiency.' *Acta Paediatrica*, **82**, 610–613.

Peliowski, A., Finer, N.N. (1992) 'Birth asphyxia in the term infant.' *In:* Sinclair, J.C., Bracken, M.B. (Eds) *Effective Care of the Newborn Infant*. Oxford: Oxford University Press, pp. 249–279.

Pellegrino, P.A., Milanesi, O., Saia, O.S., Carollo, C. (1987) 'Congestive heart failure secondary to cerebral arterio-venous fistula.' *Child's Nervous System*, **3**, 141–144.

Perez-Fontan, J.J., Herrera, M., Fina, A., Peguero, G. (1982) 'Periventricular calcifications in a newborn associated with aneurysm of the great vein of Galen.' *Pediatric Radiology*, **12**, 249–251.

Perlman, J.M. (1989) 'Systemic abnormalities in term infants following perinatal asphyxia.' *Clinics in Perinatology*, **16**, 475–484.

—— (1992) 'Acute neurological (neuro)manifestations in newborn infants following delivery complicated by severe fetal acidemia.' *Pediatric Research*, **31**, 352A. (*Abstract*.)

—— Nelson, J.S., McAlister, W.H., Volpe, J.J. (1983) 'Intracerebellar hemorrhage in a premature newborn: diagnosis by real-time ultrasound and correlation with autopsy findings.' *Pediatrics*, **71**, 159–162.

Pickering, L.K., Hogan, G.R., Gilbert, E.F. (1970) 'Aneurysm of the posterior inferior cerebellar artery: rupture in a newborn.' *American Journal of Diseases of Children*, **119**, 155–158.

Pierre-Kahn, A., Renier, D., Sainte-Rose, C., Flandin, C., Hirsch, J.F. (1985) 'Les hématomes intracrâniens aigus du nouveau-né à terme.' *Annales de Pédiatrie*, **32**, 419–425.

Plauché, W.C. (1979) 'Fetal cranial injuries related to delivery with the Malmström vacuum extractor.' *Obstetrics and Gynecology*, **53**, 750–757.

209

—— (1980) 'Subgaleal hematoma: a complication of instrumental delivery.' *Journal of the American Medical Association*, **244**, 1597–1598.
Ponté, C., Remy, J., Christiaens, J-L., Bonte, C., Lacombe, A., Lefebvre, P. (1971) 'Hématome intracérébral et sous-dural chez un nouveau-né.' *Archives Françaises de Pédiatrie*, **28**, 267–276.
Prensky, A.L., Gado, M. (1973) 'Angiographic resolution of a neonatal intracranial cavernous hemangioma coincident with steroid therapy.' *Journal of Neurosurgery*, **39**, 99–103.
Prian, G.W., Wright, G.B., Rumack, C.M., O'Meara, O.P. (1978) 'Apparent cerebral embolization after temporal artery catheterization.' *Journal of Pediatrics*, **93**, 115–118.
Pryds, O. (1991) 'Control of cerebral circulation in the high-risk neonate.' *Annals of Neurology*, **30**, 321–329.
—— Greisen, G., Lou, H., Friis-Hansen, B. (1990) 'Vasoparalysis is associated with brain damage in asphyxiated term infants.' *Journal of Pediatrics*, **117**, 119–125.
Pryse-Davies, J., Beard, R.W. (1973) 'A necropsy study of brain swelling in the newborn with special reference to cerebellar herniation.' *Journal of Pathology*, **109**, 51–73.
Pulsinelli, W.A., Brierley, J.B., Plum, F. (1982) 'Temporal profile of neuronal damage in a model of transient forebrain ischemia.' *Annals of Neurology*, **11**, 491–498.
Quinn, C.M., Wigglesworth, J.S., Heckmatt, J. (1991) 'Lethal arthrogryposis multiplex congenita: a pathological study of 21 cases.' *Histopathology*, **19**, 155–162.
Rabe, E.F., Flynn, R.E., Dodge, P.R. (1968) 'Subdural collections of fluid in infants and children.' *Neurology*, **18**, 559–570.
Raine, J., Davies, H., Gamsu, H.R. (1989) 'Multiple idiopathic emboli in a full term neonate.' *Acta Paediatrica Scandinavica*, **78**, 644–646.
Ralis, Z.A. (1975) 'Birth trauma to muscles in babies born by breech delivery and its possible fatal consequences.' *Archives of Disease in Childhood*, **50**, 4–13.
Rand, J.C., Burton, E.M., Tonkin, I.L.D., DiSessa, T.G. (1990) 'The hyperdense choroid plexus: a CT finding associated with aortic obstruction in the newborn.' *Pediatric Radiology*, **21**, 2–4.
Raybaud, C.A., Livet, M-O., Jiddane, M., Pinsard, N. (1985) 'Radiology of ischemic strokes in children.' *Neuroradiology*, **27**, 567–578.
—— Hald, J.K., Strother, C.M., Choux, M., Jiddane, M. (1987) 'Les anévrysmes de la veine de Galien: étude angiographique et considérations morphogénétiques.' *Neurochirurgie*, **33**, 302–314.
Reeder, J.D., Sanders, R.C. (1983) 'Ventriculitis in the neonate: recognition by sonography.' *American Journal of Neuroradiology*, **4**, 37–41.
—— Setzer, E.S., Kaude, J.V. (1982) 'Ultrasonographic detection of perinatal intracerebellar hemorrhage.' *Pediatrics*, **70**, 385–386.
Reid, H. (1983) 'Birth injury to the cervical spine and spinal cord.' *Acta Neurochirurgica*, **32**, 87–90.
Remillard, G.M., Ethier, R., Andermann, F. (1974) 'Temporal lobe epilepsy and perinatal occlusion of the posterior cerebral artery.' *Neurology*, **24**, 1001–1009.
Rempen, A., Kraus, M. (1991) 'Pressures on the fetal head during normal labor.' *Journal of Perinatal Medicine*, **19**, 199–206.
Revesz, T., Geddes, J.F. (1988) 'Symmetrical columnar necrosis of the basal ganglia and brainstem in an adult following cardiac arrest.' *Clinical Neuropathology*, **7**, 294–298.
Richardson, B.S. (1991) 'Metabolism of the fetal brain: biological and pathological development.' *In:* Hanson, M.A. (Ed.) *The Fetal and Neonatal Brain Stem.* Cambridge: Cambridge University Press, pp. 87–105.
—— Patrick, J.E., Abduljabbar, H. (1985) 'Cerebral oxidative metabolism in the fetal lamb: relationship to electrocortical state.' *American Journal of Obstetrics and Gynecology*, **153**, 426–431.
Rigamonti, D., Drayer, B.P., Johnson, P.C., Hadley, M.N., Zabramski, J., Spetzler, R.F. (1987) 'The MRI appearance of cavernous malformations (angiomas).' *Journal of Neurosurgery*, **67**, 518–524.
Ritschl, E., Auer, L.M. (1987) 'Endoscopic evacuation of an intracerebral and intraventricular haemorrhage.' *Archives of Disease in Childhood*, **62**, 1163–1165.
Robinson, D., Hambleton, G. (1977) 'Cutaneous and hepatic haemangiomata.' *Archives of Disease in Childhood*, **52**, 155–157.
Robinson, R.J., Rossiter, M.A. (1968) 'Massive subaponeurotic haemorrhage in babies of African origin.' *Archives of Disease in Childhood*, **43**, 684–687.
Roche, C., Velez, A., Sanchez, P.G., Castroviejo, I.P. (1990) 'Occipital osteodiastasis.' *Acta Paediatrica Scandinavica*, **79**, 380–382.

Roden, V.J., Cantor, H.E., O'Connor, D.M., Schmidt, R.R., Cherry, J.D. (1975) 'Acute hemiplegia of childhood associated with coxsackie A9 viral infection.' *Journal of Pediatrics*, **86**, 56–58.

Rodriguez, J., Claus, D., Verellen, G., Lyon, G. (1990) 'Periventricular leukomalacia: ultrasonic and neuropathological correlations.' *Developmental Medicine and Child Neurology*, **32**, 347–355.

Roessmann, U., Miller, R.T. (1980) 'Thrombosis of the middle cerebral artery associated with birth trauma.' *Neurology*, **30**, 889–892.

Rohyans, J.A., Miser, A.W., Miser, J.S. (1982) 'Subgaleal hemorrhage in infants with hemophilia: report of two cases and review of the literature.' *Pediatrics*, **70**, 306–307.

Roland, E.H., Hill, A., Norman, M.G., Flodmark, O., MacNab, A.J. (1988) 'Selective brainstem injury in an asphyxiated newborn.' *Annals of Neurology*, **23**, 89–92.

—— Flodmark, O., Hill, A. (1990) 'Thalamic hemorrhage with intraventricular hemorrhage in the full-term newborn.' *Pediatrics*, **85**, 737–742.

Rolland, M., Fouché, S., Sevely, A., Manelfe, C., Régnier, C., Trémoulet, M. (1982) 'Hématomes de la fosse postérieure chez le nouveau-né à terme.' *Nouvelle Presse Médicale*, **11**, 1317–1320.

Romodanov, A.P., Brodsky, Y.S. (1987) 'Subdural hematomas in the newborn. Surgical treatment and results.' *Surgical Neurology*, **28**, 253–258.

Roodhooft, A.M., Parizel, P.M., Van Acker, K.J., Deprettere, A.J.R., Van Reempts, P.J. (1987) 'Idiopathic cerebral arterial infarction with paucity of symptoms in the full-term neonate.' *Pediatrics*, **80**, 381–385.

Rosenberg, E.M., Nazar, G.B. (1991) 'Neonatal vein of Galen aneurysm: severe coagulopathy with transtorcular embolization.' *Critical Care Medicine*, **19**, 441–443.

Rosenberg, H.S., Bernstein, J. (1981) *Perspectives in Pediatric Pathology. Vol. 6: Infectious Diseases.* New York: Masson.

Rosman, N.P., Wu, J.K., Caplan, L.R. (1992) 'Cerebellar infarction in the young.' *Stroke*, **23**, 763–766.

Ross, D.A., Walker, J., Edwards, M.S.B. (1986) 'Unusual posterior fossa dural arteriovenous malformation in a neonate. Case report.' *Neurosurgery*, **19**, 1021–1024.

Rothman, S., Olney, J. (1987) 'Excitotoxity and the NMDA receptor.' *Trends in Neurological Science*, **10**, 299–302.

Roy, S., Sarkar, C., Tandon, P.N., Banerji, A.K. (1987) 'Cranio-cerebral erosion (growing fracture of the skull) in children. Part I: pathology.' *Acta Neurochirurgica*, **87**, 112–118.

Roy, C., Noseda, G., Azimanogeou, A., Harpey, J.P., Binet, M.H., Vaur, C., Caille (1990) 'Maladie de Rendu–Osler révélée par la rupture d'un anévrysme artériel cérébral chez un nourisson.' *Archives Françaises de Pédiatrie*, **47**, 741–742.

Ruchoux, M.M., Renjard, L., Monegier du Sorbier, C., Raybaud, C., Santini, J.J., Lhuintre, Y. (1987) 'Histopathologie de la veine de Galien.' *Neurochirurgie*, **33**, 272–284.

Ruff, R.L., Shaw, C.M., Beckwith, J.B., Iozzo, R.N. (1979) 'Cerebral infarction complicating umbilical vein catheterization.' *Annals of Neurology*, **6**, 85. *(Letter.)*

Rumack, C.M., Guggenheim, M.A., Rumack, B.H., Peterson, R.G., Johnson, M.L., Braithwaite, W.R. (1981) 'Neonatal intracranial hemorrhage and maternal use of aspirin.' *Obstetrics and Gynecology*, **58**, 52S–56S.

Rushton, D.I., Preston, P.R., Durbin, G.M. (1985) 'Structure and evolution of echo dense lesions in the neonatal brain.' *Archives of Disease in Childhood*, **60**, 798–808.

Rutherford, M.A., Pennock, J.M., Murdoch-Eaton, D.M., Cowan, F.M., Dubowitz, L.M.S. (1992) 'Athetoid cerebral palsy with cysts in the putamen after hypoxic–ischaemic encephalopathy.' *Archives of Disease in Childhood*, **67**, 846–850.

Rydberg, E. (1932) 'Cerebral injury in the new-born children consequent on birth-trauma.' *Acta Pathologica et Microbiologica Scandinavica*, Suppl. 10.

Sachs, B.P., Acker, D., Tuomala, R., Brown, E. (1987) 'The incidence of symptomatic intracranial hemorrhage in term appropriate-for-gestation-age infants.' *Clinical Pediatrics*, **26**, 355–358.

Saku, Y., Choki, J., Waki, R., Masuda, J., Tamaki, K. (1990) 'Hemorrhagic infarct induced by arterial hypertension in cat brain following middle cerebral artery occlusion.' *Stroke*, **21**, 589–595.

Sainte-Anne Dargassies, S. (1957) 'Hématome extradural diagnostiqué, opéré et guéri chez un nouveau-né à terme.' *Etudes Néo-natales*, **6**, 165–179.

Salazar, J., Eiras, J., Mengual, J., Felipe, J., Carcarilla, L.I., Garcia, M.D. (1987) 'Anévrysme de la veine de Galien avec insuffisance cardiaque néonatale: succès de traitement neurochirurgical précoce.' *Pédiatrie*, **42**, 167–170.

211

Saliba, E., Santini, J.J., Chantepie, A., Pottier, J.M., Cheliakine, C., Gold, F., Bloc, D., Laugier, J. (1987a) 'Rétentissement cardiaque et cérébral de l'anévrysme de l'ampoule de Galien (AAG).' *Neurochirurgie*, **33**, 296–301.

—— —— Pottier, J.M., Chergui, A., Billard, C., Laugier, J. (1987b) 'Diagnostic et surveillance de l'anévrysme de l'ampoule de Galien (AAG) du nourisson par les ultrasons.' *Neurochirurgie*, **33**, 291–295.

Sänger, H. (1924) 'Über die Entstehung intrakranieller Blutungen beim Neugeborenen.' *Monatsschrift für Geburtshilfe*, **65**, 257–274.

Sarnat, H.B. (1987) 'Disturbances of late neuronal migrations in the perinatal period.' *American Journal of Diseases of Children*, **141**, 969–980.

Saunders, C. (1948) 'Intracranial haemorrhage in the newborn.' *Journal of Obstetrics and Gynaecology of the British Empire*, **55**, 55–61.

Schellinger, D., Grant, E.G., Manz, H.J., Patronas, N.J. (1988) 'Intraparenchymal hemorrhage in preterm neonates: a broadening spectrum.' *American Journal of Roentgenology*, **150**, 1109–1115.

Scher, M.S., Wright, F.S., Lockman, L.A., Thompson, T.R. (1982) 'Intraventricular hemorrhage in the full-term neonate.' *Archives of Neurology*, **39**, 769–772.

Schlegel, N., Beaufils, F. (1988) *Hémorragies et Thromboses en Pédiatrie*. Paris: Arnette.

Schmidt, B.K., Muraji, T., Zipursky, A. (1986) 'Low antithrombin III in neonatal shock: DIC or non-specific protein depletion?' *European Journal of Pediatrics*, **145**, 500–503.

Schneider, H., Ballowitz, L., Schachinger, H., Hanefeld, F., Dröszus, J-U. (1975) 'Anoxic encephalopathy with predominant involvement of basal ganglia, brain stem and spinal cord in the perinatal period.' *Acta Neuropathologica*, **32**, 287–298.

Schranz, D., Jüngst, B.K., Golla, G., Schwind, A., Vogel, K., Schmitt, T., Zimmer, B., Huth, R., Stopfkuchen, H. (1988) 'Kongestive Herzinsuffisienz bei einem Neugeborenen mit arteriovenöser Malformation der Vena Galeni: Diagnose mittels farbkodierter Doppler-Bild-Echographie.' *Monatsschrift für Kinderheilkunde*, **136**, 47–49.

Schreiber, M.S. (1959) 'Acute subdural haematoma in the newborn.' *Medical Journal of Australia*, **46**, 157–158.

Schubiger, G., Schubiger, O., Tönz, O. (1982) 'Thrombose des sinus sagittalis superior beim Neugeborenen—Diagnose durch Computertomographie.' *Helvetica Paediatrica Acta*, **37**, 193–199.

Schum, T.R., Meyer, G.A., Grausz, J.P., Glaspey, J.C. (1979) 'Neonatal intraventricular hemorrhage due to an intracranial arteriovenous malformation: a case report.' *Pediatrics*, **64**, 242–244.

Schwartz, P. (1964) *Geburtsschäden bei Neugeborenen*. Jena: Gustav Fisher.

Scott, R.M., Barnes, P., Kupsky, W., Adelman, L.S. (1992) 'Cavernous angiomas of the central nervous system in children.' *Journal of Neurosurgery*, **76**, 38–46.

Scotti, L.N., Goldman, R.L., Hardman, D.R., Heinz, E.R. (1974) 'Venous thrombosis in infants and children.' *Radiology*, **112**, 393–399.

Scotti, G., Flodmark, O., Harwood-Nash, D.C., Humphries, R.P. (1981) 'Posterior fossa hemorrhages in the newborn.' *Journal of Computer Assisted Tomography*, **5**, 68–72.

Segall, H.D., Ahmadi, J., McComb, J.G., Zee, C., Becker, T.S., Han, J.S. (1982) 'Computed tomographic observations pertinent to intracranial venous thrombotic and occlusive disease in childhood.' *Radiology*, **143**, 441–449.

Seidenwurm, D., Berenstein, A., Hyman, A., Kowalcki, H. (1991) 'Vein of Galen malformation: correlation of clinical presentation, arteriography and MR imaging.' *American Journal of Neuroradiology*, **12**, 347–354.

Seitz, L. (1907) 'Ueber Hirndrucksymptome bei Neugeborenen in Folge intrakranieller Blutungen und mechanische Hirninsulte.' *Archiv für Gynäkologie*, **82**, 528–618.

Serfontein, G.L., Rom, S., Stein, S. (1980) 'Posterior fossa subdural hemorrhage in the newborn.' *Pediatrics*, **65**, 40–43.

Sharpe, W., Maclaire, A.S. (1924) 'Further observations of intracranial hemorrhage in the newborn; significance of yellow spinal fluid and of jaundice in these cases.' *American Journal of Obstetrics and Gynecology*, **8**, 172–186.

Shaw, C-M. (1987) 'Correlates of mental retardation and structural changes of the brain.' *Brain and Development*, **9**, 1–8.

Shen, E.Y., Huang, C.C., Chyou, S.C., Hung, H.Y., Hsu, C.H., Huang, F.Y. (1986) 'Sonographic finding of the bright thalamus.' *Archives of Disease in Childhood*, **61**, 1096–1099.

212

Shewmon, D.A., Fine, M., Masden, J.C., Palacios, E. (1981) 'Postischemic hypervascularity of infancy: a stage in the evolution of ischemic brain damage with characteristic CT scan.' *Annals of Neurology*, **9**, 358–365.

Schipke, R., Riege, D., Scoville, W.B. (1954) 'Acute subdural hemorrhage at birth.' *Pediatrics*, **14**, 468–473.

Shortland-Webb, W.R. (1968) 'Proteus and coliform meningoencephalitis in neonates.' *Journal of Clinical Pathology*, **21**, 422–431.

Shulman, S.T., Madden, J.D., Esterly, J.R., Shauklin, D.R. (1971) 'Transection of spinal cord.' *Archives of Disease in Childhood*, **46**, 291–294.

Siesjö, B.K. (1992) 'Pathophysiology and treatment of focal cerebral ischemia. Part I: Pathophysiology.' *Journal of Neurosurgery*, **77**, 169–184.

Simmons, M.A., Adcock, E.W., Bard, H., Battaglia, F.C. (1974) 'Hypernatremia and intracranial hemorrhage in neonates.' *New England Journal of Medicine*, **291**, 6–10.

Simmons, M.A., Levine, R.L., Lubchenco, L.O., Guggenheim, M.A. (1978) 'Warning: serious sequelae of temporal artery catheterization.' *Journal of Pediatrics*, **92**, 284.

Singer, D.B. (1991) 'Infections of fetuses and neonates.' *In:* Wigglesworth, J.S., Singer, D.B. (Eds) *Textbook of Fetal and Perinatal Pathology*. Cambridge, MA: Blackwell Scientific, pp. 525–591.

Slovis, T.L., Shankaran, S., Bedard, M.P., Poland, R.L. (1984) 'Intracranial hemorrhage in the hypoxic–ischemic infant: ultrasound demonstration of unusual complications.' *Radiology*, **151**, 163–169.

Snyder, L.H., Doan, C.A. (1944) 'Studies in human inheritance. XXV. Is the homozygous form of multiple telangiectasia lethal?' *Journal of Laboratory and Clinical Medicine*, **29**, 1211–1219.

Snyder, R.D., Stovring, J., Cushing, A.H., Davis, L.E., Hardy, T.L. (1981) 'Cerebral infarction in childhood bacterial meningitis.' *Journal of Neurology, Neurosurgery and Psychiatry*, **44**, 581–585.

Sorbe, B., Dahlgren, S. (1983) 'Some important factors in the molding of the fetal head during vaginal delivery. A photographic study.' *International Journal of Gynaecology and Obstetrics*, **21**, 205–212.

Sran, S.K., Baumann, R.J. (1988) 'Outcome of neonatal strokes.' *American Journal of Diseases of Children*, **142**, 1086–1088.

Stanbridge, R.D.L., Westaby, S., Smallhorn, J., Taylor, J.F.N. (1983) 'Intracranial arteriovenous malformation with aneurysm of the vein of Galen as cause of heart failure in infancy. Echocardiographic diagnosis and results of treatment.' *British Heart Journal*, **49**, 157–162.

Stehbens, W.E., Sahgal, K.K., Nelson, L., Shaher, R.M. (1973) 'Aneurysm of the vein of Galen and diffuse meningeal angiectasia.' *Archives of Pathology*, **95**, 333–335.

Stein, R.L., Rosenbaum, A.E. (1974) 'Normal deep cerebral venous system.' *In:* Newton, T.H., Potts, D.G. (Eds) *Radiology of the Skull and Brain. Vol. 2, Book 3. Angiography*. St. Louis: C.V. Mosby, pp. 1904–1927.

Stein, B.M., Wolfert, S.M. (1980) 'Arteriovenous malformations of the brain. I: Current concepts. II: Treatment.' *Archives of Neurology*, **37**, 1–5; 69–75.

Steinlin, M., Dirr, R., Martin, E., Boesch, C., Largo, R.H., Fanconi, S., Boltshauser, E. (1991) 'MRI following severe perinatal asphyxia: preliminary experience.' *Pediatric Neurology*, **7**, 164–170.

Stern, L., Ramos, A.D., Wiglesworth, F.W. (1968) 'Congestive heart failure secondary to cerebral arteriovenous aneurysm in the newborn infant.' *American Journal of Diseases of Children*, **115**, 581–587.

Stewart, A.L., Reynolds, E.O.R., Hope, P.L., Hamilton, P.A., Baudin, J., Costello, A.M.deL., Bradford, B.C., Wyatt, J.S. (1987) 'Probability of neurodevelopmental disorders estimated from ultrasound appearance of brains of very preterm infants.' *Developmental Medicine and Child Neurology*, **29**, 3–11.

Stewart, K.S., Philpott, R.H. (1980) 'Fetal response to cephalopelvic disproportion.' *British Journal of Obstetrics and Gynaecology*, **87**, 641–649.

Stockman, J.A., Pochedly, C. (1988) *Developmental and Neonatal Hematology*. New York: Raven Press.

Strauss, S., Weinraub, Z., Goldberg, M. (1991) 'Prenatal diagnosis of vein of Galen arteriovenous malformation by duplex sonography.' *Journal of Perinatal Medicine*, **19**, 227–230.

Strong, T.H., Feldman, D.B., Cooke, J.K., Greenspoon, J.S., Barton, L. (1990) 'Congenital depression of the fetal skull.' *Obstetrical and Gynaecological Survey*, **45**, 284–289.

Stutchfield, P.R., Cooke, R.W.I. (1989) 'Electrolytes and glucose in cerebrospinal fluid of premature infants with intraventricular haemorrhage: role of potassium in cerebral infarction.' *Archives of Disease in Childhood*, **64**, 470–475.

Sulamaa, M., Vara, P. (1952) 'An investigation into the occurrence of perinatal subdural haematoma: its diagnosis and treatment.' *Acta Obstetricia et Gynaecologica Scandinavica*, **31**, 400–412.

Suzuki, S., Hathaway, W.E., Bonnar, J., Sutor, A.H. (1991) *Perinatal Thrombosis and Hemostasis.* Tokyo: Springer Verlag.

Svenningsen, L. (1989) *Measurement of the Forces During Spontaneous Delivery and Under Vacuum Extraction.* (Thesis: University of Oslo.)

—— Eidal, K. (1988) 'Retinal hemorrhages and traction forces in vacuum extraction.' *Early Human Development*, **16**, 263–269.

Sylvester, P.E. (1960) 'Marbling and perinatal anoxia.' *Acta Paediatrica Scandinavica*, **49**, 338–344.

Szymonowicz, W., Schafler, K., Cussen, L.J., Yu, V.H.Y. (1984) 'Ultrasound and necropsy study of periventricular haemorrhage in preterm infants.' *Archives of Disease in Childhood*, **59**, 637–642.

—— Walker, A.M., Cussen, L., Cannata, J., Yu, V.Y.H. (1988) 'Developmental changes in regional cerebral blood flow in fetal and newborn lambs.' *American Journal of Physiology*, **254**, H52–H58.

—— —— Yu, V.Y., Stewart, M.L., Cannata, J., Cussen, L. (1990) 'Regional cerebral blood flow after hemorrhagic hypotension in the preterm, near-term and newborn lamb.' *Pediatric Research*, **28**, 361–366.

Taft, T.A., Chusid, M.J., Sty, J.R. (1986) 'Cerebral infarction in *Hemophilus influenzae* type B meningitis.' *Clinical Pediatrics*, **25**, 177–180.

Takagi, T., Nagai, R., Wakabayashi, S., Mizawa, I., Hayashi, K. (1978) 'Extradural hemorrhage as a result of birth trauma.' *Child's Brain*, **4**, 306–318.

—— Fukuoka, H., Wakabayashi, S., Nagai, H., Shibata, T. (1982) 'Posterior fossa subdural hemorrhage in the newborn as a result of birth trauma.' *Child's Brain*, **9**, 102–113.

Takashima, S., Becker, L.E. (1985) 'Basal ganglia calcification in Down's syndrome.' *Journal of Neurology, Neurosurgery and Psychiatry*, **48**, 61–64.

—— Armstrong, D.L., Becker, L.E. (1978) 'Subcortical leukomalacia: relationship to development of the cerebral sulcus and its vascular supply.' *Archives of Neurology*, **35**, 470–472.

—— Ando, Y., Mito, T., Yokota, K., Kondo, I., Iwao, H. (1984) 'Ultrasonography and brain pathology of periventricular hemorrhage and subependymal cyst in the preterm neonate.' *Brain and Development*, **6**, 311–316.

—— Mito, T., Ando, Y. (1986) 'Pathogenesis of periventricular white matter hemorrhages in preterm infants.' *Brain and Development*, **8**, 25–30.

—— Ohno, K., Ando, M. (1987) 'Pathogenesis of perinatal leukomalacia.' *In:* Yabuuchi, H., Watanabe, K., Okada, S. (Eds) *Neonatal Brain and Behaviour.* Nagoya: University of Nagoya Press, pp. 45–52.

Tan, K.L. (1974) 'Elevation of congenital depressed fractures of the skull by the vacuum extractor.' *Acta Paediatrica Scandinavica*, **63**, 562–564.

Tanaka, Y., Sakamoto, K., Kobayashi, S., Kobayashi, N., Muraoka, S. (1988) 'Biphasic ventricular dilatation following posterior fossa subdural hematoma in the full-term neonate.' *Journal of Neurosurgery*, **68**, 211–216.

Tank, E.S., Davis, R., Holt, J.F., Morley, G.W. (1971) 'Mechanisms of trauma during breech delivery.' *Obstetrics and Gynecology*, **38**, 761–765.

Terplan, K.L. (1973) 'Patterns of brain damage in infants and children with congenital heart disease.' *American Journal of Diseases of Children.* **125**, 175–185.

Thiery, M. (1985) 'Obstetric vacuum extraction.' *In:* Wynn, R.M. (Ed.) *Obstetrics and Gynecology Annual.* Norwalk, CN: Appleton–Century–Crofts, pp. 73–111.

Thompson, J.B., Mason, T.H., Haines, G.I., Cassidy, R.J. (1973) 'Surgical management of diastatic linear skull fractures in infants.' *Journal of Neurosurgery*, **39**, 493–497.

Thompson, R.A., Pribram, H.F.W. (1969) 'Infantile cerebral aneurysm associated with ophthalmoplegia and quadriparesis.' *Neurology*, **19**, 785–789.

Thorn, I. (1969) 'Cerebral symptoms in the newborn. Diagnostic and prognostic significance of symptoms of presumed cerebral origin.' *Acta Paediatrica Scandinavica*, Suppl. 195.

Till, K. (1968) 'Subdural hematoma and effusion in infancy.' *British Medical Journal*, **3**, 400–402.

Toma, P., Cariati, M., Dell'acqua, A.M., Magnano, G.M. (1990) 'Diagnosi ecotomografica di emorragia cerebellare nel neonato.' *Minerva Pediatrica*, **42**, 161–164.

214

Tomlinson, F.H., Piepgras, D.G., Nichols, D.A., Rüfenacht, D.A., Kaste, S.C. (1992) 'Remote congenital cerebral arteriovenous fistulae associated with aortic coarctation.' *Journal of Neurosurgery*, **76**, 137–142.

Torrance, S.M., Wittnich, C. (1992) 'The effect of varying arterial oxygen tension on neonatal acid–base balance.' *Pediatric Research*, **31**, 112–116.

Towbin, A. (1964) 'Spinal cord and brain stem injury at birth.' *Pediatrics*, **77**, 620–632.

—— (1969) 'Cerebral hypoxic damage in fetus and newborn.' *Archives of Neurology*, **20**, 35–43.

—— (1971) 'Organic causes of minimal brain dysfunction.' *Journal of the American Medical Association*, **217**, 1207–1214.

—— (1977) 'Trauma in pregnancy—injury to the fetus and newborn.' *In:* Tedeschi, C.G., Eckert, W.G., Tedeschi, L.G. (Eds) *Forensic Medicine*. Philadelphia: W.B. Saunders, pp. 436–486.

Trauner, D.A., Mannino, F.L. (1986) 'Neurodevelopmental outcome after neonatal cerebrovascular accident.' *Journal of Pediatrics*, **108**, 459–461.

Trounce, J.Q., Fawer, C-L., Punt, J., Dodd, K.L., Fielder, A.R., Levene, M.I. (1985) 'Primary thalamic haemorrhage in the newborn: a new clinical entity.' *Lancet*, **1**, 190–192.

—— Fagan, D., Levene, M.I. (1986) 'Intraventricular haemorrhage and periventricular leukomalacia: ultrasound and autopsy correlation.' *Archives of Disease in Childhood*, **61**, 1203–1207.

Turkel, S.B. (1990) 'Autopsy findings associated with neonatal hyperbilirubinemia.' *Clinics in Perinatology*, **17**, 381–396.

Uno, M., Ueta, H., Ohshima, T., Matsumoto, K., Izumidani, T., Miyaka, H. (1990) 'A case of arteriovenous malformation in a neonate.' *No Shinkei Geka*, **18**, 953–958.

Uvebrant, P. (1988) 'Hemiplegic cerebral palsy: aetiology and outcome.' *Acta Paediatrica Scandinavica*, Suppl. 345.

Vacca, A., Keirse, M.J.N.C. (1989) 'Instrumental vaginal delivery.' *In:* Chalmers, I., Enkin, M., Keirse, M.J.N.C. (Eds) *Effective Care in Pregnancy and Childbirth*. Oxford: Oxford University Press, pp. 1216–1233.

Valdes-Dapena, M.A., Arey, J.B. (1970) 'The causes of neonatal mortality: an analysis of 501 autopsies on newborn infants.' *Journal of Pediatrics*, **77**, 366–375.

Valkeakari, T. (1973) 'Analysis of serial echoencephalograms in healthy newborn infants during the first week of life.' *Acta Paediatrica Scandinavica*, Suppl. 242.

Vanhaesebrouck, P. (1986) 'Mogelijke perinatale sequelae van vacuum extractie.' *Tijdschrift voor Geneeskunde*, **42**, 615–617.

—— Poffijn, A., Caemaert, J., De Baets, F., Van de Velde, E., Thiery, M. (1990) 'Leptomeningeal cyst and vacuum extraction.' *Acta Paediatrica Scandinavica*, **79**, 232–233.

Vannucci, R.C. (1990*a*) 'Current and potentially new management strategies for perinatal hypoxic–ischemic encephalopathy.' *Pediatrics*, **85**, 961–968.

—— (1990*b*) 'Experimental biology of cerebral hypoxia–ischemia: relation to perinatal brain damage.' *Pediatric Research*, **27**, 317–326.

—— Christensen, A., Yager, J.Y. (1992) 'Cerebral edema and perinatal hypoxic–ischemic (H-I) brain damage.' *Pediatric Research*, **31**, 355A. *(Abstract no. 2116.)*

Varga-Khadem, F., O'Gorman, A.M., Watters, G.V. (1985) 'Aphasia and handedness in relation to hemispheric side, age at injury and severity of cerebral lesion during childhood.' *Brain*, **108**, 677–696.

Velut, S. (1987) 'Embryologie des veines cérébrales.' *Neurochirurgie*, **33**, 258–263.

—— Santini, J-J. (1987) 'Anatomie microchirurgicale de l'ampoule de Galien.' *Neurochirurgie*, **33**, 264–271.

Vermylen, J., Blockmans, D. (1989) 'Acquired disorders of platelet function.' *Baillière's Clinical Haematology*, **2**, 729–748.

Vinazzer, H. (1983) 'Antithrombin III substitution in septicemia.' *Biomedical Progress*, **2**, 3–6.

Voet, D., Govaert, P., Caemaert, J., De Lille, L., D'Herde, K., Afschrift, M. (1992) 'Leptomeningeal cyst: early diagnosis by color Doppler imaging.' *Pediatric Radiology*, **22**, 417–418.

Voit, T., Lemburg, P., Neven, E., Lumenta, C., Stork, W. (1987) 'Damage of thalamus and basal ganglia in asphyxiated full-term neonates.' *Neuropediatrics*, **18**, 176–181.

Volpe, J.J. (1981) 'Neonatal intraventricular hemorrhage.' *New England Journal of Medicine*, **304**, 886–891.

—— (1987) *Neurology of the Newborn. 2nd Edn.* Philadelphia: W.B. Saunders.

215

—— (1990) 'Brain injury in the premature infant: is it preventable?' *Pediatric Research*, **27**, S28–S33.
—— Herscovitch, P., Perlman, J.M., Kreusser, K.L., Raichle, H.E. (1985) 'Positron emission tomography in the asphyxiated term newborn: parasagittal impairment of cerebral blood flow.' *Annals of Neurology*, **17**, 287–296.
Vomberg, P.P., Breederveld, C., Fleury, P., Arts, W.F.M. (1987) 'Cerebral thromboembolism due to antithrombin III deficiency in two children.' *Neuropediatrics*, **18**, 42–44.
Von Bucke, B., Pohl, M. (1964) 'Die sogenannte wachsende Schädelfraktur als Komplikation der Vakuumextraktion.' *Monatsschrift für Kinderheilkunde*, **111**, 424–426.
Von Gontard, A., Arnold, D., Adis, B. (1988) 'Posterior fossa hemorrhage in the newborn—diagnosis and management.' *Pediatric Radiology*, **18**, 347–348.
Von Issel, E.P., Bilz, D. (1978) 'Empfehlungen zur Registrierung geburtsmechanischer Einwirkungen am Neugeborenenschädel.' *Zeitblatt für Gynäkologie*, **100**, 65–68.
Voorhies, T.M., Lipper, E.G., Lee, B.C.P., Vannucci, R.C., Auld, P.A.M. (1984) 'Occlusive vascular disease in asphyxiated newborn infants.' *Journal of Pediatrics*, **105**, 92–96.
Wakai, S., Andoh, Y., Nagai, M., Teramoto, C., Tanaka, G. (1990) 'Choroid plexus arteriovenous malformation in a full-term neonate.' *Journal of Neurosurgery*, **72**, 127–129.
Walker, C.H.M. (1985) 'Birth trauma.' *In:* Crawford, J.W. (Ed.) *Risks of Labour*. Chichester: John Wiley, pp. 71–93.
Walters, B.C., Burrows, P.E., Musewe, N., Chuang, S.H., Armstrong, D. (1990) 'Unilateral megalencephaly associated with neonatal high output cardiac failure.' *Child's Nervous System*, **6**, 123–125.
Watkins, A., Szymonowicz, W., Jin, X., Yu, V.Y.H. (1988) 'Significance of seizures in very low-birthweight infants.' *Developmental Medicine and Child Neurology*, **30**, 162–169.
Wehberg, K., Vincent, M., Harrison, B. (1992) 'Intraventricular hemorrhage in the full-term neonate associated with abdominal compression.' *Pediatrics*, **89**, 327–329.
Welch, K., Strand, R. (1986) 'Traumatic parturitional intracranial hemorrhage.' *Developmental Medicine and Child Neurology*, **28**, 156–164.
Whitelaw, A., Rivers, R.P.A., Creighton, L., Gaffney, P. (1992) 'Low-dose intraventricular fibrinolytic treatment to prevent posthaemorrhagic hydrocephalus.' *Archives of Disease in Childhood*, **67**, 12–14.
Wigger, H.J. (1991) 'Influence of perinatal management.' *In:* Wigglesworth, J.S., Singer, D.B. (Eds) *Textbook of Fetal and Perinatal Pathology*. Cambridge, MA: Blackwell Scientific, pp. 49–76.
Wigglesworth, J.S. (1984) *Perinatal Pathology*. Philadelphia: W.B. Saunders.
—— (1988) 'Trauma and the developing brain.' *In:* Kubli, F., Patel, N., Schmidt, W., Linderkamp, O. (Eds) *Perinatal Events and Brain Damage in Surviving Children*. Berlin: Springer, pp. 64–69.
—— (1991) 'Pathology of intrapartum and early neonatal death in the normally formed infant.' *In:* Wigglesworth, J.S., Singer, D.B. (Eds) *Textbook of Fetal and Perinatal Pathology*. Cambridge, MA: Blackwell Scientific, pp. 285–306.
—— Husemeyer, R.P. (1977) 'Intracranial birth trauma in vaginal breech delivery: the continued importance of injury to the occipital bone.' *British Journal of Obstetrics and Gynaecology*, **84**, 684–691.
—— Keith, I.H., Girling, D.J., Slade, S.A. (1976) 'Hyaline membrane disease, alkali and intraventricular haemorrhage.' *Archives of Disease in Childhood*, **51**, 755–762.
Williams, C.E., Gunn, A.J., Synek, B., Gluckman, P.D. (1990) 'Delayed seizures occurring with hypoxic–ischemic encephalopathy in the fetal sheep.' *Pediatric Research*, **27**, 561–565.
—— —— Gluckman, P.D. (1991) 'Time course of intracellular edema and epileptiform activity following prenatal cerebral ischemia in sheep.' *Stroke*, **22**, 516–521.
—— Mallard, C., Tan, W., Gluckman, P.D. (1993) 'Pathophysiology of perinatal asphyxia.' *Clinics in Perinatology*, **20**, 305–325.
Williams, P.L. (1989) *Gray's Anatomy, 37th Edn*. Edinburgh: Churchill-Livingstone.
Wyatt, J.S., Edwards, A.D., Azzopardi, D., Reynolds, E.O.R. (1989) 'Magnetic resonance and near infrared spectroscopy for investigation of perinatal hypoxic–ischaemic brain injury.' *Archives of Disease in Childhood*, **64**, 953–963.
Yamasaki, T., Handa, H., Yamashita, J., Paine, J.T., Tashiro, Y., Uno, A., Ishikawa, M., Asato, R. (1986) 'Intracranial and orbital cavernous angiomas.' *Journal of Neurosurgery*, **64**, 197–208.
Yang, D.C., Sohn, D., Anand, H.K. (1969) 'Thrombosis of the superior longitudinal sinus during

infancy. Report of two cases.' *Journal of Pediatrics*, **74**, 570–575.

Yates, P.O. (1959) 'Birth trauma to the vertebral arteries.' *Archives of Disease in Childhood*, **34**, 436–441.

—— (1973) 'Cerebral birth injury.' *In:* Fox, H., Langley, F.A. (Eds) *Postgraduate Obstetrical and Gynaecological Pathology.* Oxford: Pergamon Press.

Ylppö, A. (1919) 'Pathologisch-anatomische Studien bei Frühgeborenen. Makroskopische und mikroskopische Untersuchungen mit Hinweisen auf die Klinik und mit besonderer Berücksichtigung der Hämorrhagien.' *Zeitschrift für Kinderheilkunde*, **20**, 212–431.

Yoffe, G., Buchanan, G.R. (1988) 'Intracranial hemorrhage in newborn and young infants with hemophilia.' *Journal of Pediatrics*, **113**, 333–336.

Young, R.S.K., Zalneraitis, E.L. (1980) 'Retroauricular cephalhematoma as a sign of posterior fossa subdural hematoma.' *Clinical Pediatrics*, **19**, 631–632.

—— Hernandez, M.J., Yagel, S.K. (1982) 'Selective reduction of blood flow to white matter during hypotension in newborn dogs: a possible mechanism of periventricular leukomalacia.' *Annals of Neurology*, **12**, 445–448.

Younkin, D.P., Wagerle, L.G., Chance, B., Maria, J., Delivoria-Papadopoulos, M. (1987) '^{31}P-NMR studies of cerebral metabolic changes during graded hypoxia in newborn lambs.' *Journal of Applied Physiology*, **62**, 1569–1574.

Yousefzadeh, D.K., Naidich, T.P. (1985) 'US anatomy of the posterior fossa in children: correlation with brain sections.' *Radiology*, **156**, 353–361.

Zelson, C., Lee, S.J., Pearl, M. (1974) 'The incidence of skull fractures underlying cephalhematomas in newborn infants.' *Journal of Pediatrics*, **85**, 371–373.

Zimmerman, R.D., Haimes, A.B. (1989) 'The role of MR imaging in the diagnosis of infections of the central nervous system.' *Current Clinical Topics in Infectious Diseases*, **10**, 82–108.

Znamenacek, K., Horsky, J., Melichar, V., Benesova, D. (1957) 'A clinical study of perinatal trauma in newborn infants. Part II. Analysis of infants dying during the neonatal period.' *Etudes Néo-natales*, **6**, 89–95.

Zorzi, C., Angonese, I., Zaramella, P., Benini, F., Dalla Barba, B., Cavedagni, M., Melli, R., De Carolis, G. (1988) 'Periventricular intraparenchymal cystic lesions: critical determinant of neurodevelopmental outcome in preterm infants.' *Helvetica Paediatrica Acta*, **43**, 195–202.

217

INDEX